Evidence-based Child Health Care

Challenges for Practice

Edited by

Edward Alan Glasper and Lorraine Ireland

palgrave

Published by
PALGRAVE
Houndmills, Basingstoke, Hampshire RG21 6XS and
175 Fifth Avenue, New York, N.Y. 10010
Companies and representatives throughout the world

PALGRAVE is the new global academic imprint of
St. Martin's Press LLC Scholarly and Reference Division and
Palgrave Publishers Ltd (formerly Macmillan Press Ltd).

ISBN 0–333–80230–6 paperback

This book is printed on paper suitable for recycling and made from fully managed and sustained forest sources.

10 9 8 7 6 5 4 3 2
09 08 07 06 05 04 03 02 01

Editing and origination by
Aardvark Editorial, Mendham, Suffolk

Printed and bound in Great Britain by
Creative Print & Design (Wales), Ebbw Vale

Contents

List of Figures   vii

List of Tables   viii

The Contributors   ix

Foreword   xii

Preface   xiv

1   Challenging issues facing children's nurses in their quest to deliver evidence-based practice
Edward Alan Glasper and Lorraine Ireland   1

2   Demonstrating evidence-based clinical nursing practice: providing the evidence
Tony Long and Jill Asbury   13

3   The legacy of a paediatric nursing degree course
Annette Dearmun   26

4   The role of professional journals in promoting evidence-based care
Anne Casey   42

5   Parental participation in the care of hospitalised children: a review of the research evidence
Eileen Savage and Peter Callery   57

6   Being a mother of a critically sick child: issues for nursing practice and research
Jane Noyes   90

7   Children's voices in health care planning
Eva Elliott and Alison Watson   110

8   The surveillance of childhood accidents: providing the evidence for accident prevention
Laura King, Anna Gough, Iain Robertson-Steel and Donald Pennington   128

9   Children's knowledge of their internal anatomy
Claire Gaudion   148

10   Can information leaflets assist parents in preparing their children for hospital admission?
Karen J. Stone   163

11 Promoting adolescent sexual health: enhancing
    professional knowledge and skills
    Rachael L. Smith   185

12 Added Power and Understanding in Sex Education
    (A PAUSE): a sex education intervention staffed
    predominantly by school nurses
    John Rees, Alex Mellanby, Jenny White and
    John Tripp   203

13 The critically ill children study: a prospective study
    of the provision and outcome of paediatric intensive
    care in the South West
    Siobhan Warne, Lynn Garland, Linda Bailey,
    Susan Edees, Patricia Weir and John Henderson   224

14 The lived experiences of paediatric nurses' enjoyment
    of caring for sick children
    Marie Bodycombe-James   244

15 Nurses' management of fever in children: rituals or
    evidence-based practice?
    Maureen R. Harrison   262

16 Measuring effectiveness: the paediatric diabetes
    specialist nurse role
    Lesley Lowes   285

17 Decision analysis in evidence-based children's
    nursing: a community nursing perspective
    Dorothèe J. H. O'Sullivan-Burchard   306

18 Home sweet home – examining the interface
    between hospital and home
    Margaret Lane and Sarah Baker   322

19 Intravenous antibiotics at home: a parents' perspective
    Claire Ruskin   346

20 There's a whole family hurting: the experience of
    living with a child with chronic pain
    Bernadette Carter   359

21 A collaborative approach to evidence-based child
    health nursing practice
    Sue Nagy   382

Index   395

List of Figures

2.1   The tripartite relationship   17
2.2   Sources of data for evidence   19

4.1   Evidence within a model for future nursing education   53

8.1   Age groups of survey participants   135
8.2   Bar chart to show area in school where accidents occurred   137
8.3   Bar chart showing the most serious injury   138
8.4   Suggested strategies for A&E nurses to become involved
      in accident prevention work   145

9.1   Anatomical rag doll   153
9.2   Interview schedule   154

10.1 Flow chart to summarise the recommended steps for
      designing a family information leaflet   170
10.2 A copy of the leaflet used in the main study, 'Preparing
      your child for hospital. A parents' guide'   173

14.1 Framework of analysis   247

15.1 The fever cycle   264
15.2 Temperature chart   273
15.3 Paracetamol administration questionnaire   275
15.4 Reasons identified for the administration of paracetamol   279

16.1 Number of newly diagnosed children by year   290
16.2 Length of stay pre and post the establishment of the
      paediatric diabetes specialist nurse post   291
16.3 Median age at diagnosis by year   292
16.4 Bed occupancy by year of diagnosis   293
16.5 Paediatric clinic non-attendance (DNA) rate by year   299
16.6 Adolescent clinic non-attendance (DNA) rate by year   299

17.1 Concept map   309
17.2 Decision flow diagram   311

18.1 Factors influencing the commencement of discharge planning   336
18.2 A co-ordinated approach to discharge planning   339

20.1 Model of chronic pain   370

21.1 Royal Alexandra Hospital for Children model
      for the adoption of evidence-based practice   390

List of Tables

5.1 Journals manually searched for this review   62
5.2 Overview of studies relating to the effects on parents
    of parental participation in caring for their hospitalised child   74
5.3 Overview of studies relating to the effects of parental
    participation on hospitalised children   84

8.1 Ethnic origin of the children and young adults surveyed   136

9.1 Number of internal parts mentioned   156

10.1 Steps taken when subjecting literature to SMOG testing   175
10.2 Parental responses to questions relating to the design
     of the leaflet   177
10.3 Parental opinion of the value of each section within
     the leaflet   178
10.4 Preparation methods used by parents   179

13.1 Identified areas of care for critically ill children   225
13.2 Number of children requiring intensive care   226
13.3 PRISM Score   229
13.4 Information to calculate the Pediatric Index of Mortality   230
13.5 Number of cases for each diagnosis   233
13.6 Number of children, number of deaths and PRISM score
     for BPA levels, 1, 2 and 3   234

15.1 Positive immunological role of fever   265
15.2 Signs and symptoms that indicate fever   277

16. 1 Readmissions 1.4.93–31.3.99   295
16.2 Length of hospital stay for readmission   295

20.1 Overview of stages of the study   367
20.2 Overview of the children in the study   369
20.3 Overview of interviews   369
20.4 Overview of diaries   369

21.1 Nurses' views of evidence-based practice in three countries   383

The Contributors

Jill Asbury is a Paediatric Nurse Specialist at the Leeds Teaching Hospitals NHS Trust.

Sarah Baker is a Team Leader in Croydon Community Health's Children's Hospital at Home department.

Linda Bailey is a Research Nurse at the University of Bristol.

Marie Bodycombe-James is Lecturer in Nursing at the School of Health Science, University of Wales, Swansea.

Peter Callery is Lecturer in Nursing at the School of Nursing, Midwifery and Health Visiting, University of Manchester.

Bernadette Carter is Senior Lecturer/Researcher in Health Care Studies at Manchester Metropolitan University.

Anne Casey is Editor of *Paediatric Nursing* from the RCN Publishing Company, Royal College of Nursing.

Annette Dearmun is Senior Nurse/Principal Lecturer Practitioner at the School of Health Care/Childrens Clinical Centre at Oxford Brookes University/Oxford Radcliffe Hospital, Oxford.

Susan Edees is Consultant Paediatrician at the Royal Berkshire Hospital, Reading.

Eva Elliott is a Research Fellow in the Public Health Research and Resource Centre, University of Salford.

Lynn Garland is a Research Nurse at the University of Bristol.

Claire Gaudion is a Staff Nurse, Piam Brown Ward, at Southampton University Hospitals NHS Trust.

Edward Alan Glasper is Professor of Nursing and Academic Head of Child Health Studies at the School of Nursing and Midwifery, University of Southampton.

Anna Gough is Senior Lecturer at the School of Health and Social Sciences, Coventry University.

Maureen R. Harrison is Lecturer in Child Health Studies at the Florence Nightingale Division of Nursing and Midwifery, King's College, London.

John Henderson is Senior Lecturer in Child Health at Bristol Children's Hospital.

Lorraine M. Ireland is Lecturer in Child Health Studies at the School of Nursing and Midwifery, University of Southampton.

Laura King was (at the time of writing) Research Assistant at the School of Health and Social Sciences, Coventry University.

Margaret M. Lane is Sub-Dean of Nursing, St Bartholomew School of Nursing and Midwifery, City University, London.

Tony Long is Senior Lecturer of Child Health Nursing at the School of Healthcare Studies, University of Leeds.

Lesley Lowes is Paediatric Diabetes Specialist Nurse in the Department of Child Health, University Hospital of Wales.

Alex R. Mellanby is Honorary Research Fellow at the Department of Child Health, Exeter University.

Sue Nagy is Professor of Paediatric Nursing at the Royal Alexandra Hospital for Children, Westmead, NSW, Australia and the University of Western Sydney Nepean School of Health and Nursing Studies.

Jane Noyes is Senior Lecturer in Paediatric Intensive Care and Child Health at the Department of Nursing/Institute for Health Research, University of Salford.

Dorothèe J. H. O'Sullivan-Burchard is Lecturer in the Department of Nursing and Community Health, Glasgow Caledonian University.

Donald Pennington is Dean of the School of Health and Social Sciences, Coventry University.

John B. Rees is A PAUSE Programme Manager at the Department of Child Health, Exeter University.

Iain Robertson-Steel is Consultant in Primary Care in the A&E Department at Royal Wolverhampton Hospitals NHS Trust.

Claire Ruskin is a Registered Children's Nurse.

Eileen B. Savage is Lecturer in Nursing at the Department of Nursing Studies, University College Cork, Eire.

Rachael L. Smith is Lecturer in Nursing/Director of Quality in the School of Nursing and Midwifery, University of Southampton.

Karen J. Stone is a Registered Children's Nurse.

John H. Tripp is Senior Lecturer in Child Health at the Department of Child Health, Exeter University.

Siobhan Warne is a Research Nurse at the University of Bristol.

Alison Watson is a Research Fellow at the Public Health Research and Resource Centre, University of Salford.

Patricia Weir is Consultant in Paediatric Intensive Care at Bristol Children's Hospital.

Jenny White is School Nurse at the Department of Child Health, Clyst Vale Community College, Devon.

Foreword

I was very pleased indeed to be asked to prepare a foreword for this absorbing new text for child health care professionals. The book has an interesting history as it was inspired by the First International Evidence-based Child Health Nursing Conference which took place in Jersey in 1998. It is, therefore, a good example of the efficient dissemination of evidence in support of effective practice. Child health care professionals often feel that it is very difficult to make their voice heard. We are part of a numerically small group within the health care system, and children's services represent a small part of the totality of the health services. Indeed, it has taken time and a good deal of hard work for us to achieve a position where children's issues are prominent on the agendas of public policy at all. This book allows our voice to be heard loud and clear.

As an edited text, there is, although the editors have done a careful job of unifying the text, a freshness about the differences in style between the various writers. Each chapter has its distinctive character. It is particularly significant to point out that the contributors come from a very wide range of backgrounds in clinical practice, management, research and education in the child health arena. The chapters certainly contain their theoretical perspectives, but the overall tenor is that of the viewpoint of the doer; real practical experience in dealing with the everyday practical challenges of child health care shines through in each of the chapters of this book.

This text offers us the opportunity to learn a good deal from the work and experience of our colleagues that it presents. With that learning, we are also challenged to take the same journey as the contributors: to expose to systematic examination issues that intrigue and interest us in our day-to-day professional work, and to inform our colleagues about the results of that examination. The sheer range of the topics tackled by the contributors is particularly impressive, but the emphasis is always firmly placed on the welfare of children using the health services and their families. The importance of the family for the child in the health services, the subject of so many of the chapters in this book, emerges clearly as a topic upon which child health care professionals are placing great store. This underscores an important and constructive development in our professions towards family-centred care. The voice of the health services user – the child and the family – is, to a satisfying degree, prominent throughout the book.

The growing body of specific child health professional knowledge based on valid and reliable research strengthens the credibility of the child health care professions in the eyes of other professional colleagues. This in turn enhances our confidence in engaging in the important developmental debates at all levels of health care. This book, therefore, marks our continually improved standing in professional and scholarly communities.

All these are important issues, but they must not detract from the essential point that this is a lively, stimulating and highly readable book. Child health care practitioners – from students to qualified and experienced practitioners – will all find something to inform them and inspire them in this text.

This book signals the growing maturity and professionalisation of the child health care services as it admirably demonstrates the growing evidence basis of our professions.

JIM RICHARDSON
University of Glamorgan

Preface

The UK National Health Service's drive towards clinical governance has added impetus to the pursuit of evidence-based practice. The nursing profession is at the sharp end of practice and is now mandated to deliver care based on best evidence. The audit cycle built into the criteria of clinical governance will make this a high priority on the agenda of all nurses. Children's nurses are no exception to this and their philosophy of 'the child first and always' will ensure that their evidence base for practice is commensurate with this stance.

This text aims to give readers exemplars of clinically focused research that questions existing care paradigms and makes suggestions on how research findings can be incorporated into clinical practice. In addition, all aspects of the process of delivering evidence-based care are highlighted, from initial thoughts through to implementation, from educational input to research output. The individual contributors to this book, although differing in their position and approach, have one thing in common – their excellence in care for children and their families.

The development of a global network of institutions linked through the World Wide Web, all committed to collating precise accounts of research using the process of systematic review, is a modern feature of health care. As children's nursing moves forward into the early years of the third millennium, it will need to develop the skills not only of conducting research with children and their families, but also of interpreting the work of others and how it might apply in the real world of clinical practice. This process will be helped when all practising nurses have access to the technology that harnesses the latent power of the telecommunication industry.

Soon every ward or environment where patients are cared for will have ready access to the World Wide Web. Busy practitioners, however, want easily digestible accounts and 'bottom-line' approaches to evidence-based care. They do not have the time or indeed the inclination to wade through tomes of heavy text in their search for solutions to their problems. *Evidence-based Child Health Care* attempts to provide an easily readable and focused account of contemporary child health research and its application to clinical practice.

In this first UK evidence-based textbook for children's nurses, the editors have endeavoured to include a range of chapters, each of which addresses different issues in contemporary children's nursing practice. Clearly, no textbook can encompass the full range of research activity in which children's nurses are currently involved, but the chapters do reflect the repertoire of contemporary issues that currently affect care. It must be stressed that the quest for evidence-based nursing care must be on the basis of partnership and multi-disciplinary collaboration. Children's nurses do not practise in a professional vacuum, and the introduction of a philosophy of clinical governance, which is designed to implement the very highest stand-ards of care, is based on a framework in which all health care profes-sionals can work together as a team to bring about positive change.

Within the context of health care in the UK, a number of institu-tions have been developed to augment and make easier the inherent difficulties of accessing research findings and, importantly, the sources of best evidence. The National Institute of Clinical Excellence and the NHS Centre for Reviews and Dissemination, within the University of York, both have sophisticated web sites whose remit is to provide carers with the information they need to incorporate research-based evidence into their practice.

Quality care is dependent on best evidence, and children's nurses must learn to reconcile the inherent tensions that are always present in the work environment. In a health care world where there are perennial shortages of children's nurses, coupled with earlier discharge, more acute care and a growth in ambulatory and primary health care for children, it is not difficult to appreciate the dilemmas facing the practitioner. In recognition of these difficulties, this 'evidence-based child health care' text is designed for all children's nurses who wish to be inspired by the work of their peers. The incor-poration of a strong research strand within the diploma and under-graduate child branch curricula makes this text timely.

Contemporary accounts by journalists in British newspapers, suggesting that today's nurses are somehow too educated to care properly for patients, will be revealed by the readers of this textbook to be false. The chapters included in this text are a celebration of contemporary child health care and its enduring mission to provide excellence in care for the children and families with whom the nurses work.

In Chapter 1, the authors attempt to examine the issues facing children's nurses in their quest to deliver evidence-based care. In particular, the potential ethical pitfalls of conducting research with children and their families are discussed. Chapter 2 examines the

inherent problems of providing the evidence upon which clinical
nursing practice is based. The assessment of practice must now
include evidence from a range of sources, and within educational
programmes for children's nurses, the emphasis on assessing practice
is just as crucial as that on assessing theory. Similarly, Chapter 3
investigates the legacy of an undergraduate educational programme
for children's nurses and seeks to examine the influence of the research
component of the course and its ongoing impact on care delivery.

Chapters 5 and 6 take one of children's nursing icons of care, that
is, parental participation in care, and subject it to constructive
conceptual analysis. In Chapter 5, the authors review the research
evidence that underpins parental participation in care, using the principles and procedures of systematic review. Chapter 6 examines care
from the perspective of a parent and reveals that the psychosocial
elements of care are often inconsistent.

Chapter 7 valuably addresses the issue of taking the views of children and young people seriously. The study discussed in this chapter
adds to the growing body of evidence that children should be
involved in decisions about their own treatment and, just as importantly, involved in the planning and development of child health and
welfare services.

Chapter 8 reflects the concerns that children's nurses have related
to childhood accidents, the study describes the identification of target
groups and priorities for accident prevention. In suggesting strategies
for nurses to become involved in childhood accident prevention
work, the study emphasises the important role that nurses can adopt
in the best use of evidence and its relevance to care practice.

Chapter 9 investigates how children perceive their own internal
anatomy; the study on which the chapter is based highlights the
importance of communicating information accurately to children.

In Chapter 10, the author also examines the necessity of ensuring
good communication between families and health care professionals.
This study investigates the use of parent information leaflets and how
effective they are in helping parents to prepare their children for
hospital admission.

Chapters 11 and 12 examine the sexual health needs of young
people. In Chapter 11, the author explores the development of
young people's sexual health through interviews with a sample of
young student nurses. In Chapter 12, the authors report on an innovative study related to service provision to secondary schools. Both
studies highlight the continuing need for effective health education
for young people.

Chapter 13 is related to the growth and increasing recognition of paediatric intensive care provision for children. The chapter details the pilot work of a prospective large-scale study that aims to identify the facilities available for critically ill children and ascertain outcomes using a range of scoring tools and other measures. The authors believe the information generated through this study will form a rational basis on which to provide the most effective service for critically ill children.

Chapter 14 describes a study in which the author attempts to ascertain whether some children are more popular as patients than others. Factors associated with being unpopular are discussed, as is the importance of children's nurses recognising their own value and belief systems.

Chapter 15 reports on an investigative study undertaken to audit how children's nurses manage fever in hospital, with particular reference to the administration of antipyretics. An evaluation of a specially designed fever chart and a survey of children's nurses from ten units reveals that fever management is based on tradition rather than evidence, thus highlighting the problems of practising nurses accessing the information they need in order to care appropriately.

In Chapter 16, the author emphasises the importance of a multi-disciplinary team approach in the management of children with diabetes. The study reports the evaluation of a paediatric diabetes specialist nurse position and demonstrates positive outcomes for the children concerned.

Chapters 17, 18 and 19 adopt a community perspective on evidence-based care for children, examining in particular the interface between hospital and home. Given the emphasis on developing paediatric community services, these chapters help to illuminate some of the difficulties facing the parents of sick children in the home environment.

Chapter 20 explores the evidence related to chronic childhood pain. This study discusses the experiences of families when living with children with chronic pain and recommends strategies that professionals might use when caring for similar children.

Chapter 21 is a fitting conclusion to the text in that it provides a detailed analysis of the process of collaborative approaches to evidence-based child health nursing practice. Readers should be able to emulate the process in their own clinical environments.

The primary goal of this text is to challenge children's nurses to understand, appreciate and use best evidence when planning the care of individual children and their families. The chapters contained therein utilise a variety of research, methods, some quantitative and some qualitative, all, however, following the same mission.

We hope you enjoy using this text and find it valuable in your day-to-day work.

The painting on the front cover, 'The Doctor' by Fildes, graphically shows the futility of working in an environment in which the evidence base for care is unknown. Child health care professionals in the nineteenth century had little access to evidence on which to base practice. In this the dawn of the twenty-first century we are surrounded by evidence but we must learn to harness it for the benefit of the children and families we care for.

ALAN GLASPER
LORRAINE IRELAND

1   *Challenging issues facing children's nurses in their quest to deliver evidence-based practice*

Edward Alan Glasper and Lorraine M. Ireland

Introduction

This chapter seeks to address the challenging issues facing children's nurses when attempting to change practice based on best evidence. The expansion of nursing roles in recent years is not always underpinned by sound research, and it is argued that children's nurses need to emulate their medical colleagues if they are to achieve effective practice.

The transfer of nursing education from hospital-based schools to the world of higher education provides new opportunities for nursing academics to work in partnership with their clinical colleagues to promote nursing care that is underpinned by research evidence. There remain, however, some misgivings among children's nurses that the benefits of engaging in research with children might not always be in the children's best interest. Despite these worries, the introduction of clinical governance as a strategic quality initiative by the UK National Health Service (NHS), will necessitate the development of nursing protocols and interventions based on evidence-based research.

It is argued that the role of the lecturer practitioner will be pivotal in bridging the theory–practice gap that has for so long bedevilled the nursing profession. Although the process of incorporating high-quality research findings into clinical practice is not straightforward, there is some optimism that the new nursing programmes will effectively address the issue and thus facilitate multiprofessional working with children and their parents in the promotion of excellence in care.

The UK NHS Executive directive *Achieving Effective Practice* (1998a) asks nurses to consider practice that is undertaken in the right way to achieve the right results. The whole quest for evidence-based care by nurses, fuelled by recent government White Papers (DoH, 1997, 1998), follows a path similar to that taken by the medical

1

profession, who are endeavouring to implement evidence based medi
cine. Sackett *et al.* (1996) state that evidence-based medicine can be
defined as the conscientious, explicit and judicious use of the best
evidence in making decisions about the care of individual patients. In
striving for the source of best evidence in an attempt to deliver
evidence-based care, there is a need for individual professionals,
including children's nurses, to examine both the conceptual basis of
this movement and the sources of best evidence.

Expanded nursing roles

Evidence-based care and the expanding role of the nurse are inexorably linked as the growth of the clinical nurse specialism has
followed advances in care delivery based on research findings. Some
areas of nursing have proliferated specialist nurses, the child health
field being no exception. Children's nurses have proved their commitment to family-centred care over a period of many years. It can be
postulated, however, that this commitment has been based on patri-
archal principles of empowerment rather than true partnership as
described by Casey (1993).

It must be acknowledged that the relative youthfulness of nursing
when compared with that of medicine is evident in that there is a
limited body of research-generated knowledge on which to base practice. This is particularly true of children's nurses, who make up only
about 15 per cent of the registered UK nursing workforce.

In addition, when compared with adult nursing, undergraduate and
Master's programmes to prepare children's nurses are a recent
phenomenon. Despite this, the proactive stance of this group is such
that their activity within the field of research is out of all proportion to
their relatively small number. Indeed, the UK's first International
Evidence-based Child Health Nursing Conference, held on the island
of Jersey in November 1997, was oversubscribed with research papers.

Although there is a paucity of nursing research on which to base
practice when compared with medicine, it must be acknowledged
that the foundation stones of modern scientific nursing were laid on
those founding principles of care first articulated by Florence
Nightingale. As a highly regarded empirical health care researcher in
contemporary Victorian society, it is Florence Nightingale who is
credited with that famous nursing quotation 'First do the patient no
harm.' It is perhaps this poignant message from the past that underpins the whole drive towards evidence-based care based on the
premise that some custom and practice might actually harm patients.

This is especially true for children's nurses, who, faced with past tragedies such as the deaths and injuries on the children's ward at Grantham and Kesteven General Hospital in 1991, are endeavouring to remain true to Nightingale's legacy to the profession. This cardinal tenet, which lies at the very heart of the nursing profession, must similarly be the guiding principle for those who seek to undertake research involving children and their families.

New tensions

Changes in the provision of UK education for nurses have seen the demise of hospital-based nursing colleges. The move of these essentially monotechnic institutions into the wider stream of the British universities has many benefits, not least the adoption of research-led culture by the ranks of nurse educationalists now employed by universities rather than the NHS. New tensions have, however, emerged. The research-led ethos of the universities demands that nurse educators demonstrate prowess in the field of scientific enquiry. Although the philosophies of caring and research are not incongruent, there might exist the potential that family empowerment will take a back seat to academic kudos sought through research (Glasper and Ireland, 1997).

The randomised controlled trial as the gold standard of research

The evidence-based care movement adheres to the randomised controlled trial as the gold standard in research. This methodology is seen as the only legitimate method through which best practice can be scientifically elicited. Such a stance fundamentally denigrates other research strategies. There is a fear expressed by many nurses that the 'rules' as followed by medical research may limit nursing development and in particular fail to reflect the perceptions of the consumers of health care, in this case sick children and their families (Kitson, 1997).

Although the UK NHS has for many years promoted practice that is effective, efficient and economical, it is the utilitarian approach advocated by the research and development arm of the service, squeezed, as most western economies, by a shrinking health care currency, that is exacerbating an already precarious moral situation.

McSherry and Haddock (1999) discuss why quality improvements have been placed at the forefront of the NHS agenda. They highlight the emphasis that is being placed on cost-effectiveness and how this is evaluated and measured against national indicators of success. The development in the UK of The National Institute for Clinical Excellence (NICE) can only accelerate the drive towards a nursing profession that is research based.

It must not be assumed that children's nurses are excessively enthusiastic in embracing care based on best evidence, but neither are they academic Luddites, seeking to delay progress. Instead, children's nurses are somewhat wary of research undertaken for research's sake. They need to be reassured that the hoped-for benefits of engaging in research with children outweigh any negative sequelae.

Clinical governance

As part of its mission to modernise the NHS, the UK government has introduced the concept of clinical governance. In essence, clinical governance makes clinical nurses, doctors and managers accountable for the care they deliver. This, more than any other factor, will necessitate the development of clinical protocols based on sound research; much contemporary child health nursing practice is currently based on little more than 'custom and practice', 'myths and rituals'.

Clearly, if clinical governance is going to reflect current nursing practice, the curricula of all nursing courses must reflect how nurses are able to translate the rhetoric of taught research into sound practice development. In such a climate of change, nurses must develop the confidence to play a major role in the articulation of clinical governance as it cascades throughout the service. Evidence-based practice is such a key feature of clinical governance that eventually all nursing practice will be subject to the research process. This is essential if the steps that are required, in order to facilitate and promote clinical governance, are to occur. The catastrophic events at the Bristol Children's Hospital, where a much higher number of children with a cardiac abnormality died when compared with other centres in the UK, are a timely reminder of the necessity of using best evidence when making decisions about patient and, in this case, child treatments (Smith, 1998).

The theory–practice gap

The 'theory–practice gap' has become a euphemism to describe apparent failures by nursing educational establishments to teach what trained nurses need to know and practise in the real world of clinical nursing. Ironically, the major changes in the way in which the

UK has educated its nurses under the Project 2000 initiative, aimed specifically at addressing and resolving the issue, have failed significantly to alter the perceptions of the nursing workforce that the gap remains. Strident debates at nursing conferences and prolific correspondence within the nursing literature have only fuelled the fire of this internecine conflict.

Increasing concern about the theory–practice gap in nursing has led to the UK's Chief Nursing Officer commissioning an investigation to throw more light and less heat onto the subject (NHS Executive, 1998b). The most important message of the Chief Nursing Officer's report is that a consideration of how theory and practice can be better interpreted is both desirable and achievable. The role of nurse lecturers in both the generation and dissemination of research-derived best evidence for practice is stressed. However, in order to achieve this, lecturers need to move from the perceived ivory towers of the universities into the world of the practising nurse. The growth in the number of lecturer practitioners is beginning to address this controversial issue and is refocusing research questions away from educational issues and more towards patient-centred activities. One consequence of these debates is the growing number of nurses who are actively seeking to undertake clinically related research.

It is within this multifaceted environment that nursing has embraced the culture of higher education within a structure no longer stratified by a binary line that once separated universities from polytechnics. As a result of this transfer, there has been a major shift in emphasis from teaching to research. Nurse educators have had to adopt the university maxim of 'publish or perish' within the new environment, those who do not being at a disadvantage; there is little if any reward in the university culture for those who teach but do not research. In a university climate, dominated by quadrennial research assessments in which individual academics are measured by their publishable research output, it is not difficult to appreciate the fervour for patient-centred research, which in turn liberates the data so necessary to develop the publications. The adoption of the research-led philosophy of the universities is a cause of the dichotomy so obviously manifest among many nurse educators, fearful for their own jobs but also fearful of the new gods of 'data first' and, implicitly, 'patient second'. This is not surprising as consequent to the reordering of priorities comes the real risk that the advocacy role of the children's nurse, long recognised as a pivotal component of family-centred care, will be threatened.

Despite the Chief Nursing Officer's optimism, Cullum (1997) has indicated that the process of incorporating high-quality research findings into clinical nursing practice is not straightforward. Year on year, crises related to nurse recruitment and retention ensure that trained nurses working in clinical environments are constrained by the reality that action must take precedence over reflection. In a nursing world where early discharge, high patient throughput and staff shortages are the norm, the well-educated nurse struggles to get through the work and maintain minimal standards of care. In addition, these same nurses, no matter how well motivated, have difficulties in accessing digestible accounts of nursing and other health care research. The challenge of illuminating the relevance of research findings to nurses at the forefront of clinical practice has been described by Akinsanya (1994). He suggests that an appreciation of research needs to be firmly rooted in the educational processes of all registered practitioners. In fact, this now underpins all pre-registration diploma/advanced diploma and undergraduate nursing programmes.

However, nurse educators are well aware of the large number of registered nurses who trained prior to the Project 2000 initiative. It is for this group that post-registration pathways of education have been developed. Such pathways, leading to a variety of National Board awards, now include mandatory research modules whose aim is to inculcate a culture of care based on best evidence. It must be recognised, however, that the enormity of the task is beyond a quick-fix solution, and other methods of rolling out the UK government's clinical governance agenda must be sought.

In addition, it is the belief of the university academics that only through close contact with those who are conducting research will nurses recognise the benefits to care practice. It is for this reason that nurse lecturers are expected to participate and be actively involved with research. However, the quest for evidence-based practice is founded not solely on a diet of empiricism, other less measurable criteria for determining the efficiency of care existing, despite the ascendancy of the randomised controlled trial. There are other stakeholders, that is, parents and guardians, whose views on the provision of child care are rarely sought, and their inclusion may not be commensurate with the prescriptive stance of the evidence-based medicine movement.

Conducting research with children and their families

Callery (1997) notes that the traditional evidence-based medicine approach focuses on the patient rather than the whole family. It is, therefore, important for those who seek to undertake research involving children that the various users of the child health services and their differing interests need to be taken into account, both in the questions asked and in consideration of the evidence.

Children are one of the most vulnerable groups of potential research participants. Alderson (1993), in her text *Listening to Children – Ethics and Social Research*, has clearly highlighted the difficulties of safeguarding the rights of the child, pointing out that much research is carried out *on* children but seldom *with* children. As a consequence, children are often just passive bystanders in the whole process of health care research. Despite the higher profile of ethical principles and issues in research that have been hard fought for since the post-war Nuremberg Trials and the Declaration of Helsinki, there continue to be flagrant abuses of the rights of children in the field of research.

Gaining consent from parents or guardians does not always equate to gaining consent from the child. Ascertaining whether or not a child is 'Gillick competent' is an over-simplistic method of determining whether a child should be asked for consent. Hendrick (1998) believes that children's competence tends to be underestimated and that this has ramifications for consent, although Alderson (1993) firmly believes that children of all ages can be helped to participate in the decision-making processes. No-one suggests that it is easy to involve children in the consenting process, and it is perhaps because it involves more time and resource that researchers are happy to have the proxy consent of the parents or guardians. Many ethical committees, in vetting research proposals, will specifically request copies of all consenting letters, forms, protocols and so on before making a decision to grant ethical approval.

It is the individual's right to informed consent failing to be operationalised within the field of child care that is a source of worry for so many children's nurses. As there is no universal agreement on the way in which research subjects should give their consent, the nurse researcher should endeavour to give maximum rather than minimum information to families. Behi (1995) believes that the medium for communicating issues related to consent must be appropriate to the target subjects. This will prove challenging to children's nurses and will require greater ingenuity to accomplish the task. It should not, however, be beyond the realms of possibility for a nursing workforce, used to operating in a multicultural society, to develop appropriate child-centred strategies for gaining informed consent. This is echoed in the United Nations Convention (DoH, 1991), which states that children should be able to get hold of a wide range of information, especially anything that would make life better for them (Article 17).

The academic aspirations of the nursing profession

As the UK nursing profession stands on the brink of becoming all-graduate at the point of registration, it must be appreciated that this meets the academic aspirations of its members. In a climate of lifelong learning, nurses are increasingly encouraged to undertake further education. As nursing moves inexorably towards an all-graduate status, this is focusing the attention of non-graduate, experienced pre-project 2000 practitioners on studies that are perceived to be essential in safeguarding their own future employment. The over-robustness of some university accreditation of prior learning schemes does little to ease this rite of passage for the non-graduate, experienced children's nurse, who may be mandated to conduct a research project that may have no future beyond being a vehicle for academic attainment.

The number of pre- and post-registration students now wishing to conduct research in clinical environments is such that some hospital ethical committees have been forced to make major decisions on who may or may not access patients for the purposes of research. It is not uncommon in some children's units to find that the majority of patients are in one or more research cohorts. Alderson (1995) reminds would-be researchers that the topic of research should be worthwhile, with clear hoped-for benefits for children and their families. Students should be encouraged to look to other sources of data if they are unable to answer these straightforward questions.

In addition to the large volume of undergraduates wishing to access patients, there are now appreciable numbers of graduate nurses who wish to undertake an MSc, MPhil or PhD. Such qualifications have become the new gold standard in nursing, and the changing role of nurse educators within higher education will only exacerbate this situation.

There is no doubt that 'doing research' conveys an aura of academic respectability. The 'publish or perish' *raison d'être* of the university system is directly channelling the efforts of nurse lecturers towards research and the achievement of higher degrees where these are called for. The percentage of nurse lecturers with a PhD is much smaller than that seen in similar academic subjects, and the acquisition of a doctorate will, for the foreseeable future, continue to be the perceived pinnacle of some careers. The pressure to gain a doctorate, which in the near future is likely to be the minimal entry qualification for a lectureship in nursing in a British university, is, for expediency's sake, forcing some nurses to chose a project not of their own making. This may or may not be the source of evidence on which to base best practice.

In such a climate, the voice of the family or sick child is less likely to be taken into consideration in the commissioning or writing of research and development bids to funding bodies. This is especially true if the funding body is the research and development arm of the NHS, which is increasingly driven by health economics and other fiscal forces. Kitson (1997) reminds nurses that the drive for clinical effectiveness is undoubtedly medically led and that this in turn shapes the whole profile of the evidence-based practice movement, which is in reality geared to a national sickness service rather than a service that puts health and the prevention of ill-health on the top of its list of priorities. This should not, however, deter nurses from the advantages of interprofessional collaboration, and they must continue to strive for a voice that articulates nurse-led, family-focused initiatives.

UK university research assessment exercises clarify and reinforce the academic reality that nursing is now fully integrated into higher education. It is perhaps salutary to note that academic success in research is measured on a scale of 1–5, 5* being an international accolade of excellence. During the 1996 assessment exercise, only one nursing department in the UK was awarded a mark of 5 (Watson, 1997).

Ethical dimensions of research related to children

It is perhaps understandable that the fervour for research among nurse academics is blurring the parameters of what is and what is not ethical when working with children. Children, being one of the most vulnerable groups of research participants, need powerful advocates. The special role of the children's nurse in the support and education of parents and children can only be considered in the light of research findings (Glasper *et al.*, 1996).

Despite this, research studies involving children must not liberate data that actually or potentially harm the subjects for whom the research was intended. The whole history of empirical research in children is littered with examples of studies with questionable ethical standards. The work of the German Dr Josef Mengele in the concentration camps during the Second World War is often quoted as an example of how children's rights have been in some cases obscenely abused. The German pharmaceutical giant Bayer, once part of the pre-war industrial conglomerate I.G.Farben, which manufactured the gas used in the Holocaust, is currently being sued for co-operating with Nazi doctors such as Mengele who deliberately infected children with a series of diseases to test out drugs manufactured by Bayer (Borger and Kundani, 1997).

The fervent media reports surrounding the use of continuous negative extra thoracic pressure (CNEP) ventilators to treat premature babies requiring respiratory support is a timely warning that families need full information before giving their consent (Wainright, 1999). In this randomised controlled trial, the parents of those premature babies who died in the experimental group receiving CNEP felt 'hoodwinked and duped', believing that the steps taken by the doctors to gain consent were totally inadequate. As a result of this inquiry, the consent procedure for research involving children and their families is likely to be improved.

In a similar case, the negative media reports surrounding the research of a nurse lecturer at the University of Birmingham into the experience of those families bereaved following the Dunblane massacre (Cloustron, 1997) attest to the insensitivity of some research projects. Such was the gravity of this poorly thought-out research project that it demanded personal apologies from the vice-chancellors at the universities of Birmingham and Wolverhampton to the families concerned.

The report in the *Lancet* (1997), which disclosed that the US Center for Disease Control had supported unethical trials of drugs for the treatment of human immuno-deficiency virus (HIV) (women in a placebo group being allowed to transmit HIV infection perinatally to their children) is a reminder that all researchers must abide by those principles first stated during the Nuremberg trials (United States Government, 1949). Children's nurses must endeavour to be constantly vigilant in order to represent families whose voice may be too weak to articulate concerns related to research affecting their children.

The role of professional bodies

Professional bodies such as the Royal College of Nursing and the Royal College of Paediatrics and Child Health are beginning to voice a fundamental commitment to the inclusion of children within the decision-making process of research (RCPCH, 1997).

Given the perennial problems associated with consent and research, it would be timely for the professional bodies to unite in giving more explicit guidance to would-be investigators. Such guidance is necessary as, unlike adults who are able to give their own consent, children who are not Gillick competent must rely on others to give proxy consent (BPA, 1992). This is usually given by a parent, and a presumption is made that he or she will always act in the child's best interest. This should not negate the moral responsibility to respect fully children's rights, including that of giving their own agreement, perhaps by giving their own consent or at the very least their assent (Ireland and Holloway, 1996).

Conclusion

The quest by children's nurses to base their care on best evidence is only just beginning, but gaining access to systematic reviews that reveal best practice is becoming easier.

The University of York's NHS Centre for Reviews and Dissemination is now available on the World Wide Web (http://nhscrd.york. ac.uk/dbhelp.htm) and regularly publishes bulletins presenting material in a digestible format.

The bulletin *Getting Evidence into Practice* (NHS Centre for Reviews and Dissemination, 1999) highlights some of the steps to be taken by health care professionals before they attempt to bring about change in a clinical environment. If children's nurses are to be successful in bringing about change, they themselves will need to be equipped with the appropriate knowledge and skills.

The chapters in this book reflect this tenet and are a tribute to children's nurses and their desire to base care on best evidence. The motto of the UK's first children's hospital, founded in 1852 in Great Ormond Street, London – 'The child first and always' – is as pertinent today as it was then.

References

Akinsanya J. (1994) 'Making research useful to the practising nurse', *Journal of Advanced Nursing* **19**: 174–9.

Alderson P. (1995) *Listening to Children – Ethics and Social Research*, Ilford, Barnardos.

Behi R. (1995) 'The individual's right to informed consent', *Nurse Researcher* **13**(1): 14–23.

Borger J. and Kundani H. (1999) 'Drugs firm sued by Auschwitz guinea pig', *Guardian*, 19 February, p. 12.

British Paediatric Association (1992) *Guidelines for the Ethical Conduct of Medical Research Involving Children*, London, BPA.

Callery P. (1997) 'Using evidence in children's nursing', *Paediatric Nursing* **9**(16): 13–17.

Casey A. (1993) 'Development and use of the partnership model of nursing care' In Glasper E. A. and Tucker A. (eds) *Advances in Child Health Nursing*, London, Scutari Press.

Cloustron B. (1997) 'Dunblane anger at naïve questions on killings' (editorial). *Guardian*, 15 January, p. 5.

Cullum N. (1997) 'Evidence-based nursing: an introduction', *Evidence Based Nursing* (pilot edn), pp. 3–4.

Department of Health (1991) *The Rights of the Child – A Guide to the UN Convention*, DoH, Children's Rights Development Unit.

Department of Health (1997) *The New NHS: Modern, Dependable*, London, HMSO.

Department of Health (1998) *A First Class Service: Quality in the New NHS*, London, HMSO.

Glasper E. A. and Ireland L. (1997) 'Is the quest for evidence-based care detrimental to children's nursing?', *British Journal of Nursing* 6(21): 1253–5.

Glasper E. A., Powell C., Darbyshire P. *et al.* (1996) 'Children's nursing as a research-based profession', *British Journal of Nursing* 5(7): 420–1.

Hendrick J. (1998) 'Legal and ethical issues'. In Moules T. and Ramsay J. (eds) *The Textbook of Children's Nursing*, Cheltenham, Stanley Thornes.

Ireland L. M. and Holloway I. (1996) 'Qualitative health research with children', *Children and Society* 10: 155–64.

Kitson A. (1997) 'Using evidence to demonstrate the place of nursing', *Nursing Standard* 11(28): 34–9.

Lancet (1997) 'The ethics industry' (editorial), *Lancet*, 350: 297.

McSherry R. and Haddock J. (1999) 'Evidence-based health care: its place within clinical governance', *British Journal of Nursing* 8(2): 113–17.

NHS Executive (1998a) *Achieving Effective Practice*, London, DoH.

NHS Executive (1998b) *Integrating Theory and Practice in Nursing – A Report Commissioned by the Chief Nursing Officer/Director of Nursing*, London, NHS Executive.

NHS Centre for Reviews and Dissemination (1999) 'Getting evidence into practice', *Effective Health Care* 5(1): 1–16

Royal College of Paediatrics and Child Health (1997) *Withholding or Withdrawing Life Saving Treatment for Children: A Framework for Practice*, London, RCPCH.

Sackett D. L., Rosenberg W. M. C., Gray J. A. M., Haynes R. D. and Richardson W. S. (1996) 'Evidence-based medicine: what it is and what it isn't', *British Medical Journal* 312: 71–2.

Smith R. (1998) 'All changed, changed utterly. British Medicine will be transformed by the Bristol Case', *British Medical Journal* 316: 1917–18.

United States Government (1949) *Trials of War Criminals for the Nurenberg Military Tribunals*, Washington, DC, US Government Printing Office.

Wainright M. (1999) 'Inquiry into experiment on babies', *Guardian*, 13 February, p. 4.

Watson R. (1997) 'United Kingdom universities assessment exercise, 1996. Critique, comment and concern', *Journal of Advanced Nursing* 26(4): 641.

2 Demonstrating evidence-based clinical nursing practice: providing the evidence

Tony Long and Jill Asbury

Introduction

Our ability to assess practice at degree level is just as crucial as our ability to assess theory. What, it is suggested, differentiates degree-level practice is the intellectual process associated with the practice in question. A key element of the effective assessment of practice is that evidence must be collected from a range of sources. Examples of such sources that have been exploited within a programme of study are discussed, including critical incident analysis, commentary in practice, prescribed specific outcomes, the documentation of care, the observation of practice, written evidence, spontaneous discussions of practice, and extracts from a reflective diary. The process of providing and evaluating the evidence was conducted within a tripartite arrangement involving the practitioner or student, the supervising practitioner and a lecturer. The net result was an overall assessment of the degree of competence.

This chapter addresses one means of providing evidence of achievement in clinical nursing, particular emphasis being laid on level 3 (graduate) practice. Although the assessment of theory for undergraduates is well established, the assessment of differing levels of practice, by self-assessment in the case of clinical supervision, or as a formal part of a programme of study, remains a major challenge. Since nursing is a practice-based discipline, this is a challenge that cannot be ignored. While the key function of the framework suggested in this chapter refers to the individual practitioner providing evidence of achievement for his or her own purposes (perhaps for application for regrading, for appraisal or for role justification), there are also applications for programmes of study. In addition to the burgeoning of undergraduate pre-registration

13

programmes, the development of programmes leading to specialist
[practitioner] status with a stated emphasis on practice within
programmes of study (UKCC, 1994) highlights the need for new
approaches to undergraduate assessment strategies. The processes
discussed here have been developed for use in a Graduate Diploma in
Child Health Nursing. This programme is designed for registered
nurses wishing to complete a further specialist registration in child
health nursing. In the UK, such specialist registration is expected for
professional practice in the field of child health nursing.

The need for nursing as graduate activity

Several factors have caused an acceleration and broadening of the
movement towards graduate-level practice, the first qualification
through undergraduate preparation and corresponding requirements
for further study for qualified nurses being located at least at undergraduate level. It is important to realise that the driving force behind
this is the development of nursing practice into ever more complex,
high-level, intellectual intervention. Not only advances in medical
technology and science, but also, perhaps more importantly, advances
in nurses' understanding of the nature, scope and potential of nursing
have thrown back the boundaries of nursing practice. Areas of patient
needs and treatment that were previously within the sole remit of
other professionals are frequently being subsumed into holistic
nursing practice. The incorporation of such skills and interventions
into nursing requires the sort of intellectual ability and approaches
normally considered to be characteristic of a graduate. A convincing
argument on this issue has been put forward by Clark (1992).

A longer-term expectation flows from attention given to undergraduate preparation, ably expressed by the Royal College of
Nursing (RCN, 1996). As nursing strives to establish its own discrete
knowledge base, it must look towards future practitioners being
primed from the point of qualification to understand, support or lead
this endeavour. While much of the work in advancing nursing knowledge and theory will occur at higher levels (Master's and doctoral
research), the foundation of such work is to be established in undergraduate achievement (RCN, 1996). The call for nursing to be
learned through undergraduate study has been repeated by a number
of other relevant bodies (Commission of the European Communities,
1989; ICN, 1989; Council of Europe, 1994).

Many nurses cherish the notion of nursing being an essentially
practice-based discipline. However, our ability to provide evidence of

achievement at degree level has largely been limited to theoretical rather than practical perspectives. While valuing 'experience' of varying nature and intensity, we have little to show for our efforts to demonstrate the level of achievement in that crucial aspect of nursing: practice. Within programmes of study too, the equivalence of practice to theory has been highlighted (ENB, 1993, 1994) with regard to value, study time and assessment. Consequently, our ability to provide evidence of practice at degree level is just as crucial as our ability to assess theory.

The tripartite relationship

The assessment of competence has historically been an issue for nurse education to address but for clinical nurses to undertake. Given that a significant proportion of the activity in question will continue to be related to programmes of study, it is worthwhile reviewing the relative roles of clinical practitioners and academic staff in assessing practice.

The issue of the 'theory–practice gap' has been evident in the debate and discussion surrounding the clinical supervision of nurses for several decades (see, for example Wong, 1979). Certainly, since the beginning of nurse education, there has been a perceived discrepancy between what is taught in the classroom and what is experienced in the clinical area (Elliot, 1993). The issues contributing to this state of affairs have been the subject of a working group set up by the National Health Service (NHS) Executive (NHS Executive, 1998a). The reasons for nursing knowledge failing to be expressed in nursing practice are legion and include fear, lack of understanding and a lack of confidence to challenge existing practices. The gap will remain as long as nurses concern themselves with the origin of theories rather than their relevance to practice (Jolley and Allen, 1991). As higher education and the health service continue to undergo review and reform, the potential exists further to separate the theoretical and the practical aspects of nursing. This may be accentuated as nurses and lecturers strive to stay abreast of organisational changes and developments while delivering the current agenda.

A number of approaches have been aimed at reducing the divide, most notably the role of the clinical nurse teacher. This, however, has not been a success, Akinsanya (1993) suggesting that the separation of tutors and clinical teachers proved to be both 'divisive and costly'. More recently, the development of lecturer practitioners, who, by virtue of their combined role, have the skills to design educational programmes and act as role models during participant observation, has attracted interest. The implementation of the role of community practice teacher is another example of action to remedy this problem. Even allowing for these roles, the fact remains that the clinical assessment of nurses has been the domain of clinical nursing staff, with distant or troubleshooting support from academic staff. If the distancing of the theory from the practice of nursing is to be prevented, a proactive approach needs to be taken within the practice arena in partnership with university schools and departments.

The emergence of level 3 practice and the need to provide a consistent, higher-quality approach to clinical assessment offered the opportunity to review current practices. This led to the devising of a method to bring together elements of assessment of clinical practice – the nurse, the supervising or appraising practitioner, and the lecturer – with a view to instigating a reflective discussion of the theoretical issues and realities of evidence-based practice. This was largely dependent upon shared values, mutual respect and understanding and genuine communication. When examining the possible approaches to assessing graduate practice, it seemed most appropriate to take this collaboration further.

In the current climate of structural change and financial pressure faced by the health and educational systems, it seems inappropriate to commit to one model for achieving assessment. A pluralistic approach involving multiple models would seem to ensure a flexible and adaptable framework that could be used in any number of clinical settings depending upon the demands of the specialism and the departmental structure. This has resulted in a tripartite relationship involving the nurse, the supervising practitioner and the lecturer (Figure 2.1). This model is compatible with community-based arrangements, which include the community practice teacher, as well as with acute care settings such as hospital-based clinical areas.

In the UK, the supervision of clinical practice and the assessment of students is carried out by practitioners who have undertaken further preparation and achieved additional qualification. The student is expected to be an active participant in the assessment process, and there is usually a named clinical supervisor and a designated academic lecturer for each individual student. The relationship is based on values to which both the organisations and the individuals involved can commit: those of openness, pragmatism and mutual respect. This tripartite approach enables a depth and richness to be embodied in the assessment, through demonstrating the realities of integrating theory in practice. It uses a variety of sources for assessment, as detailed below, and allows for a more complete assessment through the complementary relationships of practitioner, supervisor and academic.

The lecturer's presence is not necessarily a component of every assessment meeting. His or her role is to facilitate reflexivity, to assist

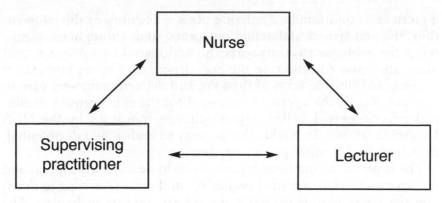

Figure 2.1 The tripartite relationship

in analysing areas of uncertainty and to offer an external view of what might otherwise be too familiar to the participants to review effectively. Should the nurse whose level of practice is being considered be a student, the academic may have additional contributions to make to the process. The contractual arrangements (for example, meeting times and levels of individual involvement) are left to the tripartite group to determine, minimum guidelines being suggested, and do not preclude informal discussions. A further benefit of this arrangement is that there is a greater variety and scope of opportunities for the nurse to demonstrate his or her achievement.

Collaborative positions involving education and service, in which the post-holder has a contractual obligation to both organisations, for example joint appointments or the lecturer practitioner role, are not uncommon, currently tending to be associated with clinical specialisms. Such positions are being actively promoted in some areas as the key to supporting and assessing students (DoH, 1997). Where such a position exists, it presents an opportunity for the individual involved to act as either the supervising practitioner or the lecturer. Alternative clinical assessors working in conjunction with the lecturer may be clinical nurse specialists, clinical nurse advisors, community practice teachers or ward managers, whichever is most beneficial to the individual circumstances. The tripartite approach allows the nurse the flexibility to approach one or both assessors when he or she feels that an appropriate or unusual intervention may provide the basis for assessment. This, however, necessitates a commitment to a change in culture from an assessor-driven model to student-led assessment.

A key area in the assessment of level 3 practice is examining episodes of nursing care and encouraging the nurse to explore, own and analyse the decisions taken in the systematic provision of care for

a given child and family. Analysing the applicability of the intervention, the anticipated and actual outcomes, and, throughout, identifying the evidence that supports the actions taken (or not taken)
allow the nurse to reflect on the experience, developing innovative,
creative and flexible ways of thinking and delivering nursing care to
children. This is the approach proposed for the enhancement of clinical effectiveness, labelled 'inform–change–monitor', by the NHS
Executive (1996). To enable this process to realise its full potential,
those involved require specific preparation.

The tripartite relationship appears to be loose in its description and
be expected to place a further burden on staff already striving to maintain the *status quo*. Fortunately, the reverse appears to be true. The
assessment process has to occur by one means or another, and this
commitment has not increased. However, the direct involvement of the
three participants has promoted an increased understanding of the
others' roles and, offered the stimulation of creative and innovative
ideas for developing evidence-based practice, the nurse being central to
and often the catalyst in questioning current approaches to care. The
process is enabling the nurse to 'live' the integration of theory and practice while increasing the dialogue, support and collaboration between
the service and educational organisations. This can only bring future
strengths to the assessment of clinical practice at level 3 and beyond.

The means of assessing practice

Certain assumptions must be made about the assessment of practice
at any given level. Below follows an explanation and justification of
the assumptions made here about degree-level practice. First, it is
assumed that the psychomotor element of what is to be achieved in a
given aspect of nursing practice is a matter of either having achieved
or not achieved, demonstrated competence or not demonstrated
competence. Some practitioners will of course demonstrate more
flair, more manual dexterity and so on, but what, it is suggested,
differentiates degree-level practice is the intellectual process associated with the activity in question. Several attributes suggest a level of
intellectual activity commensurate with graduate achievement:

- Skilled, holistic assessment and critical analysis
- The application, in creative or innovative ways, of existing theory
- An insight into wider perspectives on the issues explicit
- A conceptualisation of the nature and context of phenomena.

To achieve the goal of assessment and, eventually, the classification of degree-level practice, two major issues need to be addressed. The nature of graduate practice has not been widely debated, and there is no clear, universal understanding of what level 3 practice may mean. However, the characteristics of a graduate have been expounded in a number of centres, and there is an acceptance by universities, professional bodies and professional organisations of this work (see Davis and Burnard, 1992; RCN, 1996). Most universities have a grid of marking criteria for theoretical work in undergraduate programmes: indeed, the Higher Education Quality Council has a sample grid of assessment criteria. It has been suggested above that similar aspects of intellectual activity and the presentation of thought can (and should) be applied to the assessment of clinical practice; corresponding criteria can be devised for the assessment and classification of clinical practice at this level. While this may seem to be more directly applicable to formal programmes of study, such criteria are also useful for self-assessment and for the varied purposes outlined above.

Collecting evidence

The remaining difficulty relates to the means of collecting the data to be judged against these criteria. The crucial requirement of the ability to articulate standards of clinical practice and to communi-

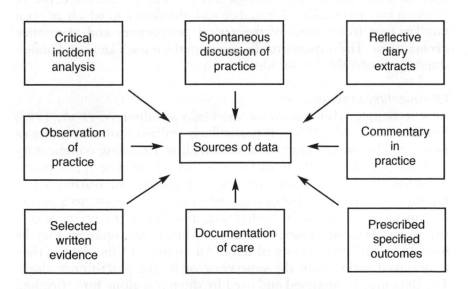

Figure 2.2 Sources of data for evidence

cate effectively on such issues is highlighted by the NHS Executive (1998b). Key elements have been identified as being crucial to the effective assessment of practice (ENB, 1993), one of these being that evidence should be collected from a range of sources. These should then form the basis for a reflective discussion of theoretical issues and the realities of practice within the tripartite arrangement. This approach is supported by Goding (1997), who justifies the need for multiple-source qualitative data for the evaluation of the many intangible facets of nursing practice at degree level. The following sources of data have been exploited by the authors for the assessment of level 3 practice (Figure 2.2).

Critical incident analysis
Critical incident technique was first described in detail by Flanagan (1954) but has an established place in nursing in the UK (see, for example Long, 1976). The application of critical incidents here is an amended version of the technique, undertaken in a location removed from patient contact but within the clinical practice area. It involves the nurse detailing a significant incident arising from clinical practice and reflecting with a supervisor or lecturer on the various perspectives that may be identified within the incident. The supervisor's role is to facilitate reflection, to challenge assumptions and interpretation, to offer alternative theoretical perspectives and to clarify meaning with the nurse. The individual practitioner may then choose whether or not to document this discussion. Through this process, the nurse's depth of thinking may be considered, together with the degree to which an open mind is kept to a variety of theoretical perspectives and alternative explanations. The response to challenges to the nurse's ideas and understanding should also be considered.

Commentary in practice
This technique, also known as 'think-aloud' (Fonteyn *et al.*, 1993; Fonteyn and Fisher, 1995), is particularly utilised during episodes of practice. This entails practitioners providing a running commentary on their thoughts and actions for brief periods of time (perhaps the duration of a single interaction with a patient, or during a few minutes of preparation for or consideration of a response to a particular incident). This can be undertaken alone or in the presence of a supervisor. Hand-held tape-recorders and lapel microphones may be used to record these bursts of data. An analysis of the data is then undertaken, either with the supervisor or by the practitioner alone. The data may be analysed and used by the nurse alone for reflection, to be reported on later to his or her supervisor. Sharing the audio-

taped data is most useful when the supervisor has been present during the interaction since a comparison can then be made between actions and reported thoughts.

Opinion varies on the value and desirability of this method, some concern being voiced that clinical performance may be adversely affected by 'thinking out loud'. This has not been the authors' experience, but Corcoran *et al.* (1988) provide a useful discussion on this topic. This means of collecting evidence is both an acquired skill and a matter of personal choice. For some it is an anxiety-provoking activity, for others a source of stimulation for their own reflection. As with other uses of audiotaped data, there is a variable time lapse before the user becomes familiar and comfortable with the process.

Reflective diary extracts
Practitioners are encouraged to record a reflective diary from which extracts may be selected for presentation and discussion with another member of the tripartite relationship. This can provide a useful vehicle for the consideration of issues arising from practice and the nurse's response to these. Such sessions are led by the nurse, who retains control over which parts of the diary are to be divulged. This strategy is supported by the work of Schön (1987). Such diaries may be not formal affairs but intermittent entries written roughly on loose sheets and often held in an A4 loose-leaf folder. In the authors' study, it very quickly became clear that maintaining and using a reflective diary is a learned skill (see Hahnemann, 1986; Lyte and Thompson, 1990) and should be routinely included in study skills sessions on formal programmes of study. Richardson and Hendrika (1995) discuss the nature of these skills.

Documentation of care
The planning and evaluation of care for individual children and families, supplementary reports and other suitable documentation is scrutinised by the supervisor or lecturer, a justification of judgements and conclusions being required. While there are normally many alternative solutions to clinical problems and needs (each possibly equally acceptable), the thoughts and knowledge that led to the decision taken in a specific case may be indicative of the level of competence. A plethora of rich material for consideration, debate and review is provided by such documentation.

Benner (1984) finds it deeply regretful that nursing, because of individuals' failure to chart their minor, common success and innovations in practice, has missed so many opportunities to advance and capture nursing knowledge. Perhaps through closer critical attention to our reports of our actions, we may not only recognise effective, graduate-level practice, but also engender and promote potential advances in practice as a profession. The grand plan of enhancing the overall quality of service in the NHS relies not only on macro-level activity such as contributing to the Cochrane Centre database, as suggested by the NHS Executive (1996), but also on micro-level inspection and reflection on interventions with individual patients, which often serves to stimulate more formal research.

Observation of the nurse in practice

While this is in any case required as part of normal clinical supervision in order to assess psychomotor competence, evidence may also be extracted of higher-level activity. An observer shadows the nurse in clinical practice for short periods, usually by agreement, concentrating not only on demonstrated skills, but also on the surrounding context and visible clues to the nature of the encounter with children or their families. Such observations serve to stimulate and structure subsequent discussion, the supervisor or lecturer, as ever, challenging assumptions, seeking justification for the nurse's actions and exploring explanations of the perceived situations.

There is a great deal of work available pertaining to the strengths and weaknesses of observation as a means of collecting data (see, for example, Hammersley and Atkinson, 1995), but the clearest difficulty so far encountered is the fear of incessant observation and assessment, which adversely affects concentration, creativity and, ultimately, competence. One response to this has been to encourage discrete periods of observation, selected by agreement, with clear indications of when the activity starts and finishes. Practitioners will usually begin by selecting non-threatening situations and work up to more challenging scenarios as their confidence grows.

Spontaneous discussion of practice in general

As part of normal professional activity, a discussion of aspects of practice is common. A practitioner's level of intellectual activity may be partly assessed (and supplemented) by spontaneous discussion. This could be initiated by any member of the tripartite relationship. It is important to clarify, once again, that this does not constitute incessant assessment, practitioners never being able to relax and concentrate on other issues. This activity is considered to be a minor part of the assessment process, but it would be foolish to assume that impressions gained at such informal moments could in practice be entirely dismissed. Nevertheless, there is a danger of undue bias affecting such judgement, the process relying heavily upon the professionalism, experience and expertise of supervisors and lecturers in recognising and minimising this.

Selected written evidence

Practitioners may chose to present a written document of whatever nature or size that helps to demonstrate their ability in clinical practice. Some of the aspects suitable for inclusion in critical incident analysis or a reflective diary could equally well be presented in this manner. The nature of such documents is very varied. Often, they take the form of hand-written pieces, sometimes presented as mind maps, occasionally as annotated copies of existing documents such as admissions protocols or ward philosophies. Alternatively, thoughts may be presented more formally in academic-style papers, more commonly word-processed and fully referenced. As it became clear in the authors' research that time needed to be allocated in a formal manner to this activity, two models were developed. In the first, there was a set period of perhaps 30 minutes in each shift for nurses to engage in producing this evidence, while in the second there was simply a formal agreement within the clinical area that it was legitimate for practitioners to remove themselves at mutually convenient times whenever they had some thoughts to write up.

Specified outcomes

This source of data often relates only to formal programmes of study in which specific outcomes are associated with each module. Predetermined outcomes help to direct students' efforts for that part of the programme. However, it is also useful in other circumstances in which formal outcomes are predetermined. This may include job descriptions or grading criteria. Should a nurse be seeking to demonstrate the attainment of a higher level of practice for such purposes, this method may prove helpful. Some of the methods detailed above are useful in establishing competence in the prescribed aspects of practice. The outcomes or criteria in themselves often provide material for reflection and discussion, and it would of course be legitimate for individuals to evaluate the outcomes with critical commentary and suggestions for improvement. Such a critique of required aspects of clinical practice could certainly demonstrate higher-level activity.

Not all of these means of data collection need be used. The crucial factors are, first, that a variety of sources is addressed, and second, that the nurse–supervising practitioner–lecturer tripartite relationship is utilised effectively. The net result should be an overall assessment of the degree of competence, including a consideration of the nurse engaging in clinical practice and reflecting upon practice.

If the practice of child health nursing needs to be evidence based (NHS Executive, 1996, 1997), the assessment or appraisal of that practice should be no less rigorous. It is useful if a system can be devised that is equally applicable and workable within a number of clinical arenas, including primary, secondary and tertiary care environments. There remains much work to be completed in establishing a means of assessment of level 3 practice that is both rigorous and effective. However, the authors' experience to date of tackling the changing culture and facing up to the numerous and disparate problems encountered has invariably been positive. The efforts discussed here represent a framework for a strategy and the beginning of an evolving repertoire for providing evidence of achievement.

References

Akinsanya J. (1993) 'Preparation of nurse teachers: a rethink', *Nursing Standard* 8(5): 28–30.

Benner P. (1984) *From Novice to Expert: Excellence and Power in Clinical Nursing Practice*, Menlo Park, CA, Addison-Wesley.

Clark J. (1992) 'Nursing: an intellectual activity', *International Nursing Review* 39(2): 60.

Commission of the European Communities (1989) *Nursing Education in the 21st Century*, proceedings of a symposium. Brussels, CEC.

Corcoran S., Narayan S. and Moreland H. (1988) '"Thinking aloud" as a strategy to improve clinical decision making', *Heart Lung* 17: 463–8.

Council of Europe (1994) *Working Party on the Role and Education of Nurses*, CDSP (94): 35, Strasbourg. Council of Europe.

Davis B. and Burnard, P. (1992) 'Academic levels in nursing', *Journal of Advanced Nursing* 17: 1395–400.

Department of Health (1997) *A Bridge to the Future: Nursing Standards, Education and Workforce Planning in Paediatric Intensive Care*, London, HMSO.

Elliot P. (1993) 'Locality based teaching', *Senior Nurse* 13(2): 35–9.

English National Board for Nursing, Midwifery and Health Visiting (1993) *Assessment of Competencies in Nursing and Midwifery Education and Training (the ACE Project)*, London, ENB.

English National Board for Nursing, Midwifery and Health Visiting (1994) *Creating Lifelong Learners – Partnerships for Care*, London, ENB.

Flanagan J. (1954) 'The critical incident technique', *Psychological Bulletin* 51(4): 327–58.

Fonteyn M. E. and Fisher A. (1995) 'Use of think aloud method to study nurse decision making in clinical practice settings', *Journal of Neuroscience Nursing* 27(2): 121–6.

Fonteyn M. E., Kuipers B. and Grobe S. J. (1993) 'A description of think aloud method and protocol analysis', *Qualitative Health Research* 3(4): 430–40.

Goding L. (1997) 'Can degree level practice be assessed?', *Nurse Education Today* 17(2): 158–61.

Hahnemann B. (1986) 'Journal writing: a key to promoting critical thinking in nursing students', *Journal of Nursing Education* 25: 213–15.

Hammersley M. and Atkinson P. (1995) *Ethnography: Principles in Practice* (2nd edn), Routledge, London.

International Council of Nurses (1989) *Development of Standards for Nursing Education and Practice: Guidelines for National Nurses Associations*, Geneva, ICN.

Jolley M. and Allen P. (1991) *Current Issues in Nursing*, London, Chapman & Hall.

Long P. (1976) 'Judging and reporting on student nurse clinical performance: some problems for the ward sister', *International Journal of Nursing Studies* 13: 115–21.

Lyte V. and Thompson I. (1990) 'The diary as a formative teaching and learning aid incorporating means of evaluation and renegotiation of clinical learning objectives', *Nurse Education Today* 10: 228–32.

NHS Executive (1996) *Promoting Clinical Effectiveness: A Framework for Action in and through the NHS*, London, DoH.

NHS Executive (1997) *The New NHS: Modern, Dependable*, Cmnd 3807, London, DoH.

NHS Executive (1998a) *Integrating Theory and Practice in Nursing*, London, DoH.

NHS Executive (1998b) *A First Class Service*, London, DoH.

Richardson G. and Hendrika M. (1995) 'Reflection-on-practice: enhancing student learning', *Journal of Advanced Nursing* 22(2): 235–42.

Royal College of Nursing (1996) *A Principled Approach to Nurse Education*, London, RCN.

Schön D. (1987) *Educating the Reflective Practitioner: Towards a New Design for Teaching and Learning in the Professions*, London, Falmer.

United Kingdom Central Council for Nursing Midwifery and Health Visiting (1994) *The Future of Professional Practice – The Council's Standards for Education and Practice Following Registration*, London, UKCC.

Wong J. (1979) 'The inability to transfer classroom learning to clinical nursing practice: a learning problem and its remedial plan', *Journal of Advanced Nursing* 4(2): 161–8.

Further reading

English National Board for Nursing Midwifery and Health Visiting (1993) *A Detailed Study of the Relationships between Teaching, Support, Supervision and Role Modelling for Students in Clinical Areas, within the Context of Project 2000 Courses*, Research Highlights 3, London, ENB.

English National Board for Nursing, Midwifery and Health Visiting (1994) *Researching Professional Education: Education, Dialogue and Assessment: Creating Partnership for Improving Practice*, London, ENB.

3   The legacy of a paediatric nursing degree course

Annette Dearmun

Introduction

If I am not happy about a certain way of doing something I'll go and read about it, get the research, talk to people and question things rather than just carry it out because I saw someone else doing it that way. (Quotation from qualified children's nursing graduate)

This chapter is based upon a longitudinal empirical study investigating paediatric nursing graduates' views of their first year of professional practice (Dearmun, 1997a). The legacy of a paediatric nursing degree programme was explored, and evidence was gathered in relation to two aspects that were relevant to this chapter and had salience for education and practice. The first was that the BA (Hons) Paediatric Nursing course appeared to have had a lasting influence on the extent to which the nurses embraced client-centred care and continued to demonstrate a commitment to research and reflection after they had qualified. Second, the milieu exerted an influence in shaping the newly qualified nurses' impressions of their graduate status and their approaches to their work. These findings have implications for the retention and recruitment of newly qualified staff and may help to inform rotational and other professional development programmes.

A perusal of some of the literature on evidence-based practice (for example, Stevens, 1997; Mulhall, 1998; Thompson, 1998) confirms an affinity between the intellectual capacity required to embrace research and that needed to engage in evidence-based practice. A commitment to research has traditionally been promoted in educational programmes at degree level. Nurses who are graduates are expected to be comfortable with the skills of critical analysis, to be conversant with the research process and to be able to use research to inform their practice (Miller, 1992). In the past decade, reflection has been introduced into the curriculum of nursing courses, and the students have been encouraged to use this analytical process as a way of weaving together theory, research and practice (Dearmun, 1997b, 1998; Harding, 1997; Wooton, 1997). There are indications that when students are introduced to this way of thinking during their educational programmes, it remains with them as a legacy during the year after they have qualified (Dearmun, 1997a). In other words, a disposition towards scrutinising practice becomes an integral part of the graduate nurses' approach to care. It is reasonable to assume that, in their quest to identify practice that is clinically effective, they may seek out the evidence and ultimately use it to challenge tradition and ritualistic approaches to care delivery.

However, if practitioners are to remain committed to developing evidence or using it to underpin their practice, it will be necessary to foster an environment that values these characteristics. Aligned to this is the influence of the milieu on the practice of newly qualified nurses and the notion that experience is gained and consolidated in the field. This may complement or conflict with what they have already learnt in the classroom (Kramer, 1974). In this respect, two types of socialisation have been distinguished by Rothman (1998). The first is 'formal classroom socialisation' (p. 240), in which individuals are exposed to the knowledge base of the profession and are urged to use this to inform their practice. The second and arguably more powerful type is 'on the job socialisation' (p. 241), which contributes the technical component and usually takes place in practice under the guidance of mentors. This gives credence to a view that the service environment and the role models to which the novice nurses are exposed are key factors in their socialisation process and are influential in shaping their attitudes and practice style.

The first part of this chapter provides the contextual background for the study and includes a review of the salient literature. The methodology and approach to data analysis are then described, and this is followed by a discussion of the main themes that emerged from the data. Finally, the conclusions and implications for practice and education are highlighted.

Background to the study of children's nursing graduates

The BA (Hons) in Paediatric Nursing was the first in an increasing number of children's nursing courses designed to reflect the changes in nursing and nurse education in the UK (Rogers, 1988). A prediction was made that the nurses educated on degree courses would be:

Academically able people, with a desire to pursue a career in clinical nursing, and an apparent aptitude for working with people, as professional practitioners in nursing. [These nurses would have]... an inquiring, analytical and creative approach to care and [the ability] to use independent judgement and critical self-awareness.

The philosophy of the course was underpinned by the tenets of client-centred care. Commensurate with this was an emphasis on the application of research, knowledge and principles to care, in contrast to being constrained by the rules and procedures that may result in ritualistic practice. It was anticipated that the nurses emerging from this course would champion the desired client-centred approach to care and be questioning and challenging, becoming the key players in translating research into practice.

Throughout the course, the students were introduced to reflection as a way of developing their intellectual capacity and analytical skills. This was fostered by encouraging them critically to appraise situations arising from their practice. It was intended that this would stimulate enquiry and encourage an approach to care planning and delivery that was more creative and responsive to client needs (Dearmun, 1996, 1997a; Wooton, 1997). There was considerable optimism among the course team that using reflection to learn from experience would be enduring and that these practitioners would be recognised by their use of this structured analytical approach.

In essence, it was envisaged that practitioners emerging from this degree course would have a professional orientation. They would have the intellectual capacity to problem solve, would be equipped with the skills to examine their own practice and that of others with new insight and would have the confidence to initiate change. It can be seen that these attributes mirror those required to work within an evidence-based practice agenda.

Literature review

An exploration of the characteristics of graduate nurses has received considerable research interest. There have been attempts to measure their ability to think critically about their practice, to problem solve and to make clinical judgements (Meleis *et al.*, 1974; Sinclair, 1987; Miller, 1992; Reed, 1992; Sanford *et al.*, 1992). Some researchers have studied the professional orientation of graduates and their influence on the way in which care is delivered (O'Brien, 1984; Giger and Davidhizar, 1990; Kelly, 1991, 1996; Bircumshaw and Chapman, 1988). In other studies, the extent to which the graduates' practice emulates the received characteristics of the professional model, namely autonomy or a desire to advocate on behalf of their patients, has been explored (Murray and Morris, 1982; Pinch, 1985; Lawler and Rose, 1987).

Overall, the evidence is suggestive of a resonance between being educated to degree level and internalising a professional orientation to work, especially in terms of being an advocate for patients. This has been characterised as an ability to assess patients' needs, an aptitude for using a problem-solving approach when planning care, an orientation towards critical thinking and research, and a proclivity to exercise autonomy and professional judgement.

However, most of these studies have failed to acknowledge another dimension influencing the nurses' approaches to care, that is, the effect of the environment. For example, Witts (1992) has suggested that the extent to which a nurse is able to exercise professional judgement and advocacy is dependent upon the organisational culture. Murray and Morris (1982) have testified to the subservience of nursing to medicine, and this was identified as a factor that often thwarted nurses in their quest to defend the rights of patients and deliver research-based care.

Methodology and data analysis

The aims of the study of newly qualified children's nurses included an exploration of the ways in which they perceived that their course had been effective in preparing them for their role and whether it had a continuing influence on their professional practice after they had qualified. An examination was made of the nurses' overall impressions of being a graduate in nursing and the influence of the course philosophy in providing a blueprint for their practice style, for example their propensity to be analytical of their practice, to search out research and to use this to inform their practice.

All the nurses from the first two cohorts of the BA (Hons) Paediatric Nursing degree, ten in total, were interviewed and encouraged to articulate their experiences of being a neophyte children's nursing graduate. Commensurate with the aims of the study, a longitudinal research design was chosen to capture changes in their perceptions over time. The data were collected on four occasions at 3, 6 and 9 months, and at 1 year after qualifying. The emphasis was upon the nurses' own reports of their experiences and supported the position that an individual's behaviour could be understood by studying the empirical world from the perspective of the informant rather than the researcher (Leininger, 1985). Informed by this stance, the study was located within a naturalistic paradigm. Using open questioning techniques, an approach popularised by Spradley (1979) and Cohen and Manion (1989), it was possible to produce detailed descriptions of situations, events and interactions and explore in depth the nurses' experiences, attitudes, beliefs and thoughts.

The interviews were tape-recorded and transcribed. Each transcribed account was 'relived in real time' (Swanson-Kauffman, 1986, p. 62). This involved reading the transcripts and listening to the tapes simultaneously. In this way, it was possible to correct errors and increase familiarity with any intonation or pauses that might ultimately affect the interpretation of the data. The data were eventually coded and analysed for themes.

Main themes

Many interesting findings emerged from the analysis, but for the purposes of this chapter three areas have been selected that have most salience for paediatric nurses. First, the newly qualified nurses' impressions of the enduring influence of their preparation for practice will be discussed. Second, the nurses' impressions and feelings about being a graduate will be given detailed attention, and finally, the influence of the milieu on the nurses' espoused practice style will be acknowledged.

The nurses' impressions of the enduring influence of their preparation for practice

During the interviews, the nurses volunteered their opinions on the ways in which they had assimilated their beliefs and values concerning children's nursing and their acquisition of the knowledge and specific skills required to deliver competent care. Their responses were illuminated by concrete examples that illustrated the legacy of the course on their practice.

Upholding child- and family-centred care: the influence of the course in shaping the nurses' beliefs and values

In common with previous studies, the evidence suggested that the course had been responsible for shaping the nurses' values. Consequently, they felt that they sometimes viewed nursing differently from their compatriots on the ward:

> I approach [each child] in a different way... Some of [the other staff] are much more [rigid] in the way they do things... I am much more prepared to see the normal child and I think that the [social] and theory side is [higher] on my list than it is... on other people's.

In other words, they felt they had inherited an analytical, humanistic, holistic, individualised family-centred care approach to nursing children.

There were several illustrations of the ways in which they had internalised these values. Mirroring the research into the nursing style of graduates (Kelly 1991, 1996), these children's nurses were orientated towards giving individualised holistic care. In this respect, they attached importance to being able to exercise autonomy because this afforded them an opportunity to deliver care tailored to meet the needs of the individual child. This was felt to affect positively the quality of care given to children and families, and contributed to increasing the nurses' job satisfaction. When making their career choices, they tended to gravitate towards those clinical areas where there had been an endeavour to maintain the integrity of the individual in the way in which care was organised.

The nurses acknowledged the harmonious relationships that resulted from other members of the team sharing a common philosophy of care. They were, however, acutely aware of the conflicts, tensions and frustrations that arose when their endeavours to approach the children as individuals were thwarted. They were also foiled because of organisational constraints, for example very rigid protocols and policies, and high workload demands:

> If you are working alongside someone else who has got very different ideas about care then you do come into conflict [and] it can cause tension... When you are working with someone else whose outlook on nursing is similar to yours then it is great.

The nurses vented their frustration when they did not have all the skills necessary to provide all the care to the children; for example, they had not initially been equipped to give intravenous drugs, and having to rely upon other nurses to perform this task for them fragmented care.

Throughout the year, they described the disenchantment that arose when care duties were allocated with little regard for continuity of care or when there was a failure of other professionals to recognise the primacy of the child and family's needs:

Whenever a child goes home you think about how things have gone, and if things have gone well and if things have gone... badly... you think about it and then try and change things... [in the] old style of training people just accepted the *status quo*.

If I am not happy about a certain way of doing something I'll go and read about it, get the research, talk to people and question things rather than just carry it out because I saw someone else doing it that way.

These comments may portray an espoused commitment to professional values and a willingness to challenge the '*status quo*'. However, there was initially little evidence to support the fact that this was a reality. This dissonance may be explained by the nurses' impressions of being a graduate, discussed later in this chapter.

Gaining experience: supporting the integration of theory and practice

The nurses held common views regarding their grounding in theory and research. Overall, they recognised that the theoretical basis of the course had been useful. Many of the nurses considered that as a result of having undertaken a degree, they valued research. They frequently referred to the way in which they had been taught to reflect on practice as instrumental in encouraging integration between practice and research. There were many examples of their avowed attempts to integrate research and theory within their practice. This is illustrated by these extracts:

I think the way we were taught to reflect encouraged me to use research to back things up.

I quite often think of research-based things, whereas sometimes you work with people who just do things; [I feel I am] able to contribute ideas by talking to people about research.

It seemed that reflection was also instrumental in encouraging them to examine their accountability by fostering the recognition of gaps in their knowledge and the identification of their learning needs. Thus, before accepting new responsibilities, they asked pertinent questions and consulted the literature in order to address deficiencies in their knowledge. The following extract is testament to this:

[Having done the degree course] you are quite quick to take new things on board... other... staff have commented on how quickly we seem to learn new skills. I think it is because we developed self-awareness and self-learning; therefore we expect to say 'Right I want to give IVs' and then go off and read about it, look at any research. I make sure I get the support [I] need rather than being spoon fed.

Consistent with previous and emerging research from new educational programmes (Buckingham, 1996; Macleod Clarke *et al.*, 1997), these children's nurses did not feel that there had been sufficient emphasis within the course on the acquisition of practical skills. This perception of the lack of practical skills has utility in this chapter because of the nurses' assertion that proficiency in practical skills was a prerequisite to integrating theory and research. In other words, they referred to a need to gain experience before they could apply theory in a meaningful way. This is illustrated in this extract from an interview conducted at 6 months:

I feel able to do the practical skills now so I am actually bringing in more of the knowledge [that] I learnt in college.

You don't think that theory and research is really going to affect you. When you first come into a job you don't think it really matters you are concentrating on the practical skills. I am working every day and, now I think back to things [I learnt on the course]... and it really relates in...

These findings are consistent with the submission that, given a sound knowledge base, nurses, with experience, rapidly acquire the necessary skills for practice (Benner, 1984), and is also consonant with the skills development model advanced by Benner (1984) and Benner *et al.* (1996).

In summary, the evidence presented so far suggests that exposure to a particular educational programme appears to have an impression upon newly qualified nurses during the early stages of their careers in four main ways. First, the course influences their thinking about nursing, and this in turn affects their approaches to care. This is manifested in the value they place upon being able to practise within an environment where there is a focus upon meeting the individual needs of the child and family, and in their avowed attempts to integrate research and theory within their practice. Second, an ability to work autonomously assumes importance. Third, there is a marked tendency to seek out knowledge and skills before taking on new responsibilities. Finally, the nurses' comments were suggestive of

their willingness to challenge practice, even though there were few
overt displays of this

Impressions of being a graduate

At the time of this study, paediatric nurses with a degree were still in
the minority, so the nurses' unsolicited comments about being a graduate were particularly interesting. These provided an insight into the
distinctions they made between themselves and other nurses, and the
effects that their graduate status had on them, on their behaviour and
on their relationships with colleagues. There appeared to be an association between the nurses' reticence to advertise their academic
skills, their need to be accepted by their peers and their reluctance
overtly to challenge practice. During the data analysis, a theme
emerged that came to be known as 'the public and private face of
being a graduate', and this is worthy of further elaboration.

Privately, the nurses themselves took pride in their graduate status
and chose to acknowledge their differences. From the comments they
made, however, it was evident that they did not want others to be able
to distinguish them from other children's nurses. Indeed, they were
embarrassed if they were set apart because they were graduates, and,
in an attempt to assuage their anxiety about being seen as different
from or, worse still, superior to the nurses who did not have a degree,
and to avoid possible alienation by their peers, they tended to underplay their qualifications until they could be sure of a positive reaction.
This finding was not surprising given that previous studies have
found that acceptance and belonging are crucial to the psychological
wellbeing of graduate nurses (see, for example Melia, 1981; Luker,
1984; Horsburgh, 1989).

When the opportunity arose to become involved in ward projects,
some of the nurses found that being a graduate inhibited their contribution. For example, they expressed a reluctance to take the lead in
case they were seen by others as being 'too clever' or 'academic'. A
conclusion could also be drawn that these inhibitions might limit
their public support for evidence-based practice.

There appeared to be a general lack of understanding concerning
nursing degree courses, and it could be argued that it was the scepti-
cism among other nurses that may have affected the novice nurses'
self-image and the way in which they perceived the being in possession of a degree:

> If I come up with a bright sparky idea, [people say] it is because I have
> done the degree course and the mickey is taken out of me… It is frus-
> trating because they haven't got degrees and they don't understand the
> degree course.

This may have led them to exaggerate the inadequacies of their
preparation in terms of the acquisition of practical skills or to undervalue the academic component of their course.

Paradoxically, in the privacy of the interviews, the same nurses
extolled some of the positive virtues that have already been
mentioned in previous research, for example their professional orientation and their motivation to seek out new knowledge and research.
Nearly all of the nurses felt that they could be distinguished from
other non-graduate nurses because these were features that they did
not perceive were quite so evident in the practice of other nurses.
There were other differences that were both unfavourable and positive. The former appeared to be short lived, evident in the first 3
months, and were associated with their limited experience and initial
lack of confidence in practical skills. However, perhaps more fundamental and enduring were the ongoing positive differences that were
attributed to the nature of the course they had undertaken:

> I think the degree [increases] your depth of knowledge… [it takes] you
> that little bit further into self-enquiry and research.

Overall, there was a belief that any distinguishing features lay in
cognitive domains and would not be immediately obvious to the
casual observer because they were related to the ways in which graduates thought about and analysed practice. Although it is acknowledged that further research is required, a proposition is made that,
with the exception of their predilection to use research and reflection, there is at this point little evidence of substantive differences in
practice style between diploma and degree nurses that can be
directly attributed to the difference in the academic level between
the two courses.

There seems to have been some ambivalence with respect to having
a degree, some nurses considering that practice and experience were
more meaningful than academic awards. Any uncertainty concerning
the reactions of other nurses led to a tendency to underplay the
degree qualification, and this may have led to the pressure that the
graduates put upon themselves to demonstrate their practical competence to other nurses in order to gain credibility.

There are, however, two areas of concern: the nurses' unease about being seen as different, and their feelings that if they made adverse comments about practice, they might be viewed by other nurses as a threat. It seemed that challenging behaviour tended to be accepted as a mark of a student but was not seen as an approved trait in a quali-fied nurse who was seeking to become accepted as part of the team:

> You have to learn... you can't question [everything] because it is not appropriate. You come up against a lot of barriers and if you start ques-tioning things fences start to go up and you could be seen as someone who is aggressive and unhappy with things as they are... It is harder ques-tioning as a staff nurse because as a student people accept it, but as a staff nurse [you are seen as] radical.

These nurses were not naïve but seemed conscious of possible adverse reactions or animosity from nurses without degrees; they were acutely aware that other nurses would be wary of them. By conforming to the group, they would reap the rewards of being popular with their peers. If they challenged practice, they would violate the group norms, and sanctions, such as rejection by their peers, might be imposed. Therefore, it might have been futile for them to persist in challenging the established norms because they would have just made themselves unpopular. The early sentiments expressed by these nurses are unfortunate given that it was anticipated that these practitioners would from the outset question the traditional subservience to entrenched bureaucratic or hierarchical structures, would be willing to challenge medical dominance and would cham-pion change. The implications of this for practice are apparent. These imaginations seem to lead to a reticence to challenge the *status quo* and may retard the introduction of evidence-based practice.

However, the supposition is made that this is only a temporary situa-tion that is characteristic of the first few months following graduation. The novice nurses are initially preoccupied with mastering practical skills, and during this time it is probable that they will feel more vulner-able. Understandably, self-preservation, rather than challenging the *status quo*, will be paramount. Encouragingly, as the year progresses and the nurses gain in confidence, their inclinations to suggest new ideas, actively lead projects, share their reflective conversations and gently challenge their colleagues and peers, especially in terms of imple-menting research into their practice, show a marked increase.

However, in conclusion, the contention is offered that nurses need to spend time in practice to gain experience and become proficient in their practical abilities because these are prerequisites to having credibility with their peers. When they have established themselves in this way, the milieu will then determine the extent to which graduate nurses are able to capitalise on their academic skills.

The nurses' practice style: the influence of the milieu

It thus seems from the discussion so far that the environment seems to influence the nurses' general acclamation of their degree and hence their possible contribution to the delivery of evidence-based practice. The public denial of having a degree was intensified when they were working in an environment in which other nurses were not sympathetic to the needs for research and academic accreditation, as illustrated here:

> I used to play it [the degree] down as if to say 'I am not pretending that I am something better than you just because I have got a degree...'.

> I don't think I really talked about it when I first started; it was more when people started to ask me... When I got an initial response that they were not hostile, I was quite willing to talk about it to them. A lot of them... probably still don't know... but those that do are very supportive, which is very encouraging...

In environments in which other nurses were receptive to degree nurses and were enthusiastic to learn and develop their practice, graduates were seen by others as a valuable resource. Furthermore, they were able to challenge practice with more confidence and might ultimately have been able to champion practice that was based upon evidence.

There is another way in which the environment directly influences the nurses' practice style, namely the organisational structures and overall culture of the ward, which could enhance or inhibit the graduates' desired approach to care. On the whole, those who worked in a progressive environment considered themselves fortunate because they felt that the child-centred philosophy they had internalised was shared by their nursing colleagues, that they could work independently and contribute ideas, and that they were encouraged in their professional development. The converse state was also reported. Nurses sometimes alluded to working in an atmosphere that was 'not orientated to improving and learning', where there were 'traditional ideas' and a lack of 'research-based practice'. It was felt that within a policy-dominated culture, ritualistic and task-orientated approaches to care were perpetuated, and that this was not conducive to recognising and enhancing an individual's potential or to encouraging the retention of staff. This is illustrated in this extract:

> [There are policies and procedures for everything] they stick rigidly to them... and there does not seem to be any leeway to take into account... the individual child or implement research. I don't feel I can nurse each child as an individual in such a structure... So I am being stopped [from nursing] the way I would want to, the way that I thought I would bring from my training... It is just the way the ward runs... It would make me want to leave.

Discussion and conclusions

This chapter has contributed to a debate on the legacy of educational programmes versus the influence of the milieu on the socialisation of nurses after they have qualified. Consistent with the predictions of the course team, the nurses, at the point of registration, confirmed that they felt well versed in the theory and proficient in interpersonal skills. However, it was not uncommon for them to undervalue their skills in this sphere. As was found in previous studies of graduate nurses (see, for example, Kramer, 1974), this contributed to a reduction in their self-confidence and self-esteem, as well as compounding their doubts surrounding their ability. The early preoccupation with mastering practical skills appeared to be supplanted by a greater synergy between research, knowledge and practice. It seemed that knowledge came from the course in terms of theory and research, and that this was complemented by the nurses' experiences in practice.

There thus seemed to be a chronological progression in the development of the nurses' confidence to challenge practice. At first, they furtively strove, within their own sphere of influence, to provide care that acknowledged the needs of individual patients and was based upon research. At this stage, they might have felt powerless to change practice on a grand scale and not sufficiently confident to tackle their colleagues. They were motivated to prevent discord and to this end conformed outwardly to preferred behaviours. Their acquiescence might have given the impression that they were tolerant of the *status quo*. Not withstanding this, they waited patiently until they had gained the practical skills because they were aware that they would then be bestowed with the confidence and credibility of their colleagues. Gradually, the powerlessness to modify practice on a wider level diminished, and they began to exert a subtle influence.

This study only lasted 1 year, and it would be intriguing to profile the practice style of these graduates 5 years on to see whether this was a continuing trend and how it would be manifested in the future.

Although this chapter has focused upon a study of graduate nurses, it is likely that diploma nurses, by virtue of the similarities in their training and the fact that they are a relatively new breed of practitioner, will share common experiences after qualifying. It is thus envisaged that the findings of this study will have broad implications for practice, management and the provision of future educational programmes.

The UKCC (1986) envisaged a different role for the nurse of the future, this requiring new approaches to nurse education that would encompass different ideologies from previous traditional courses. The aims of all pre-registration nurse education programmes are to encourage practitioners to become autonomous, articulate and critically aware. This was encapsulated in the following key outcomes for educational programmes: first, that practitioners should be able to 'Take a fresh look at past practices and find new ways of working' (UKCC, 1986, p. 13); and second, that they should be able to 'evaluate their practice and develop skills of logical argument' (UKCC, 1986, p. 20). This would culminate in nurses being 'able to carry out care and make decisions taking all relevant circumstances into account' (UKCC, 1986, p. 40).

However, given the new political agenda for health care (DoH, 1998) and the particular focus on clinical governance, it could be argued that all practitioners should strive to be self-aware, to be able to work independently, to be able to problem solve, to be equipped with the skills to examine their own practice and that of others with new insights, and to have the capacity to respond to and innovate change. However, this study has shown that an inherent fear of discrimination may affect the extent to which an individual is willing and able to do this, the organisational environment thus being a significant factor.

Perhaps the political drive towards clinical governance, the emphasis upon quality and the emerging evidence-based practice agenda (DoH, 1998) will be key determinants in establishing an optimum environment in which the educational skills that nurses have acquired can be valued, celebrated and utilised. In this respect, it is expected that questioning and challenging ritualistic practice will be an accepted part of practice in order to provide care that is in the best interests of clients, and that this will have an influence upon the future development of nursing.

References

Benner P. (1984) *From Novice to Expert: Excellence and Power in Clinical Nursing*, Menlo Park, CA, Addison-Wesley.
Benner P., Tanner C. A. and Chesla C. A. (1996) *Expertise in Nursing Practice: Caring, Clinical Judgement and Ethics*, New York, Springer.
Bircumshaw D. and Chapman C. M. (1988) 'A follow up of the graduates of the Cardiff Bachelor of Nursing Degree Course', *Journal of Advanced Nursing* 13(2): 273–9.
Buckingham S. (1996) Baseline nursing skills development in Project 2000 Child Branch Nurses: an exploratory study. King's College, London, unpublished MSc thesis.
Cohen L. and Manion L. (1989) *Research Methods in Education* (3rd edn), London, Routledge.
Dearmun A. K. (1988) 'Perceptions of stress', *Journal of Child Health* 2(3): 132–7.
Dearmun A. K. (1996) 'Reflection: continuing education series', *Paediatric Nursing* 8(3): 30–3.
Dearmun A. K. (1997a) Paediatric nurses' perceptions of their first year of professional practice. Reading University, Reading, unpublished PhD thesis.
Dearmun A. K. (1997b) 'Assessing practice at degree level', *Paediatric Nursing* 9(1): 25–9.
Department of Health (1998) *A First Class Service: Quality in the New NHS* (White Paper), London, DoH.
Giger J. N. and Davidhizar R. E. (1990) 'Conceptual and theoretical approaches to patient care: Associate versus Baccalaureate Degree prepared nurses', *Journal of Advanced Nursing* 15(9): 1009–15.
Harding R. (1997) 'Reflections on family-centred care', *Paediatric Nursing* 9(9): 19–21.
Horsburgh M. (1989) 'Graduate nurses' adjustment to initial employment: natural field work', *Journal of Advanced Nursing* 14(4): 610–17.
Kelly B. (1991) 'The professional values of English nursing undergraduates', *Journal of Advanced Nursing* 16(7): 867–72.
Kelly B. (1996) 'Hospital nursing: "It's a battle!" A follow up study of English graduate nurses', *Journal of Advanced Nursing* 24(5): 1063–9.
Kramer M. (1974) *Reality Shock: Why Nurses Leave the Profession*, St Louis, C. V. Mosby.
Lawler T. G. and Rose M. A. (1987) 'Professionalism: a comparison among generic Baccalaureate and RN/BSN nurses', *Nurse Educator* 12(3): 19–22.
Leininger M. M. (1985) *Qualitative Research Methods in Nursing*, London, W. B. Saunders.
Luker K. A. (1984) 'Reading nursing: the burden of being different', *International Journal of Nursing Studies* 21(1): 1–7.
Macleod Clarke J., Maben J. and Jones K. (1997) 'Project 2000: perceptions of the philosophy and practice of nursing: shifting perceptions – a new practitioner?', *Journal of Advanced Nursing* 26(1): 161–8.
Melia K. M. (1981) Student nurses accounts of their work and training: a qualitative analysis. University of Edinburgh, Edinburgh, unpublished PhD thesis.

Miller A. (1992) 'Outcomes evaluation: measuring critical thinking', *Journal of Advanced Nursing* 17(12): 1401–7.

Mulhall A. (1998) 'Nursing, research and the evidence', *Evidence Based Nursing* 1(1): 4–6.

Murray L. M. and Morris D. R. (1982) Professional autonomy among senior nursing students in Diploma, Associate Degree, Baccalaureate nursing programmes', *Nursing Research* 31(5): 311–13.

O'Brien D. (1984) 'Evaluation of an undergraduate nursing course', *Journal of Advanced Nursing* 9(4): 401–6.

Pinch W. J. (1985) 'Ethical dilemmas in nursing: the role of the nurse and perceptions of autonomy', *Journal of Nursing Education* 24(9): 372–6.

Rogers R. (1988) 'Nursing by degrees', *Paediatric Nursing* 1(1): 4–6.

Rothman R. A. (1998) *Working Sociological Perspectives* (2nd edn), New Jersey, Prentice Hall.

Spradley J. P. (1979) *The Ethnographic Interview*, London, Holt Rinehart & Winston.

Stevens J (1997) 'Improving integration between research and practice as a means of developing evidence based health care', *Nursing Times Research* 2(1): 7–15.

Swanson-Kauffman K. M. (1986) 'A combined qualitative methodology for nursing research', *Advances in Nursing Science* 1(2): 58–69.

Thompson M. A. (1998) 'Closing the gap between nursing research and practice', *Evidence Based Nursing* 1(1): 7–8.

UKCC (1986) *Project 2000: A New Preparation for Practice*, London, UKCC.

Witts P. (1992) 'Patient advocacy in nursing'. In Soothill K., Henry C. and Kendrick K. (eds) *Themes and Perspectives in Nursing*, London, Chapman & Hall.

Wooton S. J. (1997) 'The reflective process as a tool for learning: a personal account', *Paediatric Nursing* 9(2): 6–8.

4 The role of professional journals in promoting evidence-based care

Anne Casey

Introduction

Evidence-based care is an ideal that the health service and the clinical professions have wholeheartedly adopted (Rosenberg and Donald, 1995; NHS Executive, 1996), at the same time acknowledging that much care and treatment does not yet have an evidence base. Clinical guidelines, based on up-to-date evidence or the best expert opinion, have been hailed as a way in which to reduce the huge variation in health care that is seen throughout the UK (Duff *et al.*, 1996).

As a route to ensuring equitable health care of the best possible standard, evidence-based care must be the model of choice for a national health service. It is well known that clinical decisions are frequently based on custom and practice or the latest fashion, each clinician being free to decide what is best (Walsh and Ford, 1989). Although the concept of clinical freedom is fundamental to effective care, it can also be used as an excuse to ignore the evidence.

This chapter considers the role of professional journals in improving clinical effectiveness through the promotion of evidence-based care, within the wider context of how nurses are influenced to use evidence in their practice. Although there are a range of external and organisational factors that are thought to influence the implementation of evidence-based practice (Kitson *et al.*, 1998)[1], I have made the assumption that it is the individual professional who chooses whether or not to find and use evidence. The chapter therefore addresses individual factors such as motivation and access to evidence rather than organisational factors such as the context of change and the nature of facilitation (Kitson *et al.*, 1998).

The focus of the discussion is on nursing journals as there are issues for nursing that may not be applicable to other disciplines. These include a difference in the type of journal available and also in the factors that influence different clinicians to use evidence in their

42

practice. Although managers use clinical evidence to inform their decisions on services, nursing management journals are not included in the discussion, which concerns clinical effectiveness through evidence-based care.

Nursing journals

Professional nursing journals can be categorised into three main types: weekly magazines, clinical journals and academic journals. The weekly magazines (for example, *Nursing Standard* and *Nursing Times*) feature news, news analysis, topical comment and job vacancies. These journals also contain some clinical articles and occasional research papers on subjects with fairly general applicability. The style of writing tends to be 'newsy' and light, which makes the journals readable and accessible to a wide readership. The fact that they are sold on the high street is important as they can be read by the general public, who may also want evidence to support their decision making with regard to health care.

Clinical journals have a different role. Some (for example, the *British Journal of Nursing* and the *Journal of Clinical Nursing*) cover all areas of nursing; others (for example, *Paediatric Nursing*, *Mental Health Practice* and the *Journal of Pediatric Oncology Nursing*) focus on a specialist field. While these journals may include a small amount of news and comment, their main content is clinical. Research published in these journals tends to be practice orientated, although some theoretical and education-focused articles are to be found.

Then there are the so-called academic journals such as the *Journal of Advanced Nursing* and the *International Journal of Nursing Studies*. There is a common belief that you cannot be serious about publishing research unless it is in one of these journals, that your work is somehow not as credible if it is published in a weekly magazine or one of the clinical journals. Assessors for the Research Assessment Exercise, who review the research activity of academic institutes in order to allocate funding, count publications in these academic journals towards the assessment but are thought to view other journal publications differently. Researchers face a dilemma: wanting to publish in a clinical journal such as *Paediatric Nursing* so that their work is read by nurses in clinical practice, but being required to publish in an academic journal to maintain credibility and for the Research Assessment Exercise.

A fourth type of journal has recently emerged in direct response to the increasing amount of research being published and the large number of publications available. These are the 'evidence-based' journals (for example, *Evidence Based Nursing* and the *Journal of Child and Family Nursing* (US)), which present research abstracts and critical commentary, usually in a themed format. This approach, along with comprehensive literature reviews, will help busy clinical nurses to keep abreast of the latest research and to identify those studies which they might wish to follow up in more detail.

The role of academic nursing journals

As a recent correspondence between the editor of the *Journal of Advanced Nursing* and the editor of the *Nursing Times* suggested, each type of journal has an important role (Salvage, 1996; Smith, 1996). *The Nursing Times*' editor suggested that the publication of research is not the sole province of the academic journals. It is possible to write research reports that not only demonstrate the rigour and credibility of the research, but can also be read and understood by nurses in clinical practice. Every researcher has a duty to see that the research is not only published, but also read, evaluated and used in practice. Publishing is not an end in itself: it is a means to an end.

It sometimes appears that much of the scholarly discourse to be found in the pages of academic journals has no direct relevance to practice and is of interest mostly to other academics. However, the increasing number of studies of practice must be put into the hands of practitioners in a form that can be understood and used. This is the key role of the clinical journals and of the new 'evidence-based' journals, which publish authoritative 'state-of-the-knowledge' reviews to help practitioners to make informed decisions on the availability and adequacy of evidence on particular clinical topics.

Nurses who are undertaking systematic reviews of evidence to develop guidelines or who are carrying out literature searches on particular clinical topics will find the research wherever it has been published. It is, however, the clinical journals and the weekly magazines that will bring new research to the attention of most nurses and could assist them in deciding whether a change in practice is warranted by the findings. Implementation of the evidence requires more than it's merely published. To understand the part that the journals play, it is important to examine the wider context in which evidence may (or may not) by used by children's nurses.

Defining the evidence base for paediatric nursing

In 1992, Beal and Betz evaluated the quality of paediatric nursing research published in seven selected North American nursing journals between 1980 and 1989. Of the 319 research reports, only 53 (17 per cent) tested the effectiveness or outcome of nursing care – evidence on which to base decisions of what care to provide for children and their families. When the current author attempted a similar exercise in the UK nursing journals, it was immediately apparent that definitions of paediatric nursing and paediatric nursing research were required. Without an explicit definition, any research remotely connected with child health could be included in the review.

Paediatric nursing can be defined as:

> helping the child and family to prevent and manage the physiological, physical, social, psychological and spiritual effects of the child's health problem/condition and its treatment.

This is a simplistic definition, but it is specific enough to provide the scope and boundaries of any review of research. It is obvious that there is much overlap between nursing and medicine, particularly around the management of the physiological effects of health conditions and treatment, for example hypertension, hypoglycaemia or low oxygen saturation. Doctors are also concerned with the physical, social and emotional impact of disease and treatment. Conversely, much of what nurses do is 'medical work', that is, related to the investigation and treatment of the disease or injury. These are, however, the main focuses of medicine and nursing respectively, which can be broadly defined in these ways, providing definitions that are sufficient to select from the journals only those studies which are about nursing.

As well as the overlap between nursing and medicine, there are blurred boundaries between nursing and social work, play therapy and other disciplines, and nursing and parenting. The extent of the overlap will vary in different settings and even for different patients. Most clinical problems are managed collaboratively so an additional test is needed to identify which topics fall within the remit of nursing research. That test concerns who makes the decisions about this aspect of care. Whichever discipline makes decisions on what to do for the child and family should be responsible for the research and evidence to support those decisions.

A good example here is pain management. A doctor will usually write the prescription for analgesia if this is required, but it is generally the expert nurse who identifies the need for pain relief and recommends and delivers the appropriate management for the individual child. Pain assessment and management are nursing research issues, as well as issues for collaborative research led by nurses (or others). The question of which type of intravenous catheter should be inserted could be a nursing research issue depending on the context: the experienced nurse sees a range of children with catheters and knows which type will suit which situation – often better than the surgeon does.

If one accepts that the main focus of paediatric nursing is the *effect* on the child and family of the health problem and its treatment, it follows that evidence in paediatric nursing should seek to answer the following questions:

1. *What are the effects on the child and family of the health problem and its treatment?*
    For example: What is it like to be 3 years old and having naso-gastric feeds? How does it feel to sit with your child in out-patients waiting for test results? How do young people react to the diagnosis of cancer?

2. *How can these effects be assessed or measured (and the outcomes evaluated)?*
    For example: How can pain be assessed in neonates? How can the support needs of parents be identified? What is the best way to assess nausea and vomiting in children receiving chemotherapy?

3. *What is the best way to manage these effects?*
    What helps children newly diagnosed with diabetes to adapt to their changed lifestyle? What dressing is best for toddlers with central venous lines? How can you prevent pressure sores in children undergoing cardiac surgery?

What evidence is available in the journals?

Using these definitions of paediatric nursing research, I undertook a manual search of four UK nursing journals between January 1995 and December 1997 with the aim of identifying the kinds of clinical paediatric nursing research evidence that was becoming available. It seemed that, over the past few years, there had been an increasing number of articles reporting primary research studies, probably as a result of the increasing number of postgraduate dissertations being undertaken by children's nurses. Many of the studies follow the well-recognised pattern of nursing research in the UK, which has been mostly small scale, focused on local need or the interest of the researcher and of doubtful rigour. Nurses have lacked expertise, funding and support for a more co-ordinated and productive research agenda (DoH, 1993).

The studies published so far are, however, an important starting point in the development of the knowledge base of this branch of the profession and help us to identify future research priorities. Where there are several, well-conducted studies on the same topic, these can form the basis for decision making with respect to practice, provided that the practitioner considers the extent to which the findings can be relied upon (Callery, 1997).

The journals searched were those in which paediatric nurses would be most likely to publish their work: *Paediatric Nursing*, the *Journal of Advanced Nursing, Child: Care Growth and Development* and the *Journal of Child Health Care* (1997 only). A total of 32 reports of primary research into paediatric nursing practice were found. The published studies could be categorised under headings derived from the questions listed above:

1. understanding the effects on the child and family of the health problem or condition and its treatment – 20 studies
2. assessment methods and outcome measures – 2 studies
3. effectiveness of interventions – 10 studies.

As you would expect from a discipline that is just beginning to develop its evidence base, the majority (20) of the studies were about understanding the problems faced by the children and families. Topics ranged from stressors experienced by the parents of intubated children to children's behavioural response to pain. Only two assessment studies were found. It is possible that studies testing or validating specific tools will be published in specialist journals, for example measures for nausea and vomiting in an oncology journal.

This search was not rigorous and did not attempt to evaluate the quality of the studies as Beal and Betz (1992) did. It was, however, encouraging to see that ten of the studies addressed the effectiveness of interventions, some examples being: a randomised controlled trial looking at the effectiveness of an asthma education programme; an investigation of the infection rate in central venous lines; the outcomes of nurse prescribing; and the effects on the child of the parents' presence in the recovery room. This limited search also gives a broad picture of what nurses believe are important topics to research. As Beal and Betz (1992) concluded, the views of practitioners must be included when deciding priorities for future research, alongside the views of children and families, policy makers

and managers so that the limited resources for research are used
most appropriately

This discussion has so far centred on research into clinical nursing
practice. There are many other important topics that are researched
by paediatric nurses, including nursing roles, career paths, educational methods and evaluations of services. These also constitute
evidence and can be used to bring about improvements in health care,
albeit in less direct ways. In addition, research from other branches of
nursing and other disciplines can be used to inform paediatric practice, although it is potentially dangerous simply to apply results
without questioning and testing their applicability to children.
Pressure-relieving equipment produced for adult patients, for
example, has never been tested for use with young children and may
be unsuitable as pressure risks are different in children (Waterlow,
1998). The professional journal publishes the evidence, but it is the
nurse who decides whether and how to use that evidence.

The decision to use evidence

The extent to which any nursing journal can promote evidence-based
care depends on at least four factors that dictate whether the individual nurse will use evidence, and use it appropriately, to inform
practice. These factors are influenced by the organisational context in
which nurses work but, in a profession that aspires to professional
autonomy, appear to be the ones that should be addressed if evidence-
based practice is to become the norm. They are discussed below under
four headings: *inclination, access, ability and autonomy*.

1. **Inclination:** *I know about evidence-based practice, and I believe
    that it is important*
    Unless the nurse is aware of the importance of evidence and
    convinced of its value for patient care, he or she will neither seek
    it out nor include it appropriately when planning care. Teams or
    units that have a culture of innovation and a focus on quality
    will encourage questioning in staff, who will also be more likely
    to accept the importance of evidence, to seek it out and to bring
    it to the attention of colleagues.

2. **Access:** *I can get hold of relevant evidence, easily and in a form
    I can use*
    There is more to access than just being able to obtain articles or
    references from organisations such as the Cochrane Centre
    (Dickson and Cullum, 1996), or databases of evidence such as

that compiled by the Royal College of Nursing clinical effectiveness programme (RCN, 1995). On-line access to journal articles,
even if this is from a terminal in a ward or clinic, is useful but not
sufficient. Nurses do not have time during their working day to
take themselves out of the care situation and 'look up' evidence
sources. Evidence will only be used routinely if it is readily available at the point of care during the care process. An example of
such access is an electronic patient record system that provides
'intelligent help'. For example, as the nurse admits a baby with
respiratory syncytial virus (RSV) bronchiolitis she can click on
that diagnosis and is presented with a menu of four local guidelines: 'RSV precautions' and 'RSV tests and treatment' in both
staff and parent versions. These can be printed out then and
there and discussed with the parents.

The most successful promotion of evidence is likely to be the
use of locally developed care pathways, based on national clinical guidelines that have in turn been based on systematically
reviewed evidence. Such pathways achieve the aim of reducing
the variation in management by prompting a standard
approach. There is, however, a critical issue to be addressed
here concerning the diagnostic and decision-making abilities of
nurses, which will be discussed below.

3. **Ability:** *I am able to weigh up the evidence relevant to this situ-
    ation and decide what to do*
    It is not always possible, or indeed necessary, to have full
    systematic reviews before evidence can be used, as Callery's
    example illustrates (Callery, 1997). Most nursing courses now
    include skills for critiquing reported research to judge whether
    or not it should be used to inform practice. Guidance for nurses
    on critically appraising the literature to support clinical effec-
    tiveness has been produced by the NHS Executive (1998a). Even
    when the evidence is presented in a 'ready processed' format,
    such as clinical guidelines or care pathways, there are still clin-
    ical judgements and decisions to be made.

    As a professional group, nurses are very good at doing what
    they are told. Autonomous practitioners, however, must be able
    to justify their decisions, including the decision not to follow the
    evidence-based guideline in a particular situation. They need
    skills in weighing up what they know about a general case (the
    evidence or guideline) against what they know about this indi-
    vidual patient and his or her preferences. There is, at present
    insufficient weight given in nursing education to the skills of

making informed clinical judgements and decisions (Boney and Baker, 1997). Nursing education must face this challenge to prepare nurses for the evidence- and information-based future (see Figure 4.1 and its discussion, below).

4.   **Autonomy:** *I make the decisions and control the resources*
The final factor influencing the nurse's use of evidence in practice is that of autonomy. Nurses continue to struggle to achieve autonomy and some control over resources, the lack of which frequently constrains the delivery of good standards of care. All the evidence in the world about what should be done will not overcome the staff shortage that means there is no-one to do it. Evidence can of course be used to influence those who do make decisions concerning resources, as well as to help children and their families identify their options and contribute to the decision-making process.

Access to evidence by patients and public

Nursing must take some responsibility for ensuring that patients and the public have access to evidence in a form that they can understand so that they can participate in decision making.

Information sheets and leaflets are provided by most Trusts, but these generally relate to the child's diagnosis, investigations or operations rather than being a balanced critique of options for treatment or a patient's view of the latest national clinical guideline. Many children's units now employ information officers to develop and maintain child-friendly materials. In addition, national clinical guidelines are now being developed with input from patient organisations, and 'patient-friendly' versions are being produced, for example the national clinical *Guideline for the Recognition and Assessment of Pain in Children* (RCN Institute, 1999).

With increasing access to the World Wide Web, patients can obtain information about any aspect of health care from every conceivable source. In the world of paper, authors and journal editors take responsibility for ensuring that facts are accurate and information up to date in the articles they publish. They also publish the source of those articles so that individuals can decide how much reliance to place on the information and on the opinions expressed. The Internet, however, is a different matter: there is no editorial control and no watchdog to screen the content for inaccuracies or potentially dangerous information. The UK Department of Health and the professional bodies are considering how to support patient and public access to information of this kind (NHS Executive, 1998b). Information should not be censored or restricted, but there needs to be a way in which to inform the user which information is current, reliable and clinically safe. When the day comes that every high street has a health information access point, nurses need to be contributing both in terms of evidence-based content and as advocates for patients' rights to obtain information to support their decisions and health care choices. There are already touch-screen health advice points in hospital reception areas and on the high street (Jones, 1998). Children are generally happier using technology than are their parents. Facilitating access for children to evidence and information to help their health care decision making should be high on the nursing agenda.

Promoting evidence-based care through education

Given the context described above, the role of professional journals in promoting evidence-based care is limited but important. They have an essential role in raising awareness and providing education, particularly for those nurses who have not recently undertaken a formal course. Debate in the journals on issues related to the development and use of evidence helps to raise the profile of the concept and to educate practitioners. Another important role for the journals is as a resource for access to evidence. Information on where to obtain guidelines, summaries of guidelines, lists of resources and references are important services to readers who wish to seek out evidence. Finally, the journals themselves act as sources of evidence: research reports, meta-analyses, expert opinion, systematic reviews – this is the evidence for and about practice without which the evidence base would not exist. While journals have an important but limited role, it is education that is the critical factor in ensuring each nurse's inclination, access, ability and autonomy.

Nursing education is beginning to address the preparation of nurses to access and use evidence appropriately, but this development should be seen in the wider context of the future development of nursing. The model presented below (Casey, 1997) aims to provide direction for curriculum development towards the education of nurses who:

- will continue to work within shifting professional boundaries
- will use evidence in their practice
- will be lifelong learners.

The primary focus of the model is on autonomous *nursing* practice and it assumes a patient focus, but it applies equally to the nursing of families and communities. It assumes that future health care requires that nurses are educated:

- as users and generators of knowledge/evidence
- as users and communicators of information
- to make clinical judgements
- to make clinical decisions
- to perform clinical actions.

The components of the model are described below, the letters A–F referring to elements of the model shown in Figure 4.1.

A. *Users of knowledge/evidence*
    To care for patients, nurses use *personal knowledge* gained through education and experience. They cannot ever know all that there is to know, and the knowledge base for practice is always changing. Therefore nurses need to be able to access, evaluate and use the relevant *'body' of knowledge,* which will increasingly exist in the form of evidence and clinical guidelines.

B. *Users and communicators of information*
    Information about the patient, contained in the record, and added to by observation, measurement and interview, is the basis for decisions and judgements. It is also the basis for continuity and quality; it must be recorded and communicated effectively.

C. *Clinical processes: clinical judgements, decisions and actions*
    Autonomous clinical actions are based on clinical judgements that require the skills of diagnostic reasoning. The nurse takes what he or she knows in general, from his or her personal knowledge and the profession's 'body' of knowledge, and weighs it up with the information on the patient to answer the question: what is (probably) going on here? The results of that judgement are used to decide an appropriate course of action: what should be done, by whom and when? Clinical judgement is also required to evaluate the effectiveness of actions: was the intervention appropriate, and was it successful? Clinical actions encompass everything that is done with, for or to the patient and are strongly influenced by the philosophy and professional values of the nurse. All clinical processes are influenced or constrained by the context of care, including the resource constraints that are the reality of health services today (see F below).

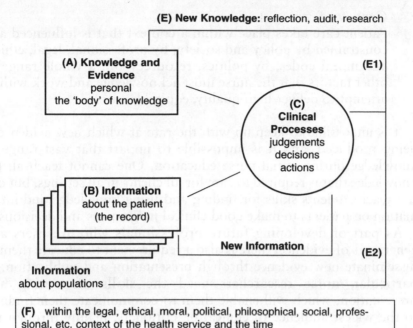

Figure 4.1 Evidence within a model for future nursing education (adapted from Casey, 1997)

D. *Generators of new information*
   During the clinical process, new information is added to the store of patient information – the record. The recording, communication and storage of this information is essential to patient care, for improving effectiveness and for the development of new knowledge: information about the patient contained in the record becomes evidence.

E. *Generators of new knowledge/evidence*
   E1 – Subconsciously or through reflection, learning takes place during every clinical encounter, adding to the personal knowledge of the nurse. Audit or research of a single case may add to the body of professional knowledge
   E2 – Data and 'stories' from populations of patients are used in audit and research to add to this body of knowledge. This new knowledge (the evidence base for practice) must be disseminated through publication and presentation so that others may evaluate it and use it in their practice.

F.   *Context of care*
      Patient care takes place within a context that is influenced and
      constrained by policy and society; by professional, legal, ethical
      and moral codes; by politics, resources and a whole range of
      other factors that the nurse must acknowledge and work with to
      attempt to deliver high-quality, equitable care.

It is impossible to keep up with the rate at which new evidence is
being produced, and it is impossible to impart that vast range of
knowledge during initial nurse education. One cannot teach all the
knowledge that is required to care for all clients in all settings, but one
can teach students skills for finding and using knowledge and information on patients to make good clinical judgements and decisions.

As part of developing future professionals who are users and
generators of evidence, there is also a requirement to educate them to
disseminate new evidence through presentation and publication. In
particular, nurse researchers need the skills of writing and
presentation, which will enable them to communicate their findings
to the widest audience of clinical practitioners, mainly through the
professional journals.

Conclusion

Research evidence to underpin the practice of children's nursing is
growing. Whether the evidence is in the form of a report of primary
research, a review of all the available evidence on a particular topic or
a national clinical guideline, its dissemination depends on the rich and
varied array of nursing journals. Practitioners face the challenge of
evaluating and using evidence in practice, researchers and academics
that of presenting evidence in a way that clinical nurses can use. The
challenge for the journals is to facilitate the process by responding to
the needs of both groups. The readers of clinical journals do not expect
to face complex academic articles, with terminology and statistics that
are outside their expertise, but they appreciate thoughtful, expert
commentary on research reports related to their area of practice. They
also expect and read evaluative literature reviews from authoritative
sources that give an overview of the current state of the research into a
specific clinical topic. The weekly 'magazines' and the clinical journals
could do more to present evidence in these accessible ways.

Although professional journals have a significant role in
promoting evidence-based care, the most important promoting influence is nursing education. Unless the ethos of evidence-based practice

is instilled into nurses along with other core professional values, there is little chance that evidence will be used in practice. It is not, however, merely the use of evidence that is the issue, but the appropriate use of evidence. The aim of using evidence is to reduce variations in practice, but these must not be replaced with standardised care that takes little account of the individual needs and preferences of patients. Again it is nursing education that must meet the challenge of preparing nurses who are able to use evidence appropriately to make informed, supportable clinical decisions.

Note

1. A conceptual framework proposed by Kitson *et al.* (1998) suggests that the successful implementation of evidence-based practice is a function of three equally important factors: the nature of the evidence, the context in which the change is implemented and the mechanisms by which the change is facilitated. Each of these factors can be further defined and evaluated in terms of whether or not it is supportive of success, providing guidance for how the implementation effort should be focused. Using real case studies, the authors illustrate that even where the evidence is high in its acceptability to patients and clinicians and is drawn from rigorous research, implementation can fail because the context is one in which leadership and a culture of learning and peer review are absent. Even when both evidence and context are highly supportive of success, implementation can still fail because facilitation is poor or absent. This framework is shown by the authors to have some degree of construct and face validity but is acknowledged to be a starting point for exploring the actual relationships between the three core elements.

References

Beal J. and Betz C. (1992) 'Intervention studies in pediatric nursing research: a decade of review', *Pediatric Nursing* 18(6): 586–90.

Boney J. and Baker J. (1997) 'Strategies for teaching clinical decision making', *Nurse Education Today* 17: 16–21.

Callery P. (1997) 'Using evidence in children's nursing', *Paediatric Nursing* 9(6): 13–17.

Casey A. (1997) A model for the future of nursing education. Unpublished paper, London, RCN.

Department of Health (1993) *Report of the Task Force on the Strategy for Research in Nursing Midwifery and Health Visiting*, London, HMSO.

Dickson R. and Cullum N. (1996) 'Systematic reviews: how to use the information', *Nursing Standard* 10: 32.

Duff L. A., Kitson A. L., Seers K. and Humphris D. (1996) 'Clinical guidelines: an introduction to their development and implementation', *Journal of Advanced Nursing* 23: 887–95.

Jones R. (1998) 'Current research in consumer heath informatics', *Information Technology in Nursing* 10(4): 11–15.

Kitson A., Harvey G. and McCormack B. (1998) 'Enabling the implementation of evidence based practice: a conceptual framework', *Quality in Health Care* 7: 149–58.

NHS Executive (1996) *Promoting Clinical Effectiveness: A Framework for Action in and through the NHS*, Leeds, NHS Executive.

NHS Executive (1998a) *Achieving Effective Practice: A Clinical Effectiveness and Research Information Pack for Nurses, Midwives and Health Visitors*, London, Stationery Office.

NHS Executive (1998b) *Information for Health: An Information Strategy for the Modern NHS 1998–2005*, London, Stationery Office.

Rosenberg W. and Donald A. (1995) 'Evidence based medicine: an approach to clinical problem-solving', *British Medical Journal* 310: 1122–6.

Royal College of Nursing (1995) *Clinical Guidelines: What you Need to Know*, London, RCN.

Royal College of Nursing Institute (1999) *Guideline for the Recognition and Assessment of Pain in Children*, London, RCN.

Salvage J. (1996) 'The danger of misusing one of British nursing's most precious assets, its lively professional press', *Journal of Advanced Nursing* 24: 883.

Smith L. (1996) 'The value of nursing journals' (editorial), *Journal of Advanced Nursing* 24: 1–2.

Walsh M. and Ford P. (1989) *Nursing Rituals, Research and Rational Action*, Oxford, Butterworth-Heinemann.

Waterlow J. (1998) 'Pressure sores in children: risk assessment', *Paediatric Nursing* 10(4): 22–3.

5 Parental participation in the care of hospitalised children: a review of the research evidence

Eileen Savage and Peter Callery

Introduction

In this chapter, principles and procedures of systematic review are applied to the question: what are the effects of parental participation in hospitalised children's care on parents, other family members and the children themselves? A search of electronic databases and nine nursing journals identified 28 papers for review. Systematic review procedures were adapted to reflect the wide range of methodologies represented. The effects of parental participation in hospitalised children's care on the parents were identified in 27 studies and concerned four themes: roles and relationships; emotional status; control and decision making; and knowledge and competence. The effects on children's physical and emotional wellbeing were identified in six studies. Recommendations are made to help practitioners to facilitate parental participation that reflects the needs of parents in caring for their hospitalised child. The need for further research is highlighted with respect to the perspectives of children, families from ethnic minority groups and family members other than mothers.

Since the 1950s, the idea of parental participation in care has become an important consideration in promoting the welfare of children in hospital. According to Brownlea (1987, p. 605), participation means 'getting involved or being allowed to become involved in a decision-making process or the delivery of a service or the evaluation of a service'. Participation is an elusive and complex concept, however, and the practice implications of implementing participation in care are not well understood. In this chapter, the authors apply principles and procedures of systematic reviews to the parental participation literature. The strengths and limitations of applying the principles and procedures of evidence-based practice to children's nursing are discussed. In addition, gaps in the current knowledge on parental participation in the care of hospitalised children are identified and recommendations are made for further research.

Literature review

Child and family-centred care is advocated as one of the cardinal principles in the provision of quality care for hospitalised children (DoH, 1991). In the interest of a child's physical and emotional well-being, it is now generally accepted that parents and other family members should be involved in their child's care while in hospital, and to this end, professionals are expected to facilitate parental and family participation in care (DoH, 1991; Audit Commission 1993).

Policies promoting parental participation in care are based on assumptions that parental participation promotes the wellbeing of children and is also beneficial to parents and other family members. The benefits to the parents and family of participating in care are assumed to be continuity of the parenting role, continuity of the family as a unit, and the development of the knowledge and competence to care for a sick child (DoH, 1991; Audit Commission 1993). Participation in care is advocated as a means of increasing the family's sense of control and decision making regarding all phases of the child's hospitalisation (Berman, 1991). It is also suggested that participation in care alleviates the parental and family distress associated with the hospitalisation of an ill child (Palmer, 1993).

Despite the claimed benefits of parental participation for hospitalised children, their parents and families, the evidence on which recommendations for parental participation is based is unclear. The effectiveness of parental participation in terms of benefiting hospitalised children, their parents and families is uncertain. Indeed, participation in care may have adverse effects on parents and other family members. Caring for a sick child in the unfamiliar environment of a hospital setting can be distressing, and there may be conflicts between the interests of different family members, including parents and their children. For example, a parental presence in the anaesthetic room may be in the best interests of the child, but it may be a source of increased distress for the parents. A clinical question arises over what level of parental distress outweighs the benefits to the child (Callery, 1997a).

In promoting the practice of parental participation, therefore, nurses are faced with the question of how to balance the conflicting interests of family members. In serving the best interests of the child, parents and family, questions arise regarding what areas of care may be suitable or unsuitable for parental participation. Although parental involvement is a matter of parental choice, nurses can be expected to advise, so they are faced with the question of what is the most appropriate level of participation for individual parents and families.

In this chapter, the authors seek to apply principles and procedures drawn from evidence-based practice to parental participation in order to examine the research literature in a systematic manner and to consider the application of evidence-based practice to children's nursing. There are problems, however, with applying the principles of evidence-based practice to nursing. Evidence-based practice is an approach to care drawn from the principles of evidence-based medicine that is designed to answer questions about individual clinical interventions (Sackett *et al.*, 1997). In formulating the question, practitioners are advised to be specific and brief, and to frame the question in the context of three essential elements – the patient or problem being addressed, the intervention and the outcome – as for example in the question 'In patients with heart failure, would long-term ACE inhibitor therapy prevent recurrences and improve the quality of life?' (Sackett *et al.*, 1997, p. 25).

This approach to questioning seems relatively easy in answering nursing problems of a physiological nature, for example concerning altered body temperature or compromised skin integrity. Many nursing problems are, however, also psychosocial in nature (involving, for example, parental role conflict and social isolation) and require the skilled integration of interpersonal, educational and supportive interventions, which cannot be readily converted into simple questions and definitive answers.

A criterion for involvement in evidence-based practice is that a profession must have a 'sufficiently sizeable and robust scientific base' from which to evaluate the effectiveness of various interventions (Kitson, 1997, p. 37). Nursing research is at a comparatively early stage of development, which narrows the availability of best evidence. Given the developmental stage of nursing research, nurses are advised to embrace a wide methodological base for evidence-based practice (Kitson, 1997). However, randomised controlled trials (RCTs) are viewed as the gold standard of best available evidence (Sackett *et al.*, 1997). This is problematic for nursing since relevant knowledge may be missed. The RCT is an appropriate design for the experimental testing of alternative clinical interventions but is less well suited to exploring patients' experiences, attitudes and relationships.

Additional problems arise with the application of evidence-based practice to children's nursing. The body of research in children's nursing is less well developed than that in other areas of nursing and the use of RCTs to test alternative interventions in children's nursing may be unethical and impractical. For example, testing the effects of parental participation using a RCT would require asking a group of parents not to participate in their children's care. The subjective experiences of parents participating in their hospitalised child's care have been studied with qualitative methods, which are usually ranked lower than RCTs in the hierarchy of evidence (NHS Centre for Reviews and Dissemination, 1996).

Finally, the approach to framing questions for evidence-based practice with an individual patient in mind is particularly difficult in children's nursing. Children's nursing has family-centred care as one of its fundamental goals. Nurses are dealing not only with the sick child, but also with parents and other family members, all of whom should be experiencing a 'seamless web' of care as part of a good-quality service (DoH, 1991).

In this chapter, the authors aim to explore the extent to which principles and procedures of the systematic literature review can be applied to the difficult case of parental participation in the care of hospitalised children. The objectives are to present a coherent review of the literature concerning parental participation and to identify difficulties in the use of systematic reviews of this type of literature, which frequently reports qualitative studies.

In any research project, including a systematic review, the research question is of central importance. The problem of focusing on an individual patient without acknowledging the family context has already been identified. Parental participation is as much a method for organising hospital care as it is a nursing procedure. The research question must, therefore, reflect the transactional nature of parental participation, which is a shared enterprise between health care staff and parents. This problem is not unique to nursing: consider the medical procedure of the prescription of an inhaler for asthma prophylaxis, which can only be effective if the patient actively co-operates in the use of the inhaler.

The research question guiding this review is: what are the effects of parental participation in hospitalised children's care on parents, other family members and the children themselves? This research question is addressed in the context of recurrent themes that emerge from the literature on parental participation. The themes with reference to parents and families are roles and relationships, emotional status, control and decision making, and knowledge and competence. These themes reflect the transactional nature and the claimed benefits and potential difficulties of parental participation in the care of hospitalised children. The research question is also addressed through an examination of the effects of parental participation in care on the emotional and physical wellbeing of hospitalised children. This is important since it is generally accepted in the literature that hospitalised children benefit from parental participation in their care.

Methods

In tracking down the best available evidence to answer the research question for this review, a search was carried out for published studies over a 14-year period (January 1984–October 1998) on parental participation in hospitalised children's care. A number of methods were used to identify relevant studies for inclusion in the review. This included searching electronic health-related databases and the manual searching of a number of journals. The NHS Centre for Reviews Dissemination (NHS CRD) was accessed via its World Wide Web site at the University of York in the UK. At the NHS CRD, both the Cochrane Database of Systematic Reviews (CDSR) and the Database of Abstracts of Reviews of Effectiveness (DARE) were searched for relevant studies. The primary search strategy was electronic, using MEDLINE, CINAHL and PSYCLIT., which were searched with the index terms: participation and child; and parents; and family; and hospital. In order to maximise the yield, the following keywords were used as free-text search terms: parent participation; parental involvement; partnership; family-centred care; family nursing; care by parents; children in hospital. These terms were also combined with free-text terms: benefits; and outcomes; and effectiveness; and evidence-based practice; and systematic reviews. No systematic reviews of the literature were found. In order to yield research papers, the index terms were combined with: quantitative study; and qualitative study; and randomised controlled trials; and clinical trials.

Since relevant studies may be missed with electronic searching alone (Droogan and Cullum, 1998), a manual search of selected journals was conducted. Journal indexes and tables of contents were scanned using the terms: parents; participation; partnership; family-centred care/nursing; children; hospitalisation (Table 5.1). In addition to searching the journals, reference lists of relevant articles and texts were scanned in order to identify other potentially relevant studies. The review was limited to published studies so does not include the 'grey literature' of unpublished studies and conference presentations. Unpublished studies were not actively sought, and the authors of published studies were not contacted for further information.

Table 5.1   Journals manually searched for this review

Journal title	Dates
Journal of Advanced Nursing	1984–1998
Journal of Clinical Nursing	1992–1998
Journal of Pediatric Nursing	1988–1998
International Journal of Nursing Studies	1984–1996
Pediatric Nursing (US)	1993–1997
Paediatric Nursing (UK)	1989–1998
British Journal of Nursing	1992–1998
Nursing Research	1984–1996
Issues in Comprehensive Paediatric Nursing	1993–1995

The inclusion criteria for the review were that studies:

• focused on parental participation in the care of hospitalised children
• were set in inpatient hospital wards/units (for example medical or surgical)
• focused on children ranging from 5 days to 18 years of age.

Both qualitative and quantitative studies were included. Individual studies were included if:

• the aim(s) of study were stated
• the methodological details of study design, sampling, study context, data collection and analysis were presented
• the study sample included parents, other family members and/or children.

In keeping with the themes already mentioned and through which the research question was addressed, individual studies on parental participation were included if the findings were of relevance to:

- the parents' and/or the family's roles and relationships; emotional status; control and decision making; and/or knowledge and competence
- hospitalised children's emotional and physical wellbeing.

Studies of parental participation in the following areas were excluded:

- short-stay hospital units – day care units, anaesthetic rooms and A&E departments
- intensive care units
- neonatal care units
- specific procedures only (for example intravenous medications and flushing central lines)
- children with mental health problems.

Studies of samples entirely composed of health professionals were excluded. However, studies that sampled nurses were not excluded if the sample also included parents, other family members and/or children.

All the studies identified for inclusion in the review were initially evaluated by one of the reviewers (ES). The second reviewer (PC) read studies that were considered to be questionable for inclusion. Subsequently, the decision to include or exclude studies in the review was reached by discussion and agreement between both reviewers.

Data were systematically extracted from each study to obtain details of the author(s), the country of origin, the aim(s) of the study, methodological issues – study sample, hospital setting, design, methods of data collection and analysis, methodological rigour/reliability and validity – and findings on the effects of parental participation in care on the parents, other family members and/or children. This approach to extraction facilitated a review of studies conducted using a variety of methods based on different epistemological assumptions. More specific quality criteria could have been used if a narrower range of study designs were reviewed. The approach selected in this review was to be inclusive and to present claims of methodological rigour rather than to apply predetermined criteria. Thus, readers are provided with details and can assess the methodological strengths and weaknesses of the studies presented in the results.

Results

The combined search strategies yielded 54 published studies, of which 28 in total met the inclusion criteria for review. Of the 28 studies reviewed, the effects of parental participation in the care of hospitalised children were gleaned from 22 studies concerning parents only, 5 studies concerning both parents and children, and 1 study concerning children only. Summaries of the studies are presented in Tables 5.2 and 5.3 at the end of the chapter as they relate to parents and children respectively.

Study characteristics

Eleven studies, which accounted for almost half of those reviewed, were conducted in the UK. Nine studies were conducted in the USA, 4 in Canada, and 2 each in Australia and Sweden. An equal number of qualitative and quantitative studies were identified for this review, with 13 studies in both categories. A combination of qualitative and quantitative approaches was used in two studies reviewed. Overall, 18 of the studies were descriptive in design, which accounts for two-thirds of the studies reviewed. None of the studies reported RCTs.

A variety of data collection methods were used across studies, interviews emerging as the dominant method, either alone (8 studies) or in combination (9 studies) with other methods. Questionnaires were used to collect data in 14 studies. Observational methods of data collection were used in 7 studies, including non-participant observation in 4 studies, and participant observation in 3 studies. Children's case notes were used as part of the data collection sources in 2 studies. Overall, a combination of methods was used in 10 studies reviewed.

Characteristics of study participants

The study participants of interest in this review were parents, other family members and hospitalised children. Out of 18 studies (Table 5.2), the participants were found to be all mothers in 6 studies and mostly mothers in the other 12. In studies that gave the breakdown of 'parents' sampled, only 7 included fathers. With the exception of the studies of Knafl and colleagues (Knafl and Dixon, 1984; Knafl *et al.*, 1988), the number of fathers sampled in these studies was far smaller than that of mothers.

In most studies, the hospitalised children for whom parents cared represented a broad age range between 1 week and 18 years. Eight studies focused specifically on parents whose children were under 5 years of age. In the majority of studies, parental participation related to children with acute medical or surgical conditions. There were only 4 studies identified that examined parental participation specifically in the care of hospitalised chronically ill children. A fifth study was identified in relation to chronically ill children, which compared parent and traditional nursing units.

Of the 6 studies relating to the effects of parental participation on hospitalised children, 5 sampled children. Children in 3 studies were under 5 years of age. Non-participant observation methods were used in 2 studies (Cleary, 1992; Jones, 1994). One study, which focused on children's weight and skin condition during hospitalisation, accordingly used assessment scales (Monahan and Schkade, 1985). Two studies sampled older children ranging from 5 to 12 years of age, all of whom were interviewed (Knafl *et al.*, 1988; While, 1992). In the sixth study, the sample represented mothers only (Caty *et al.*, 1989). However, Caty *et al.* examined how the mother's role helped hospitalised pre-schoolers to manage stressful situations.

Effects of parental participation on parents

This review highlighted four recurring themes in the literature: roles and relationships, emotional status, control and decision making, and knowledge and competence. On analysing the studies, 24 were found to present findings relating to parental 'roles and relationships'. The findings of 18 studies reported the effects of participation on parents' emotional status, 6 of these examining parents' 'stress' and 'anxiety' levels in relation to participation. Mothers' preferences for control over their hospitalised children's care were examined in 1 study. However, issues of parental control and decision making emerged in 15 studies in total. While none of the studies aimed to explore parental knowledge and competence in participating in care, this theme was evident in the findings of 19 studies.

Roles and relationships

In 16 studies that presented findings on roles and relationships, staying with the hospitalised child and continuity of parental role in the child's basic care emerged as important aspects of participation for parents. In 7 studies, the main concerns for parents were to be with their children in order to comfort, nurture and protect them (Knafl and Dixon, 1984, Algren, 1985; Knafl *et al.*, 1988; Caty *et al.*, 1989; Dearmun, 1992; Kristensson-Hallstrom and Elander, 1994; Kawik, 1996).

In 11 studies, it was revealed that some parents would have liked to participate more in their child's care. Not all parents, however, desired a greater participation in care, as was evident in 7 studies. For example, some parents preferred not to get involved and willingly handed over the care of their child to nursing staff (Knafl *et al.*, 1988; Kristensson-Holstrom and Elander, 1997a). When compared with basic care, it was found that fewer parents wished to participate in clinical and technical care activities (Algren, 1985; Lau, 1993; Coyne, 1995; Kawik, 1996; Neill, 1996b).

Irrespective of the level of participation that parents desired, it was found in 6 studies that parents felt obliged to assume a vigilant role in managing and/or monitoring their child's care. Factors contributing to the vigilant role that parents assumed were fragmentation of care (Hayes and Knox, 1984), staffing deficits and inexperienced staff (Tomlinson *et al.*, 1993), a powerful need to be with the child (Darbyshire, 1994) and the need to be the child's central person in long-term care (Perkins, 1993). The vigilant role whereby parents felt obliged to take charge of the child's care was evident in all 4 studies relating to chronically ill children (Hayes and Knox, 1984; Robinson, 1985, 1987; Burke *et al.*, 1991; Perkins, 1993).

A finding in 11 studies was that little negotiation took place between nurses and parents regarding their respective roles in caring for the hospitalised child. Nurses' expectations of the parents' role differed from the parents' own expectations of their role. These differences presented in two ways. On the one hand, parents' expectations to be increasingly involved in their child's care contrasted with nurses' expectations of parents assuming a passive role (Hayes and Knox, 1984; Robinson, 1985, 1987; Ball *et al.*, 1988; Rowe, 1996). Conversely, parents' expectations of being less involved differed from nurses' expectations, nurses taking it for granted that parents wanted more involvement in their child's care (Dearmun, 1992; Kawik, 1996; Neill, 1996b). A lack of negotiation and unacknowledged differences in expectations between nurses and parents resulted in parental role conflict (Algren, 1985; Burke *et al.*, 1991; Darbyshire, 1994) and adversarial relationships with health care professionals (Robinson, 1985, 1987).

Control and decision making

With regard to parental control and decision making, the benefits of negotiated and shared care between nurses and parents were suggested in Keatinge and Gilmore's (1996) study. Shared care afforded parents a choice in their level of involvement, increased time spent in planning their child's care with the nurses, and control over their situation in the hospital setting.

Only 1 study examined parental control over hospitalised children's care, which found the mothers of younger children to have the strongest correlation with a preference for control (Schepp, 1992). However, a further 14 studies presented findings relating to control and decision making. The dominant pattern for parents across all 14 studies was that participation in their child's care was characterised by reduced control and decision-making autonomy. For example, in Darbyshire's (1994) study, the lived experiences of parents were that they felt disempowered and perceived nursing staff to be in a greater position of power than themselves. Similarly, in Rowe's (1996) study, some parents were found to experience a sense of exclusion characterised by nurses' holding a greater degree of control, leaving parents in the position of 'bystanders'.

Initiatives by parents to increase their level of participation and thus control evolved along covert pathways, for example seeking permission (Perkins, 1993), patiently waiting for opportunities to participate (Robinson, 1985) and reluctantly taking charge (Burke *et al.*, 1991). These covert pathways that parents assumed arose from their concerns of being perceived by professionals to be 'interfering' (Robinson, 1987) and 'trouble-makers' (Burke *et al.*, 1991). Although parents' initiatives carved the way for increasing their control and decision-making autonomy, it was viewed by parents as a negative and distressing experience (Hayes and Knox, 1984; Burke *et al.*, 1991).

Knowledge and competence

Parental participation was found to be beneficial in increasing parents' knowledge and competence in carrying out basic care activities with their sick child (Sainsbury *et al.*, 1986) and in being involved in complex aspects of care (Cleary, 1992; Tan, 1993) Furthermore, the knowledge and competence acquired through participation in care was perceived by parents to enhance their readiness to continue caring for their child following discharge from hospital (Keatinge and Gilmore, 1996).

The positive experiences identified in the above 4 studies were in the context of the planned implementation of parental participation. However, the majority of studies revealed negative experiences for parents. Negative experiences unfolded in two different ways for parents depending on their status of knowledge and competence regarding their child's care. On the one hand, a lack of information and guidance from professionals was found to stifle parents' desires to engage in greater levels of participation (Coyne, 1995; Kristennson-Hollstrom and Elander, 1997a). On the other hand, parents who viewed themselves as knowledgeable, competent and expert carers felt that their endeavours to participate in their child's care were disregarded by professionals (Robinson 1985, 1987; Darbyshire, 1994).

A finding that emerged from 8 studies was that parents viewed themselves as 'experts' in their child's care. Parental expertise differed from the objective scientific basis sometimes claimed for professional knowledge. Parental expertise, especially maternal expertise, was based on intuitive judgement that rose from intimately knowing their child on an everyday basis (Callery, 1997b). The theme of parent as expert emerged from all 4 studies pertaining to chronically ill children. Parents' expert knowledge on complex chronic conditions was based on their experience of being the primary health care providers in the long-term management of their child. A lack of recognition from professionals of parents' expertise contributed to parental role conflict and adversarial relationships with professionals (Robinson 1985, 1987), lack of control and decision-making autonomy (Hayes and Knox, 1984), and emotional distress, leaving parents feeling angry and frustrated (Burke *et al.*, 1991; Callery, 1997b).

Emotional status

The findings of this review illustrate that participation in the care of a hospitalised child can be a distressing experience. In most studies that presented findings on parents' emotional status, themes of unpleasant affective states emerged. The emotional costs to parents were identified in terms of financial costs through loss of earnings, travel and subsistence, and social costs through a discontinuity of family functioning and relationships (Hayes and Knox, 1984; Callery, 1997d). However, personal costs emerged as the main source of distress for parents, relating to alterations in the parenting role, the emotional demands of caring for a sick child in hospital, a lack of control and decision-making autonomy, and a lack of recognition from professionals of parental expertise (Hayes and Knox, 1984; Darbyshire, 1994; Callery, 1997b, d).

In 5 studies regarding acutely ill children, the clinical and technical aspects of care were found to be particularly distressing for parents. For example, in Coyne's (1995) study, parents expressed 'anxiety' about hurting their child and about their abilities to perform clinical and technical tasks. For the parents of chronically ill children, the most distressing aspect of their participation was the necessity of maintaining a constant vigilance and taking charge of the management of their child's situation. The lack of recognition from professionals of parental expertise further compounded the experience of distress (Hayes and Knox, 1984; Robinson, 1985, 1987; Burke *et al.*, 1991; Perkins, 1993).

In a pilot study on the implementation of a shared care project, the stress and anxiety levels of parents were found to be significantly reduced compared with those of parents who were not part of this project (Keatinge and Gilmore, 1996). This conflicts with the findings of Monahan and Schkade's (1985) study, which found that parents in a 'care by parent' (CBP) unit experienced an increasing level of anxiety over time, in contrast to parents in a traditional 'care by nursing staff' (CBN) unit. In most studies, it appeared that parental participation occurred in an *ad hoc* manner with little regard for the emotional vulnerability of parents. Callery (1997c) highlighted the status of parents involved in their hospitalised child's care as co-clients in need of care themselves, but reported that this care was a hidden area of nursing work.

Effects of parental participation on hospitalised children

As presented in Table 5.3 at the end of the chapter, 6 studies were identified that addressed the effects of parental participation in care on hospitalised children. Five studies presented findings on children's emotional wellbeing, but only 1 study was identified that presented findings on children's physical wellbeing.

Emotional and physical wellbeing

The dominant theme that emerged from the 5 studies was that children felt secure and comforted by their parents' presence and participation in their care. The need to be comforted by parents, although particularly important for younger children (Caty *et al.*, 1989; Jones, 1994), was also important for older children when encountering unpleasant procedures (Knafl *et al.*, 1988). Another positive aspect of parental participation on hospitalised children was the social attentiveness that they received from parents and other family members (Knafl *et al.*, 1988; Cleary, 1992). In Cleary's study, for example, children in a CBP scheme were better integrated with family, received more social attentiveness and spent less time crying alone than did those children not in the scheme but with resident or non-resident mothers.

The review gleaned very little evidence to determine the effects of parental participation on children's physical wellbeing, only 1 study being identified in this regard (Monahan and Schkade, 1985). The study examined the effects of increased parental participation on the efficacy of gait training in children who were first-time ambulators and receiving orthotic management. The quality of care in parent and traditional nursing units was compared. The physical indicators of hospitalised children's wellbeing in this study were weight and skin condition. The quality of care did not appear to be compromised or improved by allowing parents in this study to assume increased responsibility for their hospitalised child's care.

Discussion

In this chapter, the authors set out to explore the extent to which the principles of evidence-based practice could be applied to children's nursing, with reference to parental participation in the care of hospitalised children. Studies that examined the effects of parental participation on parents, other family members and/or children were reviewed.

Most studies presented negative accounts of the effects of participation on parents. This could reflect a publication bias because descriptive studies that identify problems might be more likely to be published. However, a factor identified in this review that seemed to contribute to parents' negative experiences was the unplanned approach to implementing parental participation in practice. Four papers provided evidence to suggest that a planned and shared approach to parental participation in the care of hospitalised children results in positive experiences for parents (Sainsbury *et al.*, 1986; Cleary, 1992; Lau, 1993; Keatinge and Gilmore, 1996).

While the above studies support a planned and shared approach to implementing parental participation in the care of hospitalised children, it is important to take individual differences into account. A conclusion that can be drawn from this review is that parents differ in their need to participate in the care of their hospitalised child. What may be desirable and acceptable to one parent may be undesirable and unacceptable for another. This suggests that nurses would be well advised to pay particular attention to the individual needs of parents in order to avoid the negative consequences of parental participation in care that may arise for parents. In this way, parents could choose their level of participation and areas of care relative to their emotional needs, their role expectations and other commitments, their need for control and decision making, and their levels of knowledge and competence.

A question raised at the outset of this review on parental participation in hospitalised children's care was: how can nurses balance the conflicting interests of the family members? This overview goes only part of the way to answering this question. Facilitating the needs of parents, as mentioned above, can help to reduce the conflict that they may experience while caring for their hospitalised child. However, in facilitating the needs of parents, the views and experiences of children and other family members regarding parental participation in care must also be taken into account.

Apart from that on parents, the authors found very little evidence available to inform practice on facilitating other family members (for example, grandparents, siblings and significant others) in participating in a hospitalised child's care. As already mentioned in the results section, most study participants identified in this review were mothers. Fewer fathers were found to be study participants, Knafl and colleagues' studies (Knafl and Dixon, 1984; Knafl *et al.*, 1988) being the only ones identified that sampled an equal number of fathers and mothers. In 2 studies, 'families' were sampled, but most participants were noted to be parents in one study (Sainsbury *et al.*, 1986), and the breakdown of family members was not presented in the second (While, 1992). To establish a more substantial body of evidence on the specific needs of fathers and other family members, it is necessary in future research to extend sampling beyond mothers.

Evidence on the effects of parental participation concerning the wellbeing of hospitalised children was sparse in this review, with only 6 studies identified that met the inclusion criteria. As presented in Table 5.3, only 5 of the studies sampled children. Coyne (1998) notes that children have traditionally been the objects rather than the subjects of research. This was found to be the case in this review since most data on children's wellbeing were gleaned by observational methods (Cleary, 1992; Jones, 1994) and by questioning parents (Caty *et al.*, 1989). Only 2 of the studies gleaned data from the children's perspective by interviewing them (Knafl *et al.*, 1988; While, 1992). Little is thus known on children's views and experiences of parental participation in their care. There is consequently a need for further research from the children's perspective to substantiate the effectiveness of parental participation in promoting their wellbeing while in hospital.

Another group identified as marginalised in the study of parental participation was ethnic minorities, yet the countries where most studies were conducted – the UK, North America and Canada – are of a multiethnic composition. Fuller (1997) calls for ethnic minority participation in the processes of the health care system so that people from ethnic minorities are treated equally and in accordance with their individual and different needs.

In applying the principles of evidence-based practice in this review, both strengths of and limitations to this approach for children's nursing were identified. The limitations identified lie primarily with the research methodology. The rigour of a study design is a key consideration in attaching importance to the study findings. The authors found little consistency between qualitative studies in particular, which reflects methodological debates about qualitative methods. Criteria for the assessment of qualitative studies have been proposed (Popay *et al.*, 1998), but a clear consensus is not evident in the methodological literature and certainly not in the reports examined in this review. Therefore, in presenting studies as described by researchers, the authors have reported the claims of researchers about the reliability and validity of quantitative studies and about rigour in qualitative studies.

The authors' reservations about framing clinical questions with just one patient/problem, one intervention and one outcome in mind were confirmed in this review: parents and children cannot be viewed in isolation. Furthermore, facilitating the practice of parental participation in care requires a complex amalgam of skills from practitioners that serve the best interests of children, their parents and their families.

While there are limits to the application of evidence-based practice to children's nursing, there are also strengths in this approach. This review has brought together a number of studies and provides an overview of the research on parental participation in care. The authors have minimised bias through the use of systematic methods of searching and through the use of a structured system of data extraction.

Most (12) qualitative studies reported at least three or four of the themes: roles and relationships, emotional status, control and decision making, and knowledge and competence. Most (10) of the quantitative studies focused on one or two themes, roles and relationships emerging as the most dominant theme. This finding illustrates differences in the knowledge generated by different methods and suggests that a variety of methodological approaches is required in order to study parental participation. The place of qualitative research in evidence-based practice remains problematic because there is no consensus on the assessment of rigour, and it may not even be possible to achieve such a consensus. However, qualitative studies have an important contribution to make to clinical decision making.

Conclusions

This review has demonstrated that systematic principles and procedures can be adapted to a review of literature in the 'difficult case' of parental participation in children's care in hospital. Despite the problems of framing questions that arise in children's nursing and the difficulty of considering a body of literature that includes a high proportion of qualitative studies, it has been possible to reduce bias and to examine common themes. The review does not provide answers to the problem of how to balance parental distress with benefit to children, but it does provide information that can inform clinical decisions in nursing. The background knowledge provided in this review can help practitioners, in consultation and negotiation with parents, to make decisions about the areas of care and levels of participation that may be most appropriate for parents. In addition, the review provides a basis for decisions concerning future research in this area. This chapter has demonstrated that the themes of roles and relationships, emotional status, control and decision making, and knowledge and competence as they relate to parents have been examined through research. In contrast, comparatively little research effort has been focused on the perspectives of children, families from minority ethnic communities, and family members other than mothers, which represents a gap in current knowledge.

Acknowledgement

The authors wish to acknowledge An Bord Altranais (Nursing Board), Ireland, for funding this review through a Doctoral Scholarship awarded to Eileen Savage.

Table 5.2 Overview of studies relating to the effects on parents of parental participation in caring for their hospitalised child

Authors (Year) Country	Aim(s) of study (specific to parents/family)	Methodological issues		Findings
		Sample	Design, data collection and analysis, rigour/reliability and validity	(a) Roles and relationships, (b) Emotional status (c) Control and decision making (d) Knowledge and competence
Hayes and Knox (1984) Canada	To examine the experience of stress in parents related to the hospitalisation of their children with long-term disabilities	40 parents (33 mothers, 6 fathers, 1 grandparent) of 35 children who had long-term disability extending over 1 year or longer	Qualitative. Unstructured interviews. Constant comparative method of data analysis	**Roles and Relationships:** Disruption of normal family functioning and established parenting roles. Parents expected to carry out their usual tasks, which differed from professionals' expectations. Role conflict with nurses regarding the comforting, protecting part of parenting. Lack of participation experienced by parents. Hospital bureaucracy and constant change of staff made it impossible for parents to co-ordinate their child's care and keep a close watch on the overall picture of what was happening regarding their child's care **Emotional Status:** Primary sources of stress were the constant demand for adaptation of the parental role, and feeling ultimately responsible but without control over the whole, complex family situation **Control and Decision Making:** When parents perceived themselves as sharing their child's care with professionals, they viewed their experiences more positively **Knowledge and Competence:** In modifying their role, parents learned the roles of the professionals, for example preparing the child for procedures, and how to communicate with professionals about their child. Although abdicating medical matters to professionals, parents viewed themselves as 'experts' and believed they knew their child best
Knafl and Dixon (1984) and Knafl et al. (1988) USA	To investigate (a) how parenting is carried out in the hospital, (b) the nature of interaction between parents and nurses, and (c) the expectations that each group holds for the other (also included in Table 5.3)	62 sets of parents of children aged 3–13 years on three general paediatric wards	Qualitative – based on 'symbolic interactionism'. Interview guides. Direct observation. Thematic content analysis. Revision of codes and independent coding by two project members	**Roles and Relationships:** Parents constructed their participation with hospital staff. Level 1 participation: Parents willingly hand over the care to professionals. Level 2 participation: Monitoring of caregivers' actions and decisions via the ongoing evaluation of professionals; participation in interactions with professionals; initiation of care from professionals. Re fathers (1984), 76 per cent ($n = 47$) continued their usual fathering role of comforting and providing routine care; 24 per cent ($n = 15$) of fathers expanded their usual role to reflect Level 2 participation **Control and Decision Making:** Level 1 participation: Parents relinquished control to professionals and consequently rendered themselves powerless; Level 2 participation: Greater parental control by establishing co-operative relationship with professionals and seeking information. Re fathers (1984): Only 24 per cent ($n = 15$) became involved in medical decision making **Knowledge and Competence:** Level 1 participation: Parents did not actively seek out information from professionals but waited to be informed. Level 2 participation: Parents were more active in seeking information about their child's care. Re fathers (1984): most fathers (76 per cent, $n = 47$) did not actively seek information from nurses, reflecting Level 1 participation
Algren (1985) USA	To examine the way in which mothers perceive their role in caring for their hospitalised child	20 parents (18 mothers, 2 fathers, 1 set of parents) of hospitalised children under 10 years of age on a medical-surgical unit	Descriptive quantitative survey. Questionnaire (included Likert Scale). Descriptive (frequency distributions) statistical analysis. Acknowledges that the small size of the studies precludes generalising the findings	**Roles and Relationships:** Most (60 per cent) parents had 'definitely not' been asked by nurses about the role they wished to assume, and 40 per cent had been 'somewhat' asked. Seventy per cent of parents received no explanation from nurses on the role they could or should not assume, whereas 30 per cent felt that they had 'somewhat' received an explanation. Seventy per cent or more of the parents wanted to participate in basic care activities, for example feeding (1 per cent), comforting (90 per cent) and bathing (80 per cent). Fewer parents wanted to participate in clinical/technical care activities, for example taking temperatures (50 per cent), staying with the child during a painful procedure (50 per cent), bathing the child receiving IV fluids (20 per cent), changing dressings (0 per cent) and tube feeding (0 per cent). Nurses did not negotiate with parents what role they might or would prefer to assume

Table 5.2 (cont'd)

| Monahan and Schkade (1985) USA | To examine whether the quality of nursing care is compromised by allowing parents to assume total responsibility in a Care by Parent Unit (CPBU) versus a Care by Nursing (CBN) unit (part of which focused on parental anxiety and urine sample collection techniques as quality of care variables) (also included in Table 5.3) | 44 mother–child pairs ($n = 23$ CPBU; $n = 21$ CBN) of children aged 14 months to 4.5 years who were the first-time ambulators requiring gait training (for example with cerebral palsy, osteogenesis imperfecta or sacral agenesis) | 'Experimental'. Four mother–child pair groups: 1. CBPU with special physical therapy on the unit. 2. CBPU with 'regular' physical therapy in the main hospital department. 3. CBN with special therapy on the unit; 4. CBN with regular therapy in the main hospital department. Three itemed questionnaires using 'semantic differential scales with a series of bipolar adjectives' to measure parental anxiety – administered on admission, 5 days later and on discharge. The instrument yielded a possible mean score of 1 (very anxious) to 9 (not at all anxious). Urine collection from indwelling catheters or pedi-bags, or by catheterization. Descriptive (frequency distributions, means, standard deviations) and inferential (chi-squared test and ANOVA) statistical analysis. The chi-squared test was used to analyse the differences between (a) types of urine collection and (b) types of collector. ANOVA was used to analyse differential scales regarding anxiety. The validity of data analysis on catheter specimens was questioned because of the small number of specimens | **Emotional Status:** The findings did not support the hypothesis that parents with the greatest involvement in child care (Group 1) would have less anxiety over time, than parents who were less involved in care (Group 4). Parents in the CBPU expressed increasing anxiety over time, in contrast to parents in a CBN unit who were found to have decreasing levels of anxiety over time. Group means and standard deviations for the parental anxiety scale on admission and discharge were: CBPU with special therapy – M 3.75, SD 3.33 (admission), and M 2.66, SD 1.87 (discharge); CBPU with regular therapy – M 4.09, SD 3.41 (admission), and M 4.36, SD 3.61(discharge); CBN with special therapy – M 3.77, SD 3.30 (admission), and M 3.44, SD 2.45 (discharge); CBN with regular therapy – M 2.60, SD 2.11 (admission), and M 4.20, SD 2.78 (discharge)

Knowledge and Competence: For pedi-bag urine sample collections, a chi-squared analysis showed a significant difference ($\chi^2 = 4.78$, $p < 0.029$) with fewer (27 out of 29) contaminated specimens collected by nurses. The number of contaminated specimens collected by mothers was 39, with only 5 non-contaminated specimens being collected. For catheter collections, mothers were found to have collected 3 contaminated specimens and 9 non-contaminated specimens. Nurses collected 1 contaminated specimen and 8 non-contaminated specimens. The chi-squared test revealed no significant differences between mothers and nurses for urine collection by catheter ($\chi^2 = 0.643$, $p < 0.442$) |

Table 5.2 (cont'd)

Authors (Year) Country	Aim(s) of study (specific to parents/family)	Methodological issues		Findings
		Sample	Design, data collection and analysis, rigour/reliability and validity	(a) Roles and relationships, (b) Emotional status (c) Control and decision making (d) Knowledge and competence
Robinson (1985, 1987) Canada	To explore the views of the parents of hospitalised chronically ill children	9 parents from 6 families with a hospitalised chronically ill child	Qualitative – 'phenomenology' interviews. Analysis using method of constant comparison. Accuracy of researcher's understanding validated throughout interviews	**Roles and Relationships:** Adversarial relationships caused by discrepancies of viewpoint between parents and health care professionals; 'Discrepant expectations about hospitalisa▨n': with parents expecting minimal disruption to their routine and family life. Discrepant expect▨ns about family involvement, which parents thought would be grounded on negotiation and m▨al trust. Parents felt obliged to take care of the child in hospital despite 'roadblocks' from prof▨ sionals. A role of vigilant protection emerged. Over time, relationships with professionals be▨me more mutually satisfying and effective **Emotional Status:** Discrepant orientations to sickness': professionals disregarding parent▨ ▨iews of hospitalisation as predictable and contextual in their chronic illness experience promote▨ ▨▨l- ings of anger, frustration and resentment. Parents worried about what would happen to the ▨ ild in their absence **Control and Decision Making:** Lack of decision-making dialogue between parents and pr▨s- sionals resulted in 'discrepant therapeutic goals', that is, parents being committed to 'norm▨a- tion' and professionals being 'acute disease' orientated. Lack of information restricted involv▨ nent in the decision-making process. The message for parents was that professionals were in c▨ ▨e. Participation was carefully orchestrated by parents in order not to be viewed as interfering **Knowledge and Competence:** – 'Discrepant perspectives about family involvement': atte▨ ▨s to be involved in care as experts and competent health care providers was denigrated or disr▨ rded by professionals. Parental competency was questioned by professionals
Sainsbury et al. (1986) UK	To evaluate a care by parent scheme	32 family members (mostly mothers) of children under 3 years of years (23 were under 1 year) and nurses (no details)	Descriptive. Questionnaires to parents and nurses. Descriptive statistical (frequency distributions) analysis	**Roles and Relationships:** The numbers of parents varied in their success in carrying out ▨ ▨▨e- dures: monitoring temperature ($n = 27$), pulse rate ($n = 25$) and respiratory rate ($n = 24$), ch▨ ng feeding, vomiting and bowel motion ($n = 29$), collecting urine ($n = 10$), giving drugs ($n = 18$, providing nebulizer treatment ($n = 5$), and on care of IV infusion ($n = 3$). Care by parents he▨ ▨d to minimise boredom for the parents and promoted good relationships with nurses and docto▨ **Knowledge and Competence:** All parents felt greater confidence with regard to the care ▨ progress of their child
Keane et al. (1986) UK	To examine how a policy of parental admission during children's acute medical illness was implemented, and to assess the parent's response to such a policy	34 resident parents (mostly mothers) of children with a mean age of 11 months, and 23 non-resident parents of children with a mean age of 4 years, on a paediatric ward setting	Survey. Interviews and 4-point scale to measure anxiety. Descriptive (frequency distributions, and means) and inferential (chi-squared, Wilcoxon test) statistical analysis	**Roles and Relationships:** 88 per cent ($n = 30$) of resident mothers (RMs) engaged in fee▨ ▨g and changing the baby compared with 82 per cent ($n = 19$) of non-resident mothers (NRMs). M▨ ▨ ($n = 23$, 67 per cent) RMs attended special investigations than NRMs ($n = 13$, 56 per cent) **Emotional Status:** More RMs than NRMs 'expressed very high levels of anxiety'. (The sta▨ ▨cal significance of the above results was not stated)

Table 5.2 (cont'd)

Study	Aim	Sample	Method	Findings
Cleary et al. (1986) and Cleary (1992) UK	To identify parents' experiences of participation and the care by parent (CBP) scheme (also included in Table 5.3)	26 children aged 3 weeks to 2 years on a medical ward (9 in CBP, 7 with a resident mother, 10 without a resident parent), 38 parents and 36 nurses	Structured observational study using non-participant observation. Questionnaires and interviews. Descriptive (frequency distributions and means) statistical analysis. Content analysis of narrative data	**Roles and Relationships:** *CBP scheme:* The best thing was being able to stay with the child and/or visit as often as desired. Greater contact with other family members. Parents felt useful by contributing to child's recovery. Role overlap and conflict with nurses when the nurses took over the child's care without checking with the parents. *Resident parents:* Marooned and isolated from the family **Emotional Status:** *CBP scheme:* The 'worst thing' was worrying about the child's illness and/or the distresses that treatment caused. Difficult to do unpleasant things to their child. Too much responsibility for some parents, which worried them **Knowledge and Competence:** *CBP scheme:* Increased competence to carry out complex technical skills: increased time with nurses for teaching and support. Some parents were dissatisfied – would have liked more information and professional support, especially for clinical procedures
Ball et al. (1988) UK	To ascertain parents' views on the quality of their children's nursing care.	35 parents from 4 paediatric wards (75.9 per cent being resident)	Pilot study. Questionnaire. Descriptive (frequency distributions) statistical analysis	**Roles and Relationships:** Parents generally liked being able to stay with their child but would liked to have carried out more of their child's care in hospital **Control and Decision Making:** Forty per cent of parents reported that the nurses did not involve them in care planning. **Knowledge and Competence:** Parents reported lack of information /discussion about tests and procedures (11.4 per cent) and what would happen to their child (38.2 per cent); 8.6 per cent of parents received inconsistent information. 5.7 per cent of parents felt uncomfortable asking the nurses questions
Alexander et al. (1988) USA	To compare differences in anxiety levels between the rooming-in parents (RIPs) and non-rooming-in parents (NRIPs) of hospitalised children	Convenience sample of 101 parents of whom 50 (37 mothers and 13 fathers) were RIP and 51 (35 mothers and 16 fathers) were NRIP of children aged 3–8 years on two paediatric wards	Quantitative design. Self-administered Spielberger State–Trait Anxiety Inventory (STAI) (Likert scale with a possible score of 20–80 on each measure of anxiety) completed on admission (T1) and 2/3 days post-admission (T2), and the Information about your Child Questionnaire on admission. Content and construct validity of STAI was demonstrated in previous studies. Descriptive (frequency distributions, means, medians, modes and standard deviations) and inferential (Mann–Whitney U test, Stepwise regression analysis, Spearman's rho, *t* test and Wilcoxon test)	**Emotional Status:** One statistically significant difference was revealed on comparison of the NRIP and RIP groups, that of a higher state anxiety of NRIP mothers (42.41) than RIP mothers (36.27) at T2 ($Z = 2.07$, $p < 0.04$). Although not statistically significant, other trends included: higher state than trait anxiety scores in both parent subjects at T1 and T2, fathers having the greatest increase of state above trait anxiety; NRIP mothers and fathers reported higher state anxiety at T2 (mothers = 41.67–42.41; fathers = 40.36–41.62), RIP fathers being found to have little change in state anxiety (34.0 at T1 and 34.8 at T2) and RIP mothers being found to have significantly less state anxiety at T2 (43.0 at T1 and 36.27 at T2). Mothers in both groups were found to have higher trait anxiety levels than fathers

Table 5.2 (cont'd)

Authors (Year) Country	Aim(s) of study (specific to parents/family)	Methodological issues		Findings
		Sample	Design, data collection and analysis, rigour/reliability and validity	(a) Roles and relationships, (b) Emotional status (c) Control and decision making (d) Knowledge and competence
Caty *et al.* (1989) Canada	To examine mothers' perceptions of the stressful situation their children experienced during hospitalisation and how they and their children responded to these situations (also included in Table 5.3)	30 mothers of children aged 2–5 years on a medical or surgical unit	Qualitative 'exploratory descriptive' design. Open-ended interview instrument. Descriptive (frequency distributions) statistical and content data analysis. Forty-item Children's Coping Strategies Checklist was used to categorise children's behaviours as described by mothers (information seeking, direct action, inhibition of action, seeking comfort/help, growth/independence and intrapsychic). Content validity of interview questions obtained through discussions with faculty and graduate students, and affirmed by a nursing faculty member from another hospital	**Roles and Relationships:** The two dominant strategies used by mothers to help children cope were comforting (n = 26, 87 per cent) and providing information (n = 19, 63 per cent) Fewer mothers used the provision of physical care/protection (n = 8, 27 per cent) and the provision of emotional support (n = 6, 20 per cent) as strategies to help their child cope **Emotional Status:** Mothers described their response to the child's situation with more unpleasant than unpleasant affective states. The most dominant unpleasant feelings reported were distress (n = 17, 57 per cent), depression (n = 12, 40 per cent) and fear/anxiety (n = 37 per cent). Pleasant feelings were love/affection/concern (n = 13, 43 per cent) and elation/joy (n = 5, 17 per cent)
Burke *et al.* (1991) Canada	To explore the nature of the stressful process for parents surrounding the repeated hospitalisation of chronically ill children	Theoretical sampling: 30 mothers of children with disabilities, 30 mothers of healthy non-disabled children, 100 parents of children with physical disabilities at a weekend retreat, 9 mothers of children with repeated hospitalisation. Six community nurses with caseloads of physically disabled children	Qualitative – 'grounded theory'. Interviews – Visual Life Events Schedule. Participant observation (on the sample of 9 mothers). Constant comparative analysis of data	**Roles and Relationships:** Forced to 'reluctantly take charge' of the situation because of 'hazardous secrets' dangerous to the child (that is, inadequate information, variations/gaps in care and inexperienced health professionals; reluctantly taking charge involved covert 'vigilance and taking over'. Role conflict with professionals **Emotional Status:** 'Hazardous secrets' and 'reluctantly taking charge' were the most stressful aspects of hospitalisation; in increasing participation, parents were concerned about being labelled trouble makers. Invasive procedures were found to be very stressful for parents **Control and Decision Making:** As a last resort, reluctantly taking charge involved overt 'questioning of rules' and 'calling a halt to professionals' decisions. Taking charge aimed to regain control of the potentially hazardous hospital situation **Knowledge and Competence:** Parents, on the basis of their knowledge and experience, felt that they could identify variations, gaps and/or omissions in the management of their child's care. 'Polite inquiry' was found to reflect parents' first step in seeking information from professionals. In 'reluctantly taking charge', parents moved to tenaciously information seeking'
Dearmun (1992) UK	To compare the perceptions of parents and nurses towards the parents' contribution to their hospitalised children's care, and to compare the activities performed by nurses and parents	14 mothers and 21 nurses subsample of 7 children/families for observation) on a children's ward	'Descriptive' study. Semi-structured interview schedules (Likert-type scale) and non-participant structured observation schedule (checklist on 38 child care activities). Descriptive (frequency distributions) and content analysis. Acknowledges that the small sample size precludes generalising the findings	**Roles and Relationships:** Incongruent views between parents and nurses regarding the reasons why parents choose to stay with their child: the reason for parents (58 per cent) was to meet emotional needs of their child; nurses (69 per cent) reported the reasons to be maternal/paternal drive to care for the child; Only 3 parents (22 per cent) were explicitly asked whether they wanted to be involved in care. Nurses took it for granted that parents wanted to take part in care **Emotional Status:** A number of nurses reported that they should protect parents from the distress of knowing what their child's problems were **Control and Decision Making:** The 'vast majority of nurses' claimed that they gave parents a choice of staying with their child during procedures, but only 64 per cent of parents reported being asked by nurses to stay during procedures. Over half of the mothers felt that they would not be allowed to look at the nursing records

Table 5.2 (cont'd)

Schepp (1992) USA	To profile mothers who prefer control over their hospitalised children. Variables: child's age, mother's age, time spent by the mother in hospital, number of children in the family, ethnic background, and prior experience with a hospitalised child	Purposive sample of 384 mothers (Study 1 $n = 100$, Study 2 $n = 284$) of hospitalised children with mean ages of 5.4 (Study 1) and 5.2 (Study 2) from two inpatient units	Two 'instrumentation' studies using descriptive cross-sectional design. Instrument: The Parental Control Preference Scale (PCPS)(24-item Likert Scale yielding a total possible score of 96). Descriptive (frequency distributions, means medians and standard deviations) and inferential (multiple regression, residual analysis – beta coefficients and explained variance, Pearson's correlation co-efficient and t tests) statistical analysis. Instrument was found to be reliable with an alpha of 0.85 (Study 1) and 0.87 (Study 2)	**Control and Decision Making:** Significant correlation between mother's desire for control and: (1) child's age (strongest correlate, Study 1, $r = -0.43$, $p < 0.001$; Study 2, $r = -0.38$, $p < 0.001$), mothers of younger children preferring more control, (2) mother's age (Study 1, $r = 0.27$, $p < 0.001$; Study 2, $r = 0.26$, $p < 0.001$), younger mothers preferring more control, (3) length of time in hospital (Study 1, $r = 0.27$, $p < 0.001$; Study 2, $r = 0.26$, $p < 0.001$), mothers who spent more time with their child preferring more control, (4) number of children in the family (Study 1, $r = 0.19$, $p < 0.001$; Study 2, $r = -0.13$, $p < 0.001$), mothers with fewer children preferring more control, (5) ethnic background significant in Study 1 only ($r = 0.19$, $p < 0.001$), with a preference for more control by ethnic minority mothers, (6) prior hospital experience significant in Study 2 only ($r = -0.26$, $p < 0.001$), there being a preference for more control by mothers with no prior experience of hospital with their child
While (1992) UK	To study consumers' (families') views on health care: a comparison of hospital and home care (also included in Table 5.3)	40 families (parents) and some ($n = 9$) of their children	Descriptive 'evaluative' study. Semi-structured interviews	**Roles and Relationships:** Participation was helpful for 94.75 per cent of parents in that it gave them a sense of purpose and enabled them to feel useful. **Emotional Status:** It was expected that parents would participate in their child's care, which posed difficulties regarding their obligations towards other children and their work. **Knowledge and Competence:** Caring for a child in hospital, where assistance and supervision was available if necessary, helped parents to develop their confidence and therefore helped them to learn how to care for their child
Lau (1993) USA	To describe the process of implementing a Parent in Partnership (PIP) programme on two medical wards. (Pre-implementation phase involved workshops for staff)	74 parents (40 in PIP and 34 not in PIP) and 38 nurses	Descriptive; 22-item questionnaire (parents) and 12-item Likert Scale questionnaire (nurses) pre- and post-PIP implementation phase. Descriptive (means, standard deviations and frequency distributions) statistical analysis	**Roles and Relationships:** Parents in both groups participated in basic care activities, for example bathing and feeding. Only parents in the PIP group recorded fluid balance. 12 parents in the PIP group took and recorded temperature, pulse and respiration. **Emotional Status:** Nurses reported parents in the PIP group to be less anxious than those in the non-PIP group. **Control and Decision Making:** 25 parents from each group reported being very well prepared to care for the child after discharge. 11 parents from PIP group and 4 parents from the non-PIP group were moderately prepared ($p < 0.05$). Regarding confidence in special care (for example, changing central lines and dressings, nasogastric tube feeding and so on), 27 (68 per cent) parents from the PIP group indicated moderate to very much whereas only 18 (53 per cent) from the non-PIP group felt confident ($p < 0.05$)

Table 5.2 (cont'd)

Authors (Year) Country	Aim(s) of study (specific to parents/family)	Methodological issues		Findings
		Sample	Design, data collection and analysis, rigour/reliability and validity	(a) Roles and relationships, (b) Emotional status (c) Control and decision making (d) Knowledge and competence
Perkins (1993) USA	To explore the parental management of care giving for hospitalised children with physical and intellectual disabilities	23 parents of children aged 2–13 years	Qualitative – 'grounded theory'. Interviews. Constant comparative analysis of data. To increase credibility of findings: (a) parents were interviewed as two separate groups (18 during hospitalisation and 5 post-discharge), and 8 mothers were interviewed twice; (b) data excerpts and analytical memos were reviewed by experienced grounded theory researchers and by peer review	**Roles and Relationships:** 'Parents as care givers' emerged as three phases: protection, survival and the establishment of the central person. In the protective phase, involvement moves from participant observer to active participant in parenting tasks. In the survival phase is the adoption of a more assertive role in accessing and managing resources, and monitoring the child's care; overlap with professional roles. In the central person phase, parents act as co-ordinators of care and a facilitator of professionals, both inside and outside the hospital setting. Doctors and nurses viewed as assisting parents **Emotional Status:** The acquisition of knowledge alleviated fears **Control and Decision Making:** Initial involvement dependent on encouragement and permission from staff. Being knowledgeable made parents feel on an even level with professionals. In the central person phase, parents determined their personal level of participation in various activities **Knowledge and Competence:** Knowledge acquired in phases re: protective needs (basic information about the child's care), survival needs (specific problems and long-term consequences) and central person needs (knowledge about all aspects of the child's life). As the central person parents viewed themselves as experts capable of educating others; sharing of knowledge with professional was expected at central person phase
Tomlinson et al. (1993) USA	To examine the relationships between maternal perceptions of an acutely ill child, nurse care givers and contextual factors in a paediatric bone marrow transplant unit	20 mothers of children aged 18 months to 16 years on a bone marrow transplant unit. and 20 primary nurses	'Correlation' study. Instruments: Parent Satisfaction Scale (PSS) – Likert-type index of 7 questions; Parental Participation Attitude Scale – 24-item Likert Scale. Educational and Experiential Background Survey – administered to nurses. Descriptive (means and standard deviations) and Inferential (Pearson's product-moment correlation coefficient matrix) statistical analysis. Face validity, but not internal reliability or construct validity established for PSS. Face, content and construct validity. Noted that no reliability estimates have been reported for PSS	**Roles and Relationships:.** The hypothesis that maternal satisfaction with nursing care would be positively related to nursing attitudes towards parental involvement was not supported, that is, there was no significant association (-0.04, $p < 0.01$) between maternal satisfaction and nursing attitudes towards parental involvement. The hypothesis that maternal satisfaction with nursing care would be negatively related to maternal vigilance (time spent at the bedside) was not supported, that is, there was no significant association (0.15, $p < 0.01$) between maternal satisfaction and maternal vigilance. Maternal vigilance was more likely to be associated with nurse experience (-0.39, $p < 0.05$) than with child's acuity (0.12), unit acuity (0.30) and nurses' attitudes (0.02)
Kristensson-Hallstrom and Elander (1994) Sweden	To elucidate (a) the types of care task that parents perform, (b) additional care tasks that in the opinion of parents and staff parents could perform, and (c) whether parents and staff opinions coincide	40 parents (27 mothers, 9 sets of parents and 4 fathers) of children aged l week to 5 years. 44 staff members (registered nurses 24 per cent; enrolled nurses 62 per cent; doctors 14 per cent)	'Descriptive' study. Questionnaires (37 items) to parents and staff. Descriptive (frequency distributions) statistical analysis	**Roles and Relationships:** All parents spent most of the day with their child, and most (88 per cent) spent the night. There was a congruence of views between parents and nurses that: all parents generally console, comfort and entertain their child; parents generally take care of the child's personal hygiene and food and drink; parents usually draw the staff's attention when the child is in pain **Knowledge and Competence:** Significant differences ($p < 0.01$) between what parents considered what they had done in 22 items that reflected specific clinical/technical nursing situations, and what they felt they could have done, given instructions and guidance from staff. For 14 of the 22 nursing situations (for example, tube feeding and changing urine bags), the proportion of staff who felt that parents could do the tasks was greater than the proportion of parents who felt that they could do them ($p < 0.01$). For 6 of the 22 items (for example, recording blood pressure and recording fluid intake), the proportion of parents who felt that they could do the task was greater than the proportion of staff who felt that parents could perform the task ($p < 0.01$)

Table 5.2 (cont'd)

Study	Aims	Sample	Methods	Findings
Darbyshire (1994) UK	To examine the lived experiences of parents who decided to live in hospital with their child in hospital. To explore the relationship between nurses and doctors	30 parents (26 mothers and 4 fathers) and 27 qualified nurses from a paediatric medical ward and a surgical burns/plastic ward	Qualitative – 'phenomenology' and 'grounded theory'. Interviewing (a) individuals ('4 parents and 12 nurses), (b) focus groups (a 16-parent group and a 15-nurse group). Interpretative analysis. Reflexive process used for adequacy of data	**Roles and Relationships:** Uncertainty and confusion regarding what exactly they were allowed to do. Parents were found 'learning the ropes' through trial and error. Parents viewed basic mothering care as a continuation of their normal lives. There was a demarcation of care into basic (parental) and technical (nursing) care regardless of the parents' desire to get involved in technical care. Participation did not appear to be an openly negotiated arrangement. Tensions arose between nurses and parents regarding their respective roles. 'Keeping vigil' emerged as an important aspect of parenting a child in hospital and represented parents' powerful need to be with their child **Emotional Status:** Living with a hospitalised child was likened to an 'emotional roller-coaster'. Anxiety created by uncertainty was one of the most distressing aspects of the parents' stay in hospital. Uncertainty was most often related to the child's condition, as well as to their parental role **Control and Decision Making:** Disempowerment was experienced by parents, nurses being perceived to be in a greater position of power. Parents were reluctant to interrupt nurses in case of 'being a nuisance', which placed parents in a subservient position on the ward **Knowledge and Competence:** Parents felt that their knowledge and competence were questioned by professionals. In particular, 'basic mothering skills' and expertise were undervalued by professionals. Parents perceived technical skills to be outside their area of expertise. To become valued participants, parents learned the discourse of technical and highly specialised knowledge
Coyne (1995) UK	To identify reasons why parents choose to participate in the care of their hospitalised child and to identify factors that enhance or inhibit readiness to participate	18 prime resident parents (16 mothers and 2 fathers) of children aged 1 week to 16 years on a general surgical ward	Qualitative 'descriptive'. Semi-structured interview schedule. Content analysis	**Roles and Relationships:** Participation relieved boredom and allowed continuity of the parenting role. A reluctance to take on clinical care arose out of concern about trespassing on the nurses' domain of duties. A negotiation of care evolved rather than being planned and deliberate. One mother was dissatisfied with the expectation that she should do all the general care; a reluctance to get involved was an attempt to increase communication time with staff **Emotional Status:** Emotional status at seeing many sick children; 'anxiety' about hurting the child and about their ability to perform tasks on their child **Control and Decision Making:** The negotiation and sharing of care exceeded most parents' expectation of a more strict regime **Knowledge and Competence:** Parents viewed themselves as experts on their child's care. However, a lack of information inhibited their readiness to participate in care in the hospital setting
Rowe (1996) Australia	To examine nursing and parenting practice in the care of hospitalised children. To explore the nurse–parent relationship	50 sets of interactions between 18 nurses and parents of children aged up to three years, on a paediatric ward. 5 nurses	Qualitative 'interpretative'. Participant observation. Interviews (5 nurses) Informal conversations (parents). Concurrent data collection and analysis. Thematic content analysis	**Roles and Relationships:** 'Co-operative experiences' were characterised by negotiation and sharing of information. The nurse initiated co-operative experiences. Parallel experiences of working alongside nurses independently made parents feel 'just part of the system' and relieving the nursing work burden. Excluding experiences were characterised by a lack of negotiation, which made parents feel that their role was undervalued **Control and Decision Making:** Excluding experiences was characterised by nurses holding a significant degree of control, leaving parents in the position of 'bystanders'

Table 5.2 (cont'd)

| Authors (Year) Country | Aim(s) of study (specific to parents/family) | Methodological issues | | Findings |
		Sample	Design, data collection and analysis, rigour/reliability and validity	(a) Roles and relationships, (b) Emotional status (c) Control and decision making (d) Knowledge and competence
Keatinge and Gilmore (1996) Australia	To plan, implement and evaluate a shared care project. To establish whether parental anxiety was increased by participation	Nurses: 20 in pre-trial (= 64 per cent response) and 13 in post-trial (= 42 per cent response). Parents of children aged 1 month to 12 years on a paediatric medical ward. Pre-trial: 39 on admission; 30 on discharge; 26 on both admission and discharge. Shared Care Study: 35 on admission and discharge	'Pilot study' following the implementation of an educational programme on shared care to nurses. Thirteen-item questionnaire administered to nurses (pre- and post-trial). Focused group discussions with nurses. State–Trait Anxiety Inventory (STAI) (20-item Likert Scale) administered to parents (pre- and post-trial) and informal conversations with parents. Descriptive (frequency distributions, means and standard deviations) and inferential (t test) statistical analysis. Content analysis of narrative data. Claims for reliability and validity of the STAI instrument were based on previous research	**Roles and Relationships:** *Shared care:* More inclusive of families at appropriate levels of care-giving and clarifies the roles of parents and nurses **Emotional Status:** Support for the hypotheses that: (1) the anxiety levels of parents who participated in shared care will be reduced significantly from admission to discharge ($t = 5.22$, $df = 24$, $p < 0.001$), and (2) the changes in parents' anxiety level between their children's admission and discharge will be greater for parents who participated in the shared care trial than for parents whose children were hospitalised prior to the trial (change in mean score = −10.4 for shared care parents, and −5.88 for pre-trial parents) **Control and Decision Making:** *Shared care:* Increased time was spent with nurses in planning the child's care; choice in the level of involvement; more in control of the situation **Knowledge and Competence:** *Shared care: a* clearer understanding of what was happening; better prepared and educated at the time of discharge, and increased parental confidence in caring for child after discharge
Neill (1996a, b) UK	To describe parents' views and experiences of parent participation on an acute paediatric ward. To identify factors that inhibited or facilitated participation	16 parents (mostly mothers) of children aged 2–5 years discharged from an acute paediatric medical ward	Qualitative 'exploration'. Interviews. Content analysis. Transcripts returned to parents – no response. Reliability and validity of results checked by experienced researchers	**Roles and Relationships:** Presence and involvement resulted in some continuity of the parenting role. Parents wanted to be involved in all aspects of their child's basic care. care planning, evaluation and discussions on their child. Parents felt unsure about taking on clinical care and did not want to take on aspects of this. A lack of negotiation between parents and nurses resulted in a mismatch between parental desires and experiences, for example 'left to get on with it' in isolation from professionals. Parents experienced the need for 'being there' with their child 'just in case'. The relationship between the parents and the professionals was described as paternalistic **Emotional Status:** Presence and involvement resulted in better coping with hospitalisation. Parents found it distressing to witness distress in their child during procedures that hurt. Parents reported the need for physical and emotional support from others **Control and Decision Making:** Many of the nursing staff were seen by parents as being more powerful than themselves. Nurses 'take over' the parental role. The parents' locus of control perceived to be external. Parents experienced increased control when involved in care. Loss of control was experienced when information was withheld from parents **Knowledge and Competence:** Their presence and involvement resulted in parents being better informed on their child's progress and on care following discharge. Information helped parents to increase their sense of control, but some parents felt unable to ask for information. Some parents expressed the need for more, and consistent, information

Table 5.2 (cont'd)

Study	Aim	Sample	Method	Findings
Kawik (1996), UK	To determine whether parents were able to participate in the care of their hospitalised child and work in partnership with nurses	55 nurses (84.6 per cent response) from 3 children's wards, and 12 parents of discharged children	'Descriptive method triangulation'. Postal questionnaires (nurses) and interviews (parents). Descriptive statistics (frequency distribution) for nurses' responses Content analysis for parents' responses. Acknowledges the need for a larger study to validate the findings	**Roles and Relationships:** Parents were willing to provide care for their child, particularly in the areas of comforting and reassurance. Parental participation appeared to occur in an *ad hoc* way rather than being planned. Nurses assumed parental involvement but did not negotiate the extent of involvement that parents desired **Control and Decision Making:** 50 nurses (90 per cent) claimed that they involved parents in decision making. However, parents claimed that nurses assumed that they would like to be involved in care and did not always negotiate the extent of involvement desired by parents. Parents experienced reduced control over their situation. Parents reported that nurses seldom discussed nursing notes with them. The nurses were not totally comfortable with 'sharing' the care, 60 per cent (*n* = 33) disagreeing that they should attend to the child's daily needs when parents were present. Parents were often reluctant to approach nurses, implying that they felt unequal partners in care **Knowledge and Competence:** Parents felt that they lacked some nursing skills and required professional support. They were, however, reluctant to approach nurses for information
Callery 1997(a, b, and c) UK	To investigate the role of parents in the care of hospitalised children	Parents (mostly mothers) of 24 children discharged from a surgical unit, and 12 members of nursing staff	Qualitative – 'ethnography'. Participant observation and interviewing Review of medical and nursing records. Thematic content analysis (constant comparative analysis); reflexive process of categorising data aimed to limit threats to validity	**Roles and Relationships:** Parents found that they had to deviate from their usual nurturing/protective role, and behave in a way that seemed unnaturally detached **Emotional status:** Increased distress due to financial costs (loss of earnings, travel and subsistence), personal costs (for example, distress caused by unpleasant procedures on the child, deviation from the usual parenting role, the challenge to parents' ideas of themselves, and seeing other ill children and their families) and social costs (loss of privacy and autonomy in family relationships, and decisions about child care for other children at home). Parents emerged as co-clients in need of care themselves as a result of their involvement in their child's care **Control and Decision Making:** Loss of power and autonomy **Knowledge and Competence:** Co-operation and conflict between professionals and parents were identified. Conflict was explained as arising from differences in maternal and professional knowledge. Professional knowledge was described as objective and scientific, arising from the public domain of the working world. Maternal knowledge was identified as arising from the private domain of intimate contact with the child in the home, and was characterised by intuitive judgements.
Kristensson-Hollstrom and Elander (1997a, b) Sweden	To gain a deeper understanding of parents' experiences when their child is in hospital	20 parents (12 mothers and 8 fathers) of boys aged 2–14 years undergoing hypospadias repair on a paediatric surgical unit	Qualitative – 'grounded theory'. Interview guides and review of case notes. Concurrent data collection and analysis – constant comparative method	**Roles and Relationships:** All parents appreciated the opportunity to stay with their child. Hospitalisation required a great adaptation of parents, both physically and mentally. In adopting strategies for feeling secure, 8 parents chose to leave the care to staff and not get involved, and 12 parents sought increasing participation, which allowed continuity of the parenting role. Increased participation resulted in superficial contact with numerous staff **Emotional Status:** 'Anxiety' throughout hospitalisation when not involved in care. Less 'anxiety' with increased participation except for specific events. Fatigue and limited scope for privacy exacerbated parents' mental stress. Parents felt vulnerable and dependent on staff's opinions. There was a feeling of guilt and fear of harming the child (for example, when giving an enema or removing a catheter) when violating the child's right to self-determination. Upset when staff did not treat children as autonomous persons **Control and Decision Making:** For 6 parents, achieving security was through 'getting control over care' by participating directly in the child's care. Their right to self-determination was violated in instances when they were not able to influence their own situation **Knowledge and Competence:** For 6 parents, achieving security arose through knowing their child best and consequently increasing their participation in care. For the 12 parents who chose to participate, they would have like more instructions and guidelines

Table 5.3 Overview of studies relating to the effects of parental participation on hospitalised children

Authors (Year) Country	Aim(s) of study	Methodological issues		Study findings
		Sample	Design, data collection and analysis, rigour/reliability and validity	
Monahan and Schkade (1985) USA	To examine whether the quality of nursing care is compromised by allowing parents to assume total responsibility in a Care by Parent Unit (CPBU) versus a Care by Nursing Staff (CBN) unit (part of which focused on weight changes and skin condition changes during hospitalisation as quality of care variables) (also included in Table 5.2)	44 mother–child pairs ($n = 23$ CPBU; $n = 21$ CBN) of children aged 14 months to 4.5 years who were the first-time ambulators requiring gait training (for example, with cerebral palsy, osteogenesis imperfecta or sacral agenesis)	'Experimental'. Four mother–child pair groups: 1. CPBU with special physical therapy on the unit; 2. CBPU with regular physical therapy in the main hospital department; 3. CBN with special therapy on the unit; 4. CBN with regular therapy in the main hospital department. An in-bed kilogram scale was used to measure the weight. An assessment tool to score skin condition was used to include seven skin condition categories: scaly areas, rashes, diaper rashes, insect bites, blisters, erythematous area and pressure sores. Each item was given a score of 0–3, 0 representing no skin problems. The highest possible score was 21	**Physical Wellbeing:** The hypothesis that weight maintenance in children in the CBPU would significantly greater than that of children in the CBN unit was not supported. No significant difference in weight loss was found between children in the CBPU and CBN units. Significant weight loss occurred in all categories of children during hospitalisation. For the comparison between admission and Day 5, df (1,37), $F = 8.85$, $p < 0.005$. For the comparison between admission and discharge, df (1,36), $F = 9.21$, $p < 0.0044$) The hypothesis that no significant differences existed in skin condition between children in the CBPU and children in the CBN unit was supported. Improvements in skin condition were noted for all groups regardless of assignment to the CBPU or CBN unit. For the comparison between admission and Day 5, df (1,40), $F = 11.62$, $p < 0.0015$; For the comparison between admission and discharge df (1,40), $F = 5.22$, $p < 0.0277$)
Cleary et al. (1986) and Cleary (1992) UK	To monitor the effects of a care by parent scheme (CBP) on the lives of hospitalised children. To identify parents' experiences of participation and CBP (also included in Table 5.2)	26 children aged 3 weeks to 2 years on a medical ward (9 in CBP, 7 with a resident mother, 10 without a resident parent). 38 parents and 36 nurses	Structured observational study using non-participant observation. Questionnaires and interviews. Descriptive (frequency distributions and means) statistical analysis	**Emotional Well-being:** *Children in the CBP scheme:* Spent 69 per cent of the observed time in the company of their mothers and 31 per cent of the observed time with their fathers; 94 per cent of total contact was with the parents/family, 7 per cent of contact with the nurses. The total time alone was 27.5 per cent of observed time; cried alone for 2 per cent of observed time, which less than the other two groups; spent more time (68 per cent of all interactions) receiving social attentiveness, for example play and soothing *Children of resident parents not in the CBP scheme:* Spent more time (73 per cent) than the group in the company of their mothers but less time (9 per cent) than CBP in the company of fathers; 86 per cent of total contact was with the parent/family, 15 per cent of contact with the nurses. The total time alone was 26.3 per cent; cried alone for more time (4 per cent) than the CBP group but less than the non-resident parent (NRP) group; spent less time (63 per cent of all interactions) than the CBP group but more time than the NRP group, receiving social attentiveness *Children in the NRP group:* Spent less time (27 per cent) in contact with their mothers than the CBP and RM groups; 32 per cent of total contact was with the parent/family; compared with the CBP and RM groups, children had more contact time (37 per cent) with nurses – 'a bewildering series of strangers'. Spent 69.5 per cent of time alone; cried alone for more time (10.7 per cent) than the other two groups; spent less time (58 per cent) receiving social attentiveness than the other two groups.

Table 5.3 (cont'd)

Knafl *et al.* (1988) USA	To investigate: (a) how parenting is carried out in the hospital, (b) the nature of interaction among patients, parents and nurses, and (c) the expectations that each group holds for the others (also included in Table 5.2)	35 hospitalised children aged 5–12 years. 62 sets of parents	Qualitative. Interview guides. Direct observation. Thematic content analysis. Revision of codes and independent coding by two project members	**Emotional Wellbeing:** Children were found to differ in their level of adaptation. The majority (21) of children 'fell within middle range, viewing hospitalisation to have positive and negative effects. Attention from family members was a positive aspect; painful procedures and separation from family and friends negative ones. The utilisation of parental support helped these children to manage their hospitalisation experience; parental presence helped most children in this range cope with the unpleasant elements of hospitalisation. High-level adapters (8 children) viewed their experience positively and 'revelled in the attention they were given by parents, relatives'. Low-level adapters (5 children) tended to display dependence on their parents, for example, being fed by the parent and continually needing the parent nearby. For all children in the study, visitors (parents, grandparents, siblings and so on) played an important role in the child's hospitalisation, in that they helped the child to maintain ties with home life, and provided the child with undivided attention
Caty *et al.* (1989) Canada	To examine mothers' perceptions of the stressful situation their children experienced during hospitalisation and how they and their children responded to these situations (also included in Table 5.2)	30 mothers of children aged 2–5 years on a medical or surgical unit	Qualitative exploratory descriptive design. Open-ended interview instrument. Descriptive (frequency distributions) statistical and content analysis. Forty-item Children's Coping Strategies Checklist was used to categorise children's behaviours as described by mothers (information seeking, direct action, inhibition of action, seeking comfort/help, growth/independence and intrapsychic). Content validity of interview questions obtained through discussions with faculty and graduate members, and affirmed by a nursing faculty member from another hospital	**Emotional Wellbeing:** Four types of most stressful event for children were described by mothers: intrusive procedure (*n* = 12), separation (*n* = 8), pain experiences (*n* = 6) and other events (*n* = 4). The most common response from children for each stressful event was: direct action (for example, controlling and/or self-protection) and seeking comfort/help for intrusive procedures; seeking comfort/help for separation; and seeking comfort/help for surgical pain; direct action and inhibition of action for other events. Providing comforting measures (*n* = 26, 87 per cent) and providing information and explanations (*n* = 19, 63 per cent) were the two most common strategies used by mothers to help their children to cope with the stressful situation
While (1992) UK	To study consumers' (families') views on health care: a comparison of hospital and home care (also included in Table 5.2)	9 children and 40 families (parents)	Descriptive 'evaluative' study. Semi-structured interviews	**Emotional Wellbeing:** A negative aspect of hospitalisation for half of the children was injections and intravenous infusions. Although most (94.7 per cent) parents indicated that their participation in care was helpful in that the children responded better to their parents, especially for painful procedures, none of the comments from children reflected their views on parental participation

Table 5.3   cont'd

Authors (Year) Country	Aim(s) of study	Methodological issues		Study findings
		Sample	Design, data collection and analysis, rigour/reliability and validity	
Jones (1994) USA	To identify varying levels of parental participation and their relationship to the child's behaviour during hospitalisation	Voluntary sample of 13 mothers and their children aged 2–5 years with a diagnosis of leukaemia on a 25-bedded paediatric ward. Only 10 mothers were followed through in the study	Short-term longitudinal descriptive evaluation study. Instruments: (a) The Co-operation Scale (a 5-point scale indicating the degree to which the child co-operates with a procedure); interrater reliability was established. (b) The Manifest Upset Scale (a 5-point scale to reflect the emotional state at a given time in terms of verbal/non-verbal expressions of fear, anxiety/or anger); interrater reliability was established. (c) The Activity Scale (a 5-point scale applied with a 24-hour recall of the child's activity, focusing on communication with others, interest in the surroundings, and play); no reference to the rigour of the Activity Scale. (d) An adaptation of Deatrick et al.'s (1986) Parental Participation Assessment Instrument (an 18-item tool and 2 open-ended questions). Additional categories of activity included were: stimulation—entertainment, comfort measures, activities of daily living, and therapeutic measures. Interrater reliability of the original instrument was established, but no reference made to the reliability of the adapted tool. Descriptive (frequency distributions and means) and inferential (correlation co-efficients and scatter plots) statistical analysis	**Emotional Wellbeing:** The number of activities in which mothers participated had a moderate positive relationship to improved child co-operation ($r = 0.73$) and to decreased upset behaviours ($r = 0.73$) during procedures. A strong positive relationship ($r = 0.91$) was identified between the number of activities in which a mother participated and the child's increased activity level. The relationships revealed that when mothers actively and consistently participated in providing routine care, emotional nurturance and therapeutic procedures to their child, the child was more co-operative and less upset during painful procedures, and had an increased activity level th n the child whose parent did not consistently participate in the varying categories of his or her care while in hospital

References

Alexander D., Powell G., Williams P., White M. and Conlon M. (1988) 'Anxiety levels of rooming-in and non-rooming in parents of young hospitalised children', *Maternal Child Nursing Journal* 17(2): 79–99.

Algren C. (1985) 'Role perceptions of mothers who have hospitalised children', *Child Health Care* 14(1): 6–9.

Audit Commission (1993) *Children First: A Study of Hospital Services*, London, HMSO.

Ball M., Glasper A. and Yerrell P. (1988) 'How well do we perform? Parents' perceptions of paediatric care', *Professional Nurse* 4(3): 115–18.

Berman H. (1991) 'Nurses' beliefs about family involvement in a children's hospital', *Issues in Comprehensive Pediatric Nursing* 14: 141–53.

Brownlea A. (1987) 'Participation: myths, realities and prognosis', *Social Science and Medicine* 25(6): 605–14.

Burke S., Kaufmann E., Costello E. and Dillon M. (1991) 'Hazardous secrets and reluctantly taking charge: parenting a child with repeated hospitalisations', *Image: Journal of Nursing Scholarship* 23(1): 39–45.

Callery P. (1997a) 'Using evidence in children's nursing', *Paediatric Nursing* 9(6): 13–17.

Callery P. (1997b) 'Maternal knowledge and professional knowledge: co-operation and conflict in the care of sick children', *International Journal of Nursing Studies* 3(1): 27–34.

Callery P. (1997c) 'Caring for parents of hospitalised children: a hidden area of nursing work', *Journal of Advanced Nursing* 26: 992–8.

Callery P. (1997d) 'Paying to participate: financial, social and personal costs to parents of involvement in their children's care in hospital', *Journal of Advanced Nursing* 25: 746–52.

Caty S., Ritchie J. and Ellerton M. (1989) 'Helping hospitalised preschoolers manage stressful situation: the mothers role', *Child Health Care* 18(4): 209.

Cleary J. (1992) *Caring for Children in Hospital: Parents and Nurses in Partnership*, London, Scutari Press.

Cleary J., Gray O., Hall D., Rowlandson P. and Sainsbury C. (1986) 'Parental involvement in the lives of children in hospital', *Archives of Disease in Childhood* 61: 779–87.

Coyne I. (1995) 'Partnership in care: parents' views of participation in their hospitalised child's care', *Journal of Clinical Nursing* 4: 71–9.

Coyne I. (1998) 'Researching children: some methodological and ethical considerations', *Journal of Clinical Nursing* 7: 409–16.

Darbyshire P. (1994) *Living with a Sick Child in Hospital: The Experiences of Parents and Nurses*, London, Chapman & Hall.

Dearmun A. (1992) 'Perceptions of parental participation', *Paediatric Nursing* 4(7): 6–9.

Deatrick J., Stull, M., Dixon D., Puczcynski S. and Jackson S. (1986) 'Measuring parental participation', *Issues in Comprehensive Pediatric Nursing* 9(4): 239–46.

Department of Health (1991) *Welfare of Children and Young People in Hospital*, London, HMSO.

Droogan J. and Cullum N. (1998) 'Systematic reviews in nursing', *International Journal of Nursing Studies* 35: 13–22.

Fuller J. (1997) 'Multicultural health care: reconciling universalism and particularism', *Nursing Inquiry* 4(3): 153–9.

Hayes, V. and Knox J. (1984) 'The experience of stress in parents of children hospitalised with long-term disabilities', *Journal of Advanced Nursing* 9: 333–41.

Jones C. (1994) 'Effect of parental participation on hospitalised child behaviour', *Issues in Comprehensive Pediatric Nursing* 17: 81–92.

Kawik L. (1996) 'Nurses' and parents' perceptions of participation and partnership in caring for a hospitalised child', *British Journal of Nursing (British Journal of Child Nursing)* 57: 430–4.

Keane S. and Garralda, M. (1986) 'Resident parents during paediatric admissions', *International Journal of Nursing Studies* 25(3): 247–53.

Keatinge D. and Gilmore V. (1996) 'Shared care: a partnership between parents and nurses', *Australian Journal of Advanced Nursing* 14(1): 28–36.

Kitson A. (1997) 'Using evidence to demonstrate the value of nursing', *Nursing Standard* 11(28): 34–9.

Knafl K. and Dixon D. (1984) 'The participation of fathers in their children's hospitalisation', *Issues in Comprehensive Paediatric Nursing* 7: 269–81.

Knafl K., Cavallari K. and Dixon D. (1988) *Paediatric Hospitalisation: Family and Nurse Perspectives*, London, Scott, Foresman.

Kristensson-Hallstrom I. and Elander, G. (1994) 'Parental participation in the care of hospitalised children', *Scandinavian Journal of Caring Science* 8: 149–54.

Kristensson-Hallstrom I. and Elander, G. (1997a) 'Parents' experiences of hospitalisation: different strategies for feeling secure', *Pediatric Nursing* 23(4): 361–7.

Kristensson-Hallstrom I. and Elander, G. (1997b) 'The parent between the child and the professional – some ethical implications', *Child Care, Health and Development* 23(6): 447–55.

Lau C. (1993) 'Parents in partnership: a family-centred care program', *Paediatric Nursing Review* 6(2): 11–15.

Monahan G. and Schkade, J. (1985) 'Comparing care by parent and traditional nursing units', *Pediatric Nursing* 11(6): 463–8.

Neill S. (1996a) 'Parent participation. 1: Literature review and methodology', *British Journal of Nursing* 5(1): 34–40.

Neill S. (1996b) 'Parent participation. 2: Findings and their implications for practice', *British Journal of Nursing* 5(2): 110–17.

NHS Centre for Reviews and Dissemination (1996) *Undertaking Systematic Reviews of Research on Effectiveness, CRD Guidelines for those Carrying out or Commissioning Reviews*, CRD Report No. 4, University of York, NHS.

Palmer S. (1993) 'Care of sick children by parents: a meaningful role', *Journal of Advanced Nursing* 18: 185–91.

Perkins M. (1993) 'Patient–nurse collaboration: using the caregiver identity emergence to assist parents of hospitalised children with disabilities', *Journal of Paediatric Nursing* 8(1): 2–9.

Popay J., Rogers A. and Williams G. (1998) 'Rationale and standards for the systematic review of qualitative literature in health services research', *Qualitative Health Research* 8(3): 341–51.

Robinson C. (1985) 'Parents of hospitalised chronically ill children: competency in question', *Nursing Papers* 17(2): 59–68.

Robinson C. (1987) 'Roadblocks to family-centred care when a chronically ill child is hospitalised', *Maternal-Child Nursing Journal* 16(3): 181–93.

Rowe J. (1996) 'Making oneself at home? Examining the nurse–parent relationship', *Contemporary Nurse* 5(3): 101–6.

Sackett L., Richardson W., Rosenberg W. and Haynes R. (1997) *Evidence Based Medicine: How to Practice and Teach EBM*, London, Churchill Livingstone.

Sainsbury C., Gray O., Cleary J., Davies M. and Rowlandson P. (1986) 'Care by parents of their children in hospital', *Archives of Diseases in Children* 61: 612–16.

Schepp K. (1992) 'Correlates of mothers who prefer control over their hospitalised children's care', *Journal of Paediatric Nursing* 7(2): 83–9.

Tomlinson P., Kirschawm M., Tomczyk B. and Peterson J. (1993) 'The relationship of child acuity, maternal responses, nurses attitudes and contextual factors in the bone marrow transplant unit', *American Journal of Critical Care* 2(3): 246–7.

While A. (1992) 'Consumer views of health care: a comparison of hospital and home care', *Child Care, Health and Development* 18: 107–16.

6 Being a mother of a critically sick child: issues for nursing practice and research

Jane Noyes

Introduction

Having to cope with sudden and critical illness in a child is considered to be one of the most stressful of all parenting experiences, yet the nursing literature contains few qualitative accounts of how mothers cope with this crisis. This study aimed to describe ten mothers' experiences of crisis, coping and nursing following their child's emergency admission to a paediatric intensive care unit (PICU). Using a qualitative grounded theory approach, data were elicited through focused interviews with ten mothers. Four research questions were considered:

1. What are the physical needs of parents?
2. What are the psychological needs of parents?
3. To what extent are the physical and psychological needs of parents being met?
4. To what extent are parents involved in the care of their child?

Findings reveal that mothers could clearly identify their needs. They felt that their physical needs were met but that their psychological care was inconsistent. Mothers were involved in various aspects of caring for their children. Issues for nursing practice and research are highlighted.

The discussion is based on findings drawn from a study entitled 'The experiences of mothers of children admitted as an emergency to the paediatric intensive care unit: an exploratory, qualitative study' (Noyes, 1996). The voices of mothers are central to this study in providing evidence to inform nursing practice. This approach is supported by current initiatives to develop evidence-based family-centred care and partnerships in health care (DoH, 1992, 1996). Based on the findings, recommendations are made for nursing practice and research. Nursing practice issues include meeting the psychosocial needs of parents prior to and immediately after admission, the importance of therapeutic listening and counselling skills, managing 'burn-out' among nurses, the importance of holistic nursing care and breaking down the dominant medical culture in PICU. Issues for nursing research include exploring how families cope with critical illness, the long-term effects of critical illness on the child and family, and the development of advanced nursing practice.

Literature review

An in-depth critique of studies exploring the experiences and needs of parents of children admitted to paediatric intensive care units has been published elsewhere (Noyes, 1998). In considering mothers' experiences of critical illness in their child, literature is presented here that explores the general context of critical illness in children, predominant stresses and stressors encountered by their parents, and subsequent coping strategies used by parents to deal with stress.

Critical illness

Children are usually admitted to a PICU because the medical team has identified that one or more of the child's body systems cannot maintain homeostatic equilibrium without intensive therapeutic support (Paediatric Intensive Care Society, 1996). Critically sick children have an increased risk of morbidity and mortality, necessitating immediate stabilisation and life support (Gemke *et al.*, 1995). These children are usually nursed naked or with minimal clothing, and are attached to complex life support machines, monitoring systems and computerised infusion devices that emit light, sound alarms and generate heat. Because of the severity of the child's condition, paralysing and analgesic agents may be given to induce unconsciousness and remove all muscle tone.

Parents frequently define this situation as a crisis, arising from the sudden transformation of a healthy child to a critically ill or injured child (Heuer, 1993; LaMontagne *et al.*, 1995). Paediatric intensive care (PIC) nursing has evolved a philosophy that necessitates care of the emotional needs of critically sick children and their families (RCN, 1992). Critically sick children are dependent on their parents being able to cope with the crisis, some families appearing to manage this sudden transition better than others.

Stress and stressors

Following medical stabilisation, the initial crisis may be over, but stressors generated by the child's admission to PICU continue to emerge and evolve (LaMontagne *et al.*, 1995). There are many studies identifying parental stress and stressors in the PICU, revealing a degree of inconsistency in the overall findings. Quantitative studies of parental stress using the Parental Stressor Scale: PICU (PSS: PICU; Carter and Miles, 1982) dominate the literature (see, for example, Jay and Youngblut, 1991; Curley and Wallace, 1992; Heuer, 1993; Haines *et al.*, 1995). Few qualitative studies have been conducted (Carnevale, 1990). Consistency across studies, however, has supported the importance of certain features of parents' experiences, particularly the stress induced by role conflict and the need to be near their child.

Coping strategies

Families have to deal with many stressful situations relating to a child's critical illness (LaMontagne *et al.*, 1992). Although there is considerable empirical support for what aspects of the critical care situation produce parental stress, the literature reveals that very little is known about the way in which parents cope during the experience.

Aim of the study

Several research questions derived from nursing practice require addressing. These relate to the impact of an acute life-threatening illness on the child and family, and ultimately to how parents cope with this crisis and continue to function as parents. The role and ability of PIC nurses in relation to meeting the needs of families in crisis also warrants exploration. The literature supports the need for research to explore further the challenges of coping with crisis and the roles of nurses. The overall aim of the study was to elicit mothers' lived experiences of crisis and coping, and their experiences of nursing following the unexpected emergency admission of their child to a PICU. Having formulated the aim of the study, four research questions were developed:

1.   What are the physical needs of parents?
2.   What are the psychological needs of parents?

3. To what extent are the physical and psychological needs of parents being met?
4. To what extent are parents involved in the care of their child?

Methodology

An in-depth discussion of the theoretical framework underpinning this study is presented elsewhere (Noyes, 1999). A qualitative approach was used to elicit mothers' experiences of coping and their experiences of nursing following the unexpected emergency admission of their child to the PICU (Aamodt, 1991). The sample contained ten mothers of children aged between 3 months and 15 years who had been admitted to the PICU with a life-threatening condition. The participants were chosen from a non-probability, purposeful sample of parents who had undergone the experience and whose experience was considered typical (Morse, 1991). Selection was irrespective of the child's disease process, age or sex. Parents were not approached (a condition stipulated by the senior nursing staff) if their child was critically or terminally ill. They were also excluded from the sample if their child's admission had been planned as some form of pre-admission preparation might have been undertaken. In order to gain access to the field, ethical approval was obtained from the appropriate NHS Trust ethics committee. The researcher was neither known to mothers nor involved in their child's care.

A focused, reflexive interview was piloted and used to elicit mothers' experiences (Field, 1991). Interviews were conducted within a regional PICU near to where the child was being nursed. The mothers were assured of their anonymity and confidentiality, both verbally and in writing. A grounded theory approach was used as a framework for generating and analysing the data (Hammersley and Atkinson, 1992). The mothers were interviewed once and their experiences tape-recorded. The interviews lasted between 1 and 3 hours.

Discussion of findings

The concepts identified during the analysis process were drawn from detailed descriptions of the mothers' experiences and feelings. It is impossible to convey all the specific details of the study findings, the intention being to present selected key findings considered to be those most useful for nursing practice and research. Five themes emerged

relating to mothers' experiences of living through and coping with
the unexpected admission of their child to PICU: initial shock and
crisis, concern for the child; support and coping, parent as carer, and
their perception of nursing.

Initial shock and crisis

The mothers described in considerable detail the initial shock and
crisis in two contexts: the unexpected shattering of their normal lives
and the immediate role transition into the 'PICU mother' of a critically sick child. This finding is similar to studies using the PSS: PICU
data collection tool (see, for example, Miles *et al.*, 1989; Jay and
Youngblut, 1991). The mothers identified the unexpected nature of
the crisis and how it was handled as being extremely important.
During the initial hours, the mothers said that they consumed vast
amounts of emotional energy, which left them feeling totally
exhausted immediately following their child's admission.

Initial experience

The initial experience leading up to admission to the PICU also
appeared to have implications for how parents coped with the first
few hours of role transition into being the parent of a critically sick
child. Once parents had arrived at the PICU, they were usually asked
to wait in the sitting room on the unit. At this stage, the physiological
needs of the child clearly took precedence over the needs of the
parents, and this aspect is well documented in the literature (Rennick,
1995). Mother 1 described in detail the frenetic activity that
surrounded the medical stabilisation of her child, including the
arrival of many health care professionals on the unit who would
walk past the parents' sitting room en route to her child.

Waiting and reflecting

Mothers clearly expressed that they understood the need for their
child to have immediate medical and nursing intervention, but
described the experience of waiting in the sitting room as a period of
intense reflection. They generally began the reflective process of identifying themselves as being a good or a bad parent. Mother 10, whose
daughter had been admitted unconscious following ingestion of

Ecstasy, expressed feelings of guilt and disbelief. In contrast, Mother 6, whose child had been admitted with a diagnosis of croup said:

> I knew immediately that his breathing was not right. I dialled 999 and we came straight to casualty. The ambulance man said I had saved his life.

Initial stabilisation

All the mothers said they were regularly updated on their child's progress during the initial stabilisation process. This usually involved nurses intermittently visiting the sitting room with updated information. Following intubation, ventilation and stabilisation, parents were reunited with their child. Mother 3 generally described this period as one that focused on her child's clinical history and diagnosis and did not allow for the ventilation of her own experiences and feelings. During this period of enforced separation, the needs of the children take priority over the needs of parents. The present study was conducted during a very busy period, resulting in nurses working to maximum capacity. During less busy periods, nurses may be available to support and care for families, in addition to those caring for the child.

Impact on mothers

A worrying finding emerged from the data in that the majority of mothers described symptoms of acute stress in the initial period following admission. They all described feelings of emotional and physical exhaustion. Three mothers described feeling sick (one being physically sick). Two mothers had rapid-onset headaches that were made worse by the bright lighting and noise levels in the PICU. Mother 2 recounted how she physically started to shake and had difficulty walking unaided. Five mothers said that they felt numb. Four mothers expressed that they cried while waiting in the sitting room. Mother 5 could not remember familiar telephone numbers and recounted how she tried to telephone her mother but could not remember which numbers to dial.

These symptoms of acute stress are physiological responses to the traumatic circumstances surrounding the emergency admission of a child to PICU. Mothers tended to shrug off their own needs in favour of their child and appeared to be willing to accept their experiences as inevitable.

Update on care and treatment

The need for ongoing information regarding their child did not emerge as important in the data. Mothers talked about being regularly updated by nurses and the value of being resident, which allowed them access to information on a constant basis. The environment of the PICU did not feature highly in the interview transcripts. Parents had free and open access to their children 24 hours a day. All the parents expressed satisfaction with the accommodation provided, and their needs appeared to be well catered for.

Concern for the child

Mothers talked extensively of their worries and concerns for their child, his or her siblings and the family. Mothers described in detail their concerns relating to the impact of their child's illness on all family members as being very important. This was typically described by Mother 1, who said:

> My two-and-a-half-year-old is sick in ITU; my four-year-old is staying with his grandma and stayed awake crying all last night; my six-year-old is staying with a school mate.

Fear of death or permanent brain damage

The single most feared aspect of the lived experience for mothers emerged as the death or permanent brain damage of their child. These fears generally became apparent to mothers in association with the knowledge that their child was critically sick and required admission to an intensive care unit. For the majority of parents, these fears were already internalised and causing considerable worry prior to being admitted to the PICU. Mother 9 described in detail her realisation that her child might die. Uncertainty was a feeling described commonly by mothers in the present study. Mother 6 said that she was concerned with regard to the trajectory of her child's illness and the threat of long-term complications. Four mothers expressed how if their children were brain damaged, their entire lives would change, placing huge demands on the family. They appeared to sense that the burden of care would fall on their shoulders in the event of their child requiring ongoing nursing care at home. A typical view was expressed by Mother 10, who said:

I went back to work five years ago when the kids were all at school. If the worst came to the worst, we would have her home; I could never put her into care, I would never forgive myself... I just don't know how I would cope.

All the mothers said that they had discussed their fears with the nurses. Conversations of this nature generally seemed to occur as a result of nurses and parents working together for prolonged periods of time. The value of nursing care emerged as important to mothers in dealing with death. Mother 1 said:

You always know when a child dies, you can feel the atmosphere change and you cannot get into the waiting room because of all the relatives.

Mother 8 described the nurses as being aware of her need to talk about death and about her fears relating to the long-term survival of her child.

Altered body image

Children in PICU have an altered body image, which had various meanings for the mothers. Mother 9 said of her child:

I didn't think that he looked like my baby any more

whereas mother 2 said:

She's still my baby... despite all the plaster and machines.

The environment

The PIC nurses in the current study were described by mothers as taking great care to make the child's bed space, cot and general appearance as normal as possible, and this was much appreciated. Mothers were asked to bring in photographs of their children, which were then displayed by the sick child. PICU cot linen and soft furnishings were noted by mothers as being nice. When appropriate, parents were encouraged to hold and cuddle their children. Mothers said that getting close to their children helped to normalise the situation. Mother 3 represented a common view:

I couldn't wait to hold him again, I really missed our cuddles and not being able to feed him.

Support and coping

All the mothers in the sample had been or were currently resident and had assumed the main responsibility for being with their child. They looked to their partner (if present), family members and friends as a source of support. In the present study, family members were occasionally identified as assisting with caring for the sick child. For example, Mother 1 relied upon her husband to relieve her during the evenings so that she could go home and see her other two children. Mother 5 suggested that her husband acted as a great support by telephoning three times a day and bringing food, drink and fresh clean clothes to wear each evening.

Siblings

Friends and neighbours were drawn together in order to look after siblings and keep an eye on the family home. This required an enormous amount of organisation very soon after the admission of the child to PICU, and the function of normalisation as a parent appeared to be one of the main responsibilities of resident mothers. For the mothers who had mobile telephones, this task appeared to empower them, giving them a sense of control over the situation. For other mothers who had to spend considerable amounts of money in a pay phone situated in a public place, this process of organisation was viewed as a necessary burden.

Impact on the family

A common feature in the data was mothers' accounts of efforts to manage or limit the impact of critical illness on their family. Mothers described wanting to protect their sick child from the experience and include their other children in the illness, while attempting to make sure siblings attended school and sporting activities as normal. Their concern for siblings arose in the conversations of all mothers who had more than one child. Similar findings also emerged in the data of Carnevale (1990). Mothers appeared to want to talk about their entire family rather than just the critically sick child, and provided a rich insight into their experiences of having to divide their time and emotional energy between the needs of a critically sick child and the well children coping with the critical illness of their brother or sister. This need to continue being a functional parent was mediated by the

PICU staff, who encouraged siblings to visit and be an integral part of the family. Mothers talked about the management of split families located at home and in hospital. Being in contact on a daily basis was important. Partners, relatives, neighbours and friends were all called upon by mothers to care for and transport siblings to and from the hospital. This process of normalisation appeared to be very important in the data, the process mainly being facilitated and organised by the resident mothers. On the whole, the mothers mainly valued family members for their functional and protective role with respect to the crisis. This was not evident in the experiences of mothers who received inadequate support; Mother 6 described her boyfriend as 'unreliable'. It emerged from the data that quality of support was far more important than quantity of support.

Depression

Three mothers described signs and symptoms of depression. One mother said:

> I was so close to swallowing a bottle of pills. I couldn't bear the thought of going on without him [her child].

In contrast, another mother behaved in a way that might have endangered her life, by drinking beer and driving. A third mother considered not wanting to live as she thought of herself as such a bad mother and blamed herself for her teenager's admission. Although this concept does not appear in the studies of stress and coping already published, these feelings do not appear unusual in mothers, who may rehearse in their minds outcomes related to the worst scenario they could possibly think of encountering. Carnevale (1990) found that parents talked about being depressed but does not elaborate on the nature of this.

Nurses featured highly in the data relating to the support of mothers. The mothers generally expressed how if their child was stable and improving, they felt in control and emotionally stable. This could change periodically during each day or hour. Mother 2 said that she was fine until a poor blood gas result meant that her child's ventilation had to be increased. Following this episode, everything else appeared to be, in her words, 'stressful and exhausting'. Mothers described this pattern as being like riding on a roller-coaster. The ups and downs were in the main unpredictable and out of their control. A downward slide towards a depressive episode in Mother 1 was triggered by her husband not answering the telephone when she expected him to be at home.

Parent as carer

Mothers described a refocusing of their lives with different priorities, including the value of being a parent, caring for their child and the importance of the family. They described their role in various ways. Some mothers were administering medications, nasogastric tube feeds, physiotherapy techniques, massage, cleansing and mouth and eye care to their children. They were also taking an active part in play and distraction therapy. Although the data suggest that most mothers wanted to maintain control over parenting, they looked to the nurses for support and guidance during the initial stabilisation of their child. Some mothers initially withdrew from an active role and were content with a consultative role. This could reflect the fact that mothers were interviewed between 1 and 8 days after admission and had had varying periods of adjustment to the experience.

Participation in care and maintaining a parenting role was described by mothers as being a frightening but positive experience; these findings are similar to Evans' study of parental participation in the administration of intravenous antibiotics to paediatric oncology patients (Evans, 1994).

Perception of nursing

The literature generally implies that nurses and other health care professionals must play a vital role in supporting the parents of critically sick children (Cox, 1992). This attitude is also reflected by parents, whose perceptions of and interactions with nurses appeared to place an emotional strain on the nurses. Living as the parent of a critically sick child in the PICU necessitates an almost claustrophobic dependence on members of the multidisciplinary health care team. When asked about their perceptions of nursing, mothers generally described examples of nursing care or interactions with nurses that they had encountered during their child's critical illness. They were clear in their view of the positive and negative aspects of nursing that they had encountered. Common ideas emerge from the data about what mothers valued including individualised care, competent care, teaching and befriending.

Individualised nursing care

The importance of individualised care is apparent in the mothers' expressions of valuing care in which nurses and health care professionals appear alert, motivated and well informed on their child's condition; of the role played out by the mother; and of the structure and function of the family. Most mothers desired consistency and continuity of nursing care and valued having a therapeutic relationship with a nurse. A consistent theme in the data was that holistic care, considering all of the needs of the critically sick child and family members, was important (Purcell, 1993). The desire of mothers to be valued appears to be essential to the concept of individualised care. Those mothers who managed a family on a day-to-day basis valued playing an active role in the decisions to be made about their child. The mothers wanted to be part of the process of care planning and expressed a desire to care for their child, although parents appeared to have differing feelings regarding their own ability and confidence to perform hands-on care. This may be a reflection on the fact that some parents had had a longer period of adjustment and supervision than others.

Competent care

Mothers expected nurses to be competent, technically skilled and knowledgeable. They frequently compared the abilities and consistency of individual nurses and expected to be taught nursing procedures competently and correctly. Mother 5 described the trust she placed in her nurse:

> I completely trusted [nurse's name]; she's intelligent, knows her stuff and makes me feel human.

Mothers were quick to identify when nurses were not technically skilled and knowledgeable: Mother 8 suggested that 'not all nurses are the same'. Findings in the present study suggest that the management of painful procedures in children featured as an aspect that could be well or badly managed by both medical and nursing staff. All the children in the unit were receiving continuous sedation and analgesia, and the management of pain appeared to have a high priority in care planning. Mothers talked about the expertise of the majority of doctors and nurses in managing technically difficult procedures such as cannulation and the insertion of chest drains. Mother 7 summed up the feelings of the majority of mothers' views:

[Name of baby] required loads of drips to be replaced. I came to realise that with some doctors and nurses they were brilliant... One doctor was hopeless, he took loads of stabs; he was absolutely useless.

Mother 6 felt that she was at times in conflict with the nursing staff: 'I had seen many nurses do heel pricks... but this one [the nurse] was downright rough.'

Nurses

On the whole, the perceptions of nurses tended to be positive. Nurses appeared to be negotiating care with parents and engaging in an holistic approach encompassing the needs of families, the importance of which is supported by Callery and Smith (1991). The individual personalities of nurses emerged from the data as being important to parents. Mothers generally liked nurses to be honest and 'be themselves'. Mothers seemed to make many demands on nurses, and from their conversations it became clear that the needs of mothers required nurses to be highly skilled in the psychosocial as well as the physical aspects of nursing.

Parental education

Nurses generally engaged in a process of parent education and involvement immediately after admission. Teaching aspects of care tended to vary according to the needs of individual mothers. The mothers described that with good teaching and psychosocial support, they could fulfil their individual needs.

Befriending

In the present study, befriending emerged from the data as being important; it incorporates how parents view nursing, their perception of empowerment, feeling valued and the development of relationships with nurses that appear to offer parents feelings of friendship. Mother 9 summarised the positive nature of the relationship with her nurse, whom she found to be very supportive.

I like to work with our nurse, she knows I am terrified and yet is really supportive and friendly.

Humour

The role of appropriate humour emerged as an important element of befriending. The importance of nurses having a sense of humour and individuality was highlighted by the mothers. They talked about nursing that created positive energy. The mothers were also able to identify behaviours that engendered negative feelings: 'One of the worse things is being with a depressed nurse; you spend all of your energy trying to cheer them up.' Parents appeared to be identifying a small number of 'burnt-out nurses' who might have been in need of psychosocial support themselves.

Doctors

Parents expressed varied opinions regarding their experiences of doctors. Three parents named individual consultants as being excellent doctors. The daily ward round, however, featured as a major source of dissatisfaction in the data. One mother said:

> Doctors need to take more notice of you as a parent... not just see the child as a patient, especially the junior doctors who want to impress the consultant rather than speak to a mother in a language that is easily understood.

In addition, some consistent irritations bothered the mothers, for example how they were addressed by junior doctors who appeared to call all mothers 'mum'. The mothers suggested that they just wanted a bit of individual recognition. The current study appears to identify that the dominant medical culture needs to be further addressed.

Summary of findings

The results will be summarised in relation to the four research questions:

1. What are the physical needs of parents?
2. What are the psychological needs of parents?
3. To what extent are the physical and psychological needs of parents being met?
4. To what extent are parents involved in the care of their child?

Mothers interviewed in this study appeared to be ordinary people who were suddenly faced with a crisis affecting all aspects of their everyday living. They identified their physical needs as having somewhere to sleep, eat and rest in order to be close to their children, and these needs were said to be met. Mothers described psychological needs in terms of the importance of parenting their child, working alongside nurses, carrying on managing their families and being valued. They highlighted the importance of an holistic approach to nursing care and indicated in this respect that their psychological needs were generally met (with the exception of prior to and immediately after admission, and generally during medical ward rounds). The mothers suggested that the nurses helped them to cope with crisis, although some nurses were not equipped with these skills. The mothers were all involved in various aspects of caring for their children, the extent of which was highly individual. Nurses were generally engaging in care that focused on the family, and mothers could clearly describe aspects of good- and poor-quality medical and nursing care.

Implications for nursing practice

Whether this exploratory study has general relevance will depend upon future large-scale studies. In addition, in keeping with the analysis of qualitative data, it is up to the individual PIC nurse to make their own interpretation of the data and to decide how relevant findings are for their own practice settings (Williams, 1991). Thus, while findings cannot be generalised, important issues for PIC nurses as a whole can still be derived from the study.

In considering the meaning of experiences described by the mothers of critically sick children in the PICU, nurses need to recognise that, for parents, coping with crisis entails more than just being with and caring for their critically sick child. The study highlighted many positive aspects of nursing care that were said to be meeting mothers' needs, and these aspects, such as parental participation in care, teaching and befriending, should be encouraged. Mothers identified the need to maintain a role as a parent as being one of the most demanding aspects of their child's critical illness. The goal of nursing care is to identify the individual needs of parents, and nurses must make an assessment using an holistic framework. There is an obvious necessity for mothers to depend on nurses. The mothers clearly wanted help with individualised and competent care that attended to their psychosocial and educational needs. The psychosocial needs of mothers are not being met prior to and immediately after admission to PICU. This needs to be taken into account and provision made whenever possible for an additional nurse to be available for parents.

This study highlights how important listening, communication and counselling skills are when caring for parents in crisis. Three mothers were obviously depressed and appeared to be in need of therapeutic support (with their consent, support subsequently being provided). Nurses need to be competent in assessing the psychological needs of mothers and be aware that they might be clinically depressed. In order to provide support to mothers, nurses need to have the appropriate skills and clinical supervision, and recognise their limitations (UKCC, 1992).

Mothers identified that a small number of nurses required counselling as they appeared to be 'burnt out' and unable to meet the mothers' needs. This requires further investigation from a management perspective in order to implement appropriate supportive measures for nurses working in a highly stressful environment. This concept of staff burn-out is already well represented in the literature (Dewe, 1987).

Finally, mothers want to be addressed in a proper manner and treated with respect by all members of the multidisciplinary team. Nurses need to empower parents by promoting a more holistic approach to care by weakening the dominance of the medical culture in the PICU. This could be achieved by a more collaborative approach to care and seeking parents' opinions when evaluating the quality of care delivered (DoH, 1992, 1996).

Implications for nursing research

The main outcome of this study is the generation of further research questions. The experiences of parents immediately following the onset of critical illness in their child warrant further exploration. The present study elicited new areas, such as how mothers viewed themselves as parents. A further understanding of the initial crisis and reactions of individual parents may help nurses to plan therapeutic interventions. In addition, support is highlighted as a major influence in the ability of parents to cope positively. In the current study, findings indicate that some mothers are clearly in need of care during the period of their child's initial stabilisation and that some mothers were clinically depressed. Further research is required on the nature of care and support needed and the feasibility of implementing such a service.

The mothers single most feared aspect emerged in the current study as the death or permanent brain damage of their child. Little information is known regarding the long-term sequelae of children who survive following critical illness. Further medical research is warranted regarding clinical outcome, and further nursing research is required to investigate how parents cope with the death of their child, and if the child survives with brain damage, how the parents cope once their child has been discharged home.

The current study highlighted the impact of the experience on the entire family. No studies currently exist in relation to how the family unit functions during health-related crises, and this warrants further investigation. Mothers expressed concern for their partners and other children. The nursing literature does not address how siblings, grandarents and extended families cope with a crisis of this nature. The perceptions of these groups requires further exploration as it is not known whether their needs are met.

Mothers highlighted the importance of being able to participate in their child's care and continue in the role of parent. The nature and extent of the concept of collaboration requires further nursing research in order to make explicit the therapeutic role of PIC nurses. This is especially important in relation to involving parents in planning and evaluating nursing care, both of which are key aspects of *The Patient's Charter* (DoH, 1992) and *The Patient's Charter: Services for Children and Young People* (DoH, 1996).

The importance of an holistic approach to nursing care was highlighted in the present study, mothers putting a high value on the relationship that emerged between child, family and nurse. The role of the advanced practitioner in PIC nursing is currently being implemented as a mechanism for reducing junior doctors' hours and appears to be moving away from an holistic to a medical model of care (DoH, 1994). The potential effect of this radical change in nursing practice requires further research and evaluation to see whether parents' holistic needs can be met by an advanced practitioner.

Parents identified that some nurses appeared to be in need of psychosocial support. The extent of this problem is not known and warrants further investigation in order for the needs of nurses to be understood.

Little research has been conducted with parents whose children are considered to be critically unstable and, by definition, in need of intensive therapeutic support. The experiences of these parents are unknown and further study is necessary to determine whether their unique needs are being met. The present study did not provide the opportunity to talk with parents from ethnic minorities, who may have particular spiritual or cultural needs, or those parents who experience difficulty in communicating. Further research is therefore necessary.

Conclusion

This study provided an insight into mothers' lived experiences of crisis, coping and nursing following the unexpected emergency admission of their child to PICU. The findings lend some support to other mainly quantitative studies in relation to the stress of parental role alteration. The use of a qualitative methodology incorporating a grounded theory approach elicited mothers' lived experiences as evidence to underpin therapeutic nursing interventions. The study has not developed a theory but identifies issues that provide the basis for further research.

This study has further confirmed a belief that the mothers of critically sick children have a personal resilience that allows them to carry on as a mother. Their view of motherhood takes on a new perspective associated with their experiences of their child's life-threatening illness.

Acknowledgements

The author would like to thank the mothers who gave so much by participating in this study, the medical and nursing staff who welcomed the researcher into their PICU and Professor Christine Webb for her advice and supervision.

References

Aamodt A. (1991) 'Ethnography and epistemology: generating nursing knowledge'. In Morse J. (ed.) *Qualitative Nursing Research. A Contemporary Dialogue*, London, Sage.

Callery P. and Smith L. (1991) 'A study of role negotiation between nurses and the parents of hospitalised children', *Journal of Advanced Nursing* **16**: 772–81.

Carnevale F. (1990) 'A description of stressors and coping strategies among parents of critically ill children – a preliminary study', *Intensive Care Nursing* **6**: 4–11.

Carter M. and Miles M. (1982) 'Parental stressor scale', *Nursing Research* **31**(2): 121.

Cox P. (1992) 'Children in critical care: how parents cope', *British Journal of Nursing* **1**(15): 764–8.

Curley M. and Wallace J. (1992) 'Effects of the nursing mutual participation model of care on parental stress in the pediatric intensive care unit – a replication', *Journal of Paediatric Nursing* **7**(6): 377–85.

Department of Health (1992) *The Patient's Charter*, London, HMSO.

Department of Health (1994) *The Greenhalgh Report: The Interface Between Junior Doctors and Nurses. A Research Study for the Department of Health*, London, HMSO.

Department of Health (1996) *The Patient's Charter: Services for Children and Young People*, London, HMSO.

Dewe P. (1987) 'Identifying strategies nurses use to cope with work stress', *Journal of Advanced Nursing* 12: 489–97.

Evans M. (1994) 'An investigation into the feasibility of parental participation in the nursing care of their children', *Journal of Advanced Nursing* 20: 477–82.

Field P. (1991) 'Doing fieldwork in your own culture'. In Morse J. (ed.) *Qualitative Nursing Research. A Contemporary Dialogue*, London, Sage.

Gemke R., Bonsel G. and van Vught A. (1995) 'Long-term survival and state of health after paediatric intensive care', *Archives of Disease in Childhood* 73: 196–201.

Haines C., Perger C. and Nagy S. (1995) 'A comparison of the stressors experienced by parents of intubated and non-intubated children', *Journal of Advanced Nursing* 21: 350–5.

Hammersley M. and Atkinson P. (1992) *Ethnography Principles in Practice*, London, Routledge.

Heuer L. (1993) 'Parental stressors in a pediatric intensive care unit', *Pediatric Nursing* 19(2): 128–31.

Jay S. and Youngblut J. (1991) 'Parent stress associated with pediatric critical care nursing: linking research and practice', *American Association of Critical-care Nurses* 2(2): 276–84.

LaMontagne L., Hepworth J., Pawlak R. and Chiafery M. (1992) 'Parental coping and activities during pediatric critical care', *American Journal of Critical Care* 1: 76–80.

LaMontagne L., Johnson B. and Hepworth J. (1995). 'Evolution of parental stress and coping processes: a framework for critical care practice', *Journal of Pediatric Nursing* 10(4): 212–18.

Miles M., Carter M., Riddle I., Hennessey J. and Eberly T. (1989) 'The pediatric intensive care unit environment as a source of stress for parents', *Maternal Child Health Journal* 18(3): 199–206.

Morse J. (ed.) (1991) 'Strategies for sampling'. In *Qualitative Nursing Research. A Contemporary Dialogue*, London, Sage.

Noyes J. (1996) The experiences of mothers of children admitted as an emergency to the intensive care unit: an exploratory, qualitative study. Unpublished MSc thesis, University of Manchester.

Noyes J. (1998) 'A critique of studies exploring the experiences and needs of parents of children admitted to paediatric intensive care units', *Journal of Advanced Nursing* 28(1): 134–41.

Noyes J. (1999) 'The impact of knowing your child is critically ill: a qualitative study of mothers' experiences', *Journal of Advanced Nursing* 29(2): 427–35.

Paediatric Intensive Care Society (1996) *Standards for Paediatric Intensive Care*, Saldatore.

Purcell C. (1993) 'Holistic care of a critically sick child', *Intensive and Critical Care Nursing* 9: 108–15.

Rennick J. (1995) 'The changing profile of acute childhood illness: a need for the development of family nursing knowledge', *Journal of Advanced Nursing* 22: 258–66.

Royal College of Nursing (1992) *Paediatric Nursing: A Philosophy of Care*, London, RCN.

United Kingdom Central Council for Nursing, Midwifery and Health Visiting (1992) *Code of Professional Conduct* (3rd edn), London, UKCC.

Williams A. (1991) 'Practical ethics: interpretative processes in an ethnography of nursing'. In Aldridge S., Griffiths V. and Williams A. (eds) *Rethinking Feminist Research Processes Reconsidered*, Feminist Praxis, Monograph 33, Manchester, University of Manchester.

Suggested further reading

Darbyshire P. (1994*) Living with a Sick Child in Hospital: The Experiences of Parents and Nurses*, London, Chapman & Hall.

Hazinski M. (1992) *Nursing Care of the Critically Sick Child* (2nd edn), St Louis, Mosby Year Book.

Kruger S. (1992) 'Parents in crisis: helping them cope with a seriously ill child', *Journal of Pediatric Nursing* 7(2): 133–40.

Reed J. and Procter S. (eds) (1995) *Practitioner Research in Health Care: The Inside Story*, London, Chapman & Hall.

7 Children's voices in health care planning

Eva Elliott and Alison Watson

Introduction and literature review

The views of children and young people have largely been devalued as a resource for improving health care practice and developing more effective and appropriate services. However, both within the health and welfare services and in the social sciences literature, there is increasing awareness of the role that children could play in public life and in informing the ways in which services for them are provided. This chapter describes a research project, funded by a local health authority, in which children and young people were interviewed about their views of local health services. Although the research was limited by time constraints, it provided rich data about their encounters with health care professionals, their experiences of the treatment process, their concerns with consultation and treatment settings and their perceptions of the different roles that providers play. Their insights provided valuable evidence to support the view that children and young people ought to be regarded as social actors with knowledge and expertise on their own health. We conclude that, as individuals, they should be involved in any decisions about their own treatment, and that as a social group they should be involved in informing the planning and development of local health and welfare services.

The British media provides a telling commentary on our current social preoccupations and the ways in which these concerns are often articulated. A cursory glance at the national and local press would appear to reveal that we are very concerned about children. However, media reports, discussions and editorials about children often appear to make contradictory judgements. On the one hand, children are represented as vulnerable and in need of protection and guidance. These beliefs are confirmed and reinforced in the telling of stories about the abuse, neglect or abandonment of children by parents, families and institutions. Such stories talk about the need to return to 'traditional' family values and structures, and indeed often

110

to protect children from some of the media itself – the evil influences of sex and violence in films, on television and on the Internet, for example. On the other hand, there are fears about 'untamed youth' and the latent evil within children whose criminal and other exploits regularly make headline news.

A common assumption contained within these contradictory images is of a child who is essentially ignorant and non-competent, and whose status as a person has not yet been formed. Childhood is perceived as essentially a preparation for adulthood. The onus is therefore on the social institutions of the family, school and health and welfare agencies to guide, educate, develop and sustain the physical and moral well-being of children through their journeys into adulthood, and to speak for them on the basis that they are incompetent to think 'like adults' themselves until they reach a certain developmental stage in life (Mayall, 1995). The consequence of this view of children as 'future adults' rather than as present persons is that children's own forms of knowledge and beliefs are often ignored, or seen as irrelevant, as a means of understanding their actions, concerns and needs (James and Prout, 1990; Mayall, 1998).

There is, however, a growing counterview among academics and professionals that is often hidden from the debates sprung from media sensation. They believe that children are not passive subjects of social processes and structures, but social actors in themselves (James and Prout, 1990). There is an emerging sociology of childhood that sees children as actively constructing their own lives, participating in and negotiating their own health care, education and social welfare, having knowledge and skills that often go unrecognised, and being competent reporters of their own experiences (Green, 1997; Mayall 1998). This view is reflected, in Britain, in the funding of major research programmes that have focused on children's perspectives. The Joseph Rowntree Foundation, for example, supports a variety of research projects concerning the views and experiences of children and young people in a range of health and social care contexts, while the Economic and Social Research Council has funded 22 studies in a research programme that has 'children as social actors' as a common theme (Children 5–16: Growing into the 21st Century).

The importance of seeking the views of children and giving weight to the voice of the child runs alongside a recognition that children remain relatively powerless in a world shaped by the authority of adults. The UK's judicial system is one example of an institution that is undergoing change in this context. The judicial process has been, and still is, hampered by the view that children are unreliable sources of evidence. However, more recent attempts to develop techniques of allowing children to present evidence in court recognise the child as a competent reporter while acknowledging the pressures placed on children by the adult-dominated courtroom (Wyness, 1996). The legal status of children as independent citizens was officially recognised in the UK by the Children Act 1989, although the extent of its success in this context is debatable. The Act placed duties on the courts to ascertain the views of children when ruling on decisions with regard to their upbringing.

The recognition – at least in theory – that children have a right to be heard has also been extended, albeit slowly, to the health services. While *Local Voices* (NHSME, 1992), *Patient Partnership: Building a Collaborative Strategy* (NHS Executive, 1996) and *The Patient's Charter* (DoH, 1991a) all reflected parliamentary and NHS beliefs that the views of local people as consumers should inform the development and planning of health services, these documents did not refer directly to children, and consultation tended to rely on parents or carers as proxies. However, the *Welfare of Children and Young People in Hospital* (DoH, 1991b) and the more recent *Patient's Charter: Services for Children and Young People* (DoH, 1996) have made provision for children's voices to be heard, while a recent editorial in the *British Medical Journal* said that children and young people 'should have all the information they need to enable them to participate in their own health care' (Lansdown *et al.*, 1996, p. 1565). Professional organisations such as the Health Visitors' Association and the British Paediatric Association have also shown positive concerns about allowing children to participate more widely in such decisions. Moreover, there is some evidence to suggest that children who are involved in discussions on their medical condition and possible treatment are likely to co-operate more willingly and to have better health outcomes (Alderson, 1990).

It is but a short step from the recognition that children should play a part in their own health care to an acknowledgement that children's and young people's views, alongside those of other 'consumers', ought to be taken into account, on a regular and ongoing basis, in planning and policy development within local health authorities. A recent review showed, for example, that there were often discrepancies between the actual health concerns of older children and adolescents and professional assumptions regarding their needs (Jacobson and Wilkinson, 1994).

It was in recognition of the importance of listening to children's views on health services that one health authority in the North West of England initially approached the Public Health Research and Resource Centre. With the full support of the two local education authorities, two researchers were commissioned to interview local children and young people as a part of a public consultation process concerning plans to reconfigure the existing children's health services (Elliott *et al.*, 1996).

Methodology

The research project started at the beginning of October 1996 facing two major problems. First, the consultation period was due to finish at the end of that month, and second, there was a week-long school half-term holiday within this period, making access to the children more difficult. Because of the limited time available, local schools were contacted by telephone and head teachers were asked to allow their pupils to participate in the project. The value of speaking to the children themselves was rarely questioned. However, the possibility of fitting the researchers into the timetable for the following week, the week before half-term, stretched the goodwill of school staff to the limit. Despite this, visits were organised to six schools: four primary (4–11-year-olds) and two secondary (11–16-year-olds).

Altogether, 21 semi-structured group interviews were conducted, involving a total of more than 200 children and young people between the ages of 4 and 16. A topic guide was used, and the discussions were recorded on audiotape, which, for the younger groups at least, prompted much excitement. Having informed head teachers that these interviews could be carried out in whatever space happened to be available, the researchers found themselves in a variety of what would normally be considered unfavourable interviewing situations: squeezed in at the back of a busy classroom, for example, or sitting on the floor in a corridor outside the library. This may, in fact, have had a positive impact on the interview dynamics, since the younger children in particular were much less likely to see the adult researchers as authority figures under such conditions. The older respondents (for whom the term 'children' may not be appropriate) also appeared to enjoy the opportunity to talk – and perhaps to miss lessons.

Careful consideration was given to the ethical issues involved in the research, Alderson's (1995) clear and detailed discussion proving a very useful guide in this respect. The children and young people involved were provided with information about the project, told how the data from the interviews were to be used, and asked to decide for themselves whether or not they wanted to take part. Issues of confidentiality were also discussed, and they were assured that neither their own names nor the name of the school they attended would appear in any reports that were written, as well as that anything they told us individually would not be passed on to teachers or parents without permission. Group sessions concluded with a short 'debriefing' to monitor any unforeseen effects on the children raised by the discussions.

The interviews covered general issues surrounding health and illness (including who the children wanted to be with, and where they preferred to be, when they were ill); what they remembered, liked and disliked about visits to the family doctor; and their experiences of hospital consultations and/or treatment. The younger children were also asked about the things they thought kept people healthy or made them ill (primarily to get them used to speaking about health and health care), while the older age groups talked about where they would go for information and advice on health care issues.

The tape-recorded interviews were transcribed, the themes arising from the data being coded and discussed by the interviewers. It must be pointed out that although the data were rich enough to capture commonalities in the views of the children and young people, the research was not extensive enough to pinpoint the differences between children from different population groups. Although all the schools served local populations of relatively high socio-economic deprivation, one in particular having a high population of children from black minority ethnic groups, it was not possible in this study to, for example, explore the effects of material deprivation or ethnicity on the experiences and views that children had of the services they received. Nor could the differences between the views of pupils from different geographical populations be explored.

Main findings

Research commissioned to inform health service planning sometimes has to respond quickly to government-imposed timetables and deadlines. In this case, the imminent end of the local consultation period meant that the research was conducted without the benefit of time to construct more sophisticated and 'scientific' methods of approach, or to test different data collection techniques with different age groups. Nevertheless, the information that was collected was both rich and illuminating. This suggests that as long as the adults conducting the research present themselves in as unthreatening a way as possible, children are able and willing to express their views and talk about their experiences in a way that is no less 'authentic' than if they were adults themselves.

Despite these limitations, the analysis revealed several strong themes that appeared to be common to all age groups and across localities. These centred around the way in which health professionals communicated with children and young people, feelings about the treatments imposed on them, the preferred settings for treatment, access to information and advice, and their perceptions of the roles that different health professionals played.

It's good to talk: communication issues in health care settings

There were a number of concerns that children expressed about the way in which doctors in particular communicated with them, both within primary care and secondary care settings. They felt that doctors rarely spoke to them directly, used over-technical language and were sometimes authoritarian in their manner.

Children reported that doctors tended automatically to talk to the parents or other adult carers who accompanied them. It seems that little has changed since Silverman (1987) noted over a decade ago how, in three-way meetings between the doctor, the parent and the child, the latter is often completely excluded from the discussion, and/or given only limited autonomy within the decision-making process (Brannen *et al.*, 1994). Even the older children, bordering on adulthood, reported that doctors would often speak to an accompanying parent rather than to them directly. They often found this both annoying and embarrassing:

> If you're sat there with your mum and there's something wrong with you, they just stand there talking to your mum instead of you. You're just sat there like a dummy in a chair. (age 15)

Even the youngest children felt annoyed and upset if they were completely excluded from discussions about their health. They not only felt 'shut out' if doctors spoke only to their parents, but also thought that doctors could not know what was wrong with them if they failed to ask them. 'After all', said one 8-year-old, 'I'm the one in pain.' Another child felt that parents could not always know the whole of the problem that a child was experiencing and would, therefore, fail to provide sufficient information to the doctor:

> You might have told her [your mum] just one thing but you've got two things wrong with you. (age 9)

Some of the older groups said that health professionals, like their teachers, had a negative image of people their age. They felt that doctors often did not believe them, dismissing or trivialising their complaints. The young people put this down to the fact that while they were no longer seen as small and sweet, they were not considered old enough to be trusted as responsible adults. The move from being seen as a cute child to a morose adolescent was felt to shape the encounter between them and their doctor:

> When you're little they're nice to you because you're little and cute, but when you're older they don't take much notice of you.

Jacobson and Roisin (1997) point to authors who describe anecdotal reports about 'suboptimal' care for teenagers, describing how consultations with them could be used as a chance to catch up on late surgeries, while good communication might be difficult with brisk and bureaucratic staff who lacked an understanding of adolescent problems, languages and subcultures.

The issue of 'growing up' was raised in a different context in relation to patterns of prescribing. Medicine was often seen as an important comforter. Younger children enjoyed the fruit-flavoured syrups that they were given and it therefore came as a shock when this 'treat' was withdrawn and medicine was instead offered in the form of capsules or pills. Many of the respondents would have liked to have chosen for themselves; for one group of 10-year-olds in particular, this would have shown more respect to them as individuals than the assumption that they were now 'old enough' to take tablets. It is interesting to note that a previous study of the issue of long-term medication for children found that parents preferred tablet over liquid forms of medication, but the children themselves were not consulted (Manley *et al.*, 1994).

Children of all ages saw doctors as important figures with curative powers, but they were also considered authoritarian and at times judgemental. While the older respondents resented this authority being used to dismiss or trivialise their views, the younger ones were also aware of the way in which doctors judged 'bad behaviour'. One 8-year-old complained:

> Miss, I don't like going to the doctors because they tell me off... because I've done things wrong.

Another major communication issue centred around the use of language. Most children thought that doctors used over-complicated terminology and ought to explain what they meant using language everyone could understand:

> I can understand what he's saying, right, when he's talking about the body and all that. I can understand all that. But sometimes I can't. I don't know what he's talking about, what part of the body he's talking about. Like a knee or summat you can understand... but summat like ligaments, you know, I mean, where's that and all this lot? You know half of it but you don't know the rest. (age 15)

Other literature suggests that health promotion appears to recognise the importance of using appropriate terminology: Dudley (1997, p. 232), for example, notes that 'talking to infants about the damaging effect the sun has upon the skin has little meaning unless you use the appropriate language and imagery'. Children also wanted more complete explanations about diagnoses and treatment options. Incomplete explanations only increased their feelings of being 'kept in the dark'.

The implications of these issues for the ways in which health care professionals deal directly with children and young people are clear. They become particularly important when considered alongside Alderson's finding that children who are knowledgeable about their condition and prognosis are more willing to co-operate with treatment procedures, more patient when enduring pain and more likely to make a better recovery (Alderson, 1990).

What's going on?: manipulation, intrusion and invasion

The children interviewed also had a number of concerns about the ways in which treatment procedures were carried out. They disliked, and were sensitive to, being physically manipulated or having things done to them in ways that felt invasive or intrusive, especially if they could not see any point to the intervention:

> I don't like doctors prodding and poking around for no reason. (age 10)

This was particularly the case when these 'proddings' resulted in discomfort:

> I don't like it when you go to the doctors if you've got a pain and they press down on it. (age 7)

The tools that doctors used to assist their examination were often disliked and seen as invasive. One 8 year old mentioned her reservations about 'that thing that dries and freezes things like moles'. Another 7-year-old complained that the doctors 'kept shining a light in my eyes which blinds me'. A surprising number of children said that they disliked the stethoscope, which was referred to as 'that cold thing that doctors put on your belly'. Injections also provoked a strong reaction. If a child in a group said that he or she liked injections, this invariably brought a strong response from the others; some children feared going to the local practice or to the hospital simply because of their fear of injections. Older children talked about 'freaking out', while younger ones reported that they cried. Injections were seen as something that the respondents were compelled to accept and over which they had no choice.

Hospitals in particular were seen by some who had stayed there as places in which intrusive and invasive actions took place. The children's accounts uncovered feelings of fear towards the various devices to which they were attached. Operations were seen as particularly frightening. One 5-year-old poignantly articulated her feelings as she remembered her experience of being operated on:

> When I went into hospital I had a big thing and they put it on my chest to make sure that it did not go open and then I had to go home... I didn't like it when they opened my belly.

Others remembered their fears on waking and finding themselves wired up to various devices. One 8-year-old child described how 'scary' it was to have 'all these things attached to you'. With the drips, the monitors and the 'tubes in your nose', he wanted someone to be with him when he awoke.

Many children talked about hospital experiences using the language of passivity, indicating that they sensed they were the 'objects' of treatment and the recipients of technical medical procedures. This lack of involvement of children has been highlighted elsewhere in the literature on children's experiences. In her chapter in *Children's Childhoods* (Mayall, 1994a), for example, Alderson's development of the concept of children's integrity supports the right of the individual child to give, or refrain from giving, consent to medical procedures in relation to the issues of invasion and violation of the body (Brannen and O'Brien, 1995).

From the accounts that our children gave, however, it seems that, with regard to any procedure, they felt better if their fears were recognised, understood and dealt with in some way. This included letting them hold or play with an instrument such as a stethoscope, offering 'magic cream' before an injection or operation, rewarding them for acts of bravery and allowing close relatives to stay with them while they were undergoing treatment in hospital.

Feeling 'looked after': treatment settings

Children were asked where they liked to be when they were ill and whether they would prefer to be at home or in hospital to treat some of the more serious health problems that they had experienced. On the whole, children enjoyed being at home, but their reasons for this were more complex than perhaps the understandable ones of feeling 'pampered'. While hospitals were seen as more anonymous, strange and authoritarian, there was a perception that they were centres of expertise and that care at home could entail a denial of access to essential medical skills and technologies.

All the children and young people acknowledged the value of the role of 'care' in the process of 'treatment'. If they were ill, they wanted to be 'tucked up in bed' or 'wrapped up warm and pampered'. However, close relatives were seen not only as catering for their creature comforts, but also as performing vital tasks in the process of the children's recovery. Their health care skills were sometimes considered greater than those of the professionals. One 7-year-old commented, 'the doctors don't do you any good because the doctors aren't your mum'.

It was because of this need to be in a safe and caring environment that many children preferred home as the setting in which treatment took place. This applied to both primary care and care for more serious illnesses, which would normally take place in a hospital. Wanting to be on home territory also raised issues of empowerment. More familiar settings were felt to equalise the relationship between the patient and the professional carer, some children saying that they felt more confident to say what they felt and to ask questions at home.

Familiarity and comfort were considered to be very important. In contrast to hospital, the groups felt that at home they got, on the whole, better food, they could have friends and relatives round when they wanted, and they were not bound by strict hospital rules and regulations. This preference for home care was well expressed by one 15-year-old:

I prefer home, definitely, because you've got your mum and dad there and your friends come round and keep you company and all that.

You're on your own area too, aren't you? You know everyone round ᴛʜᴇʀᴇ. ɴᴏ sᴛʀᴀɴɢᴇʀs.

Brannen and O'Brien (1995), in discussing theories of childhood, note that while more and more specialist institutions and experts are focusing on children, greater importance is being placed on the home environment and the responsibility of parents, professional intervention being structured around an ideology that deems parents and families to be the primary source of children's care. However, although the children to whom we spoke largely preferred to be at home, many expressed a suspicion that home-based treatment would deny them access to expertise. This prompted some reservations concerning the value of home treatment. One 7-year-old, for example, thought it was better to be treated at hospital because 'you could die at home'. This concern about the withdrawal of access to expertise was summed up by a 15-year-old girl who had had regular hospital treatment for her asthma:

> If I had a really bad asthma attack I'd be scared so I'd want to be in hospital, but I'd want to be at home at the same time. But if there was someone at home like a nurse or something and I knew that she could deal with it, then I'd stay at home, because you'd know the surroundings and there'd be people with you.

For some children, hospital had been a positive experience. Some enjoyed the toys, especially if they had been to a hospital that provided a wide range of activities on the children's ward. Others saw hospital as an escape from annoying siblings. A few children had formed close relationships with particular nurses and wanted the opportunity to see them again. It was, however, not possible to explore these beliefs in any further depth, and it may be that such feelings were relative to both the particular hospital they attended and their own home circumstances.

Many of the children interviewed had never stayed in hospital. They were curious, some commenting that they wanted to have the experience of a hospital stay. However, in at least one group, these views were met with 'you wouldn't like it, you wouldn't' (of 4-year-olds).

On the whole, memories of hospital were of large, strange and anonymous institutions that could be both dull and frightening. This was often worse if the hospital was far from home and thereby denied them frequent contact with friends and relatives. Children hated 'not knowing anyone', which made them feel lonely or frightened. Night-time in particular brought morbid thoughts about people dying around them. This 13-year-old said:

> I don't like being with other people, because they're bleeding and they're ill and they're all joining you in one big room. It's not good that. I don't like that. I think you should be in little cubicles.

There were a range of complaints about the hospital environment. The wards were often dull, some wards did not have enough toys or activities, and there was a lack of privacy. Hospitals were also considered to be authoritarian and rule-bound. Life was not as flexible as it was at home, and children found this very restricting. The general routine was disliked, as was the insistence on finishing their food (the standard of which many complained about anyway). A number of comments expressed children's frustrations with these rules and regulations, for example:

> Everyone told me that there was computers and games there, but I didn't get to play with any of them because the doctor made me eat all me sprouts. (age 10)

Children, however, had a number of suggestions to improve the hospital wards and routines. They suggested brighter decor, a more flexible approach to visitors, more enjoyable activities and have staff who were sympathetic and would talk to them. Many children also talked about the need to be in a ward with others of the same age, which would enable friendships to take place and encourage conversation between patients.

Tell me more: access to information and advice

Children appear to have only limited direct access to information and advice about health care issues; parents and professionals alike tend to assume that they will be accompanied by an adult when approaching service providers, while younger children in particular are restricted in terms of their physical autonomy and mobility (Mayall, 1995). Our own research indicated, however, that children and young people value the opportunity to talk to a trusted and knowledgeable person in confidence about matters that they may feel unable to discuss with their parents and/or friends, supporting the findings of previous research (Bewley *et al.*, 1984).

For some children, a parent, particularly a mother, was considered to be a reliable confidant, while others had certain teachers they felt that they could trust. Previous studies have noted that the school nurse is often valued as an advisor and an advocate for children (Nash *et al.*, 1985; Mayall, 1994b), and some of our groups called for school nurses to be present and available on a more regular basis. Older children admitted that there might be some issues, such as pregnancy, for which a confidential and anonymous source of advice away from the gaze of friends, family and teachers would be needed. There were, however, concerns that professed confidential sources of help, such as the family planning clinic, might turn out not to be so.

Respondents felt that leaflets and posters could act as sources of advice, but one group of 13-year-old boys in particular pointed out that those provided in the doctor's waiting room and at school were largely irrelevant to their concerns. It was also mentioned that one had to be ill to see them anyway as in school these were only displayed in the sick room. Some respondents suggested that leaflets on personal health matters should be in places where there was guaranteed privacy (such as toilet cubicles) since others might be watching to see which ones they were picking up.

Who does what?: the roles of health care professionals

Children and young people had very clear perceptions of the different roles that doctors on the one hand, and nurses on the other, played in the delivery of their health care. As a result, they related to doctors and nurses in very different ways. They also perceived a distinct hierarchy. Doctors were seen as having higher status, but this also meant that nurses were felt to be more approachable. While many of these views concerned their understanding of primary care professionals, very similar views were expressed on the roles of hospital staff.

On the whole, doctors were seen as the medical 'experts'. They were the ones who could treat people and make them better. They were concerned with measuring and testing but were not very good at relating to their young patients. As a result, doctors were felt to be more distant. One 8-year-old said, 'They're OK [the doctors] but they don't talk to me. They just check me.' Nurses, on the other hand, were seen as having a more caring role, being more concerned with their overall wellbeing and more obviously relating to the patient through conversation rather than consultation. As one 11-year-old said, 'They [the doctors] just tell you what is going to happen to you and stuff and the nurses don't. They ask you how you're feeling and everything.'

The focus on 'cure' rather than 'care' was realised in the terminology that doctors employed. Nurses used more everyday language
to which the children could relate. Nurses were also seen as being
more able and more willing to listen to, and understand, their
concerns. As one 11-year-old said of the practice nurse, 'she listens
more than my doctor. She takes it in better.'

Connected to this idea of a difference in role was the perception of
a professional hierarchy. No-one questioned whether or not this was
desirable, but it added to the sense that they could approach the
nurses more readily since they were able to communicate on the children's level. The groups also commented on the way in which they
felt that this hierarchy impacted on doctor–nurse relationships.
'Nurses just do what the doctors tell them', one 8-year-old said, while
another 13-year-old felt that the 'nurse always agrees with what the
doctor says'.

The children did not say that they valued nurses more than
doctors, but it was evident that they did not, on the whole, see
doctors as being particularly approachable or caring. However,
although they saw nurses as more easy to relate to, the fact that they
were also seen as less powerful than doctors might have limited the
extent to which the children saw the nurses playing an advocate's role
in the treatment process. Nevertheless, the ability to communicate
and relate to patients was valued and seen as being particularly
important in a hospital setting where the environment, as pointed out
earlier, was felt to be especially alienating. Where the nurse's role is in
a process of change, particularly in community and primary care
settings, it will be important to remember, in providing many treatments traditionally provided by doctors, the value that children, and
possibly many adults, attach to less medicalised encounters. This is
not only because such relationships recognise children's needs to be
cared for: they may also enable children and young people to feel
more able to participate and make informed choices about their own
health care treatment.

Discussion and implications for practice

The aim of this research was not to make claims about the extent to
which these particular views are generalisable to children and young
people across the country, but to offer insights into how they may
experience, and what they may feel about, health care settings. The
group interviews with children and young people discussed here
focused on contexts in which their status was often disregarded and

only occasionally acknowledged. The themes generated contribute to a growing body of knowledge, referred to at the beginning of this chapter, concerning the place of children as citizens and lay experts. The findings from this local project suggest a number of implications for the roles that they should play as users of health services.

At an individual level, it highlighted the importance that children and young people attach to being treated seriously and listened to as people who are competent in talking about their own good, and ill, health (James and Prout, 1990; Mayall, 1994b), and the implications that this may have for health care professionals. They want to be given choices and control over treatment options and treatment settings, provided that their concerns about receiving the same level of care and expertise at home as in surgeries or hospitals are addressed. This places a duty on the health care services to provide children and young people with sufficient information to enable them to make an informed choice. The information should, moreover, be provided in an accessible and non-technical format. This right to choose between treatment options should extend to the right to refuse consent to treatment, as previous discussion around the issues of invasion and violation has indicated (Alderson, 1990). Interestingly, the children interviewed for this research appeared to feel less manipulated and invaded if they were actively involved in the use of the various instruments and devices by nurses and doctors.

On the whole, however, children and young people most often saw themselves as the passive recipients of medical intervention, and essentially as invisible within the medical consultation. One significant change that could improve children's experience of the health care system would, therefore, be for all health professionals, including nursing staff, to recognise children as primary reporters of their own health (Mayall, 1995). This would entail speaking to them, listening to them and negotiating with them directly rather than merely with their parents or adult carers. Indications from this research suggest that children and young people feel nurses, on the whole, to be doing this more than doctors. This may be because nurses' perception of their own role is one of caring for the whole individual rather than simply treating the patient (Williams *et al.*, 1997). It is argued that encounters between *all* health professionals and children should be informed by an understanding of children as competent persons. This may well entail some review of procedures in primary, secondary and community practice settings.

There was also a clear need for health information and advice that was accessible, confidential and relevant for children and young adults. One step forward, for older children at any rate, may be the development of 'outreach' clinics for teenagers in schools, city centre drop-in clinics and/or teenager-specific family planning clinics (Smy, 1994; Williams *et al.*, 1994). Users' views on their effectiveness and appropriateness will be an important aspect of any evaluation, since this will be a recognition of the role of young people as critical consumers. Their own views must be considered alongside other data when addressing the emerging questions from professionals about whether such clinics are the best way to access those who need them most: teenagers at the greatest 'risk' rather than the 'worried well' (see Jacobson *et al.*, 1996).

Taking a much broader view, the richness of the data collected in this project indicates that research that involves obtaining the views of children can be used as evidence to inform the development of health care policy and practice. Many of the criticisms of the reliability of data based on children's reports are issues that researchers also have to deal with when talking to adult respondents (Alderson, 1995; Mahon *et al.*, 1996). Although children and young people may not have an equal ability to discuss certain issues, there is no reason to suppose that they are unable to talk about aspects of their own experience. Within health service research, such accounts can provide a valuable insight into what children enjoy, dislike and fear about health care services and the treatment process.

The research also highlighted a number of issues that could benefit from further exploration. These included the role that children can and do play in keeping themselves healthy; the provision of more appropriate, accessible and confidential information; the changing needs of children as they 'grow up' and what effect this has on the provision of services; and the ways in which young people's needs for social support in a hospital setting could best be met.

Conclusion

The key issue remains, however, the need for health care professionals to value the expertise that children have with respect to their own health. And since they *are* capable of formulating and expressing some very clear ideas about how local services are planned and delivered, ways of accessing their views on a regular and ongoing basis should certainly be explored. As local people and users of health services are increasingly being asked to become involved in the planning of appropriate health care, there is no good reason why the views of children and young people should not also be included in this process.

References

Alderson P. (1995) *Listening to Children: Children, Ethics and Social Control*, London, Barnardos.

Alderson P. (1990) *Choosing for Children: Parents' Consent to Surgery*. Oxford, Oxford University Press.

Bewley B. R., Higgs R. H. and Jones A. (1984) 'Adolescent patients in an inner London practice: their attitudes to illness and health care', *Journal of the Royal College of General Practitioners* 34: 543–6.

Brannen J., Dodd K., Oakley A. and Storey P. (1994) *Young People, Health and Family Life*, Buckingham, Open University Press.

Brannen J. and O'Brien M. (1995) 'Childhood and the sociological gaze: paradigms and paradoxes', *Sociology* 29: 729–37.

Department of Health (1991a) *The Patient's Charter*, London, HMSO.

Department of Health (1991b) *Welfare of Children and Young People in Hospital*, London, HMSO.

Department of Health (1996) *The Patient's Charter: Services for Children and Young People*, London, HMSO.

Dudley W. (1997) 'Sun awareness and primary school children', *Health Visitor* 70: 232–3.

Elliott E., Watson A. with Tanner S. (1996) Time to put the children first: children's and young people's views of health care in Salford and Trafford. Unpublished research report, Salford, Public Health Research and Resource Centre (University of Salford).

Green J. (1997) 'Risk and the construction of social identity: children's talk about accidents', *Sociology of Health and Illness* 19: 457–79.

Jacobson L. and Roisin M. (1997) 'Critical consumers: teenagers in primary care', *Health and Social Care in the Community* 5: 55–62.

Jacobson L. and Wilkinson C. (1994) 'A review of teenage health: time for a new direction', *British Journal of General Practice* 44: 420–4.

Jacobson L., Wilkinson C., Pill R. and Hackett P. (1996) 'Communication between teenagers and British general practitioners: a preliminary study of the teenage perspective', *Ambulatory Child Health* 1: 291–301.

James A. and Prout A. (eds) (1990) *Constructing and Reconstructing Childhood*, Basingstoke, Falmer Press.

Lansdown G., Waterston T. and Baum D. (1996) 'Implementing the UN Convention on the Rights of the Child', *British Medical Journal* 313: 1565–6.

Mahon A., Glendinning C., Clarke K. and Craig G. (1996) Researching children: methods and ethics, *Children and Society* 10: 145–54.

Manley M. C. G., Calnan M. and Sheiham A. (1994) 'A spoonful of sugar helps the medicine go down? Perspectives on the use of sugar in children's medicines', *Social Science and Medicine* 39: 833–40.

Mayall B. (ed.) (1994a) *Children's Childhoods: Observed and Experienced*, London, Falmer Press.

Mayall B. (1994b) *Negotiating Health: Children at Home and Primary School*, London, Cassell.

Mayall B. (1995) 'The changing context of childhood: children's perspectives on health care resources including services'. In Botting, B. (ed.) *The Health of our Children*, Decennial Supplement. London, OPCS/HMSO.

Mayall B. (1998) 'Towards a sociology of child health', *Sociology of Health and Illness* 20: 269–88.

Nash W., Thruston M. and Baly M. (1985) *Health at School: Caring for the Whole Child*, London, Heinemann.

NHS Executive (1996) *Patient Partnership: Building a Collaborative Strategy*, London, HMSO.

NHSME (1992) *Local Voices: The Views of Local People in Purchasing for Health*, London, HMSO.

Silverman D. (1987) *Communication and Medical Practice: Social Relations in the Clinic*, London, Sage.

Smy J. (1994) 'Confidence trick to win the minds of teenagers', *Doctor*, 38–9.

Williams A., Robins T. and Sibbald B. (1997) Cultural differences between medicine and nursing: implications for primary care. Unpublished seminar presentation, Salford, Public Health Research and Resource Centre (University of Salford).

Williams E., Kirkman R. and Elstein M. (1994) 'Profile of young people's advice clinic in reproductive health, 1988–93', *British Medical Journal* 309: 786–8.

Wyness M. (1996) 'Policy, protectionism and the competent child', *Childhood* 3: 431–47.

Further reading

Botting B. (ed.) (1995) *The Health of our Children*: Decennial Supplement, London HMSO/OPCS.

Mayall B. (1996) *Children, Health and the Social Order*, Buckingham, Open University Press.

8 The surveillance of childhood accidents: providing the evidence for accident prevention

Laura King, Anna Gough, Iain Robertson-Steel and Donald Pennington

Introduction

In 1992, the Department of Health (DoH) included accidents as a key area in *The Health of the Nation* document. This reflects the vast number of children who attend accident and emergency (A&E) departments every year following an unintentional injury. The aim of this study was to identify the target groups and priorities for accident prevention for children and young adults who attend the A&E department of New Cross Hospital, Wolverhampton, West Midlands, UK. Structured interviews were conducted by a research nurse in the A&E department at various times during a 1-year period. The data presented in this chapter are those for the first month of data collection, March 1997. Health visitors, paediatric nurses, school nurses and general nurses working in A&E will be able to incorporate these specific local data into their practice. Their clinical practice will thus be underpinned by relevant, locally derived research evidence.

The Child Accident Prevention Trust (1992) estimates that, each year, approximately 2 million children under the age of 15 years attend an A&E department following an unintentional injury. This presents an exciting challenge in terms of accident prevention to nurses who have regular contact with children and their families both in the A&E department and in the community.

The intention of this chapter is to show how the provision of evidence for accident prevention strategies can influence the practice of nurses working with children. This will be achieved by discussing issues surrounding the problem of childhood accidents and the design and evaluation of an accident surveillance project at an A&E department in Wolverhampton. This study does not evaluate what does and

128

does not work in terms of nursing care but instead aims to give nurses working with children an insight into the potential accident risks and circumstances that exist. This knowledge can then be incorporated into clinical practice to enable higher-quality A&E services for children who have had accidents and helps to identify opportunities for health promotion that nurses might not previously have considered.

Background literature

Accidents in context

The Consumer Safety Unit (1996) estimates that approximately 613,000 children aged 0–4 years and 430,000 children aged 5–14 years were injured in non-fatal accidents in the home in 1994. Falls were the most frequent cause of these injuries and are, therefore, likely to be a common reason for attendance at the A&E department. While most fatal accidents before the age of 5 occur in the home, after the age of 5 they are caused by road traffic accidents, in which the child is often a pedestrian (DoH, 1995). Therefore, the complex and age-related nature of accidents needs to be comprehensively considered in order to identify areas for potential prevention strategies. At an international level, the overall death rate from accidents in the UK appears to be lower than that of most other countries, although pedestrian death rates in children exceed those of most other European countries (DoH, 1995). If this is considered alongside the large number of children attending the A&E department following an accidental injury, the complex nature of the problem can be appreciated.

In 1992 the DoH published *The Health of the Nation* document, which included accidents as a key area for action. The target identified for children was to reduce the death rate in the 0–14 year-old age group by at least 33 per cent by the year 2005. This target is, however, somewhat controversial. Pless (1991) illustrates this by emphasising the misleading nature of having one target for all these ages. As evidence is available to show that greater improvements can be made in particular age groups and for certain injuries, he argues that each should be targeted accordingly. This emphasises the need for accident research to be clearly focused so that meaningful data are generated on particular accidents, injuries and the individuals involved.

Gender and social class are also highly influential factors in the epidemiology of childhood accidents. Boys appear to have a third more accidents than girls, and children from social class V appear to have a five times greater mortality rate from accidents than those from social class I (Roberts and Power, 1996). In their comparison of class-specific mortality in children between 1981 and 1991, Roberts and Power also concluded that socio-economic inequalities in children's injury death rate had increased. This means that *The Health of the Nation* (DoH, 1992) target for accidents will probably be met for children in non-manual classes but not for those in manual classes. Although this study considered only death after accidental injury, it does illustrate the need to consider broader social influences on children's accidents than merely the cause of the accident and injury sustained.

The population of Wolverhampton resembles the national population of the UK. Although Wolverhampton appears to have fewer fatal accidents relative to national and regional figures, there was an apparent upward trend in the under-15 years age group between 1989 and 1992 (Hutchby, 1996). Stilwell and Stilwell (1995) also noted that Wolverhampton has been found to be below average for the West Midlands Regional Health Authority in terms of health status and socio-economic conditions, the authority in turn being below the average for England and Wales. As socio-economic indicators have in the past been linked to accidental injuries, this is obviously an area of great concern when considering the pattern and occurrence of both fatal and non-fatal injuries.

By identifying the risk factors for a local community, relevant strategies for accident prevention may be identified. This information can then be utilised by local policy makers, such as in the Strategy for Children, which is currently being developed by the community Trust in Wolverhampton. However, for this policy to be effective, realistic outcome measurements need to be incorporated into the design, as for any meaningful evaluative research. The lack of specific information about accidents in Wolverhampton has acted as the impetus for this study since a comprehensive assessment of the most common accidents and injuries for children attending the A&E department involved could not be made.

Data collection issues

When an individual attends an A&E department following an accident, only the minimum data set required in the UK for recording purposes is collected in the majority of instances (DoH, 1995). Therefore, the nature of accidents in terms of their circumstances and resulting injuries is very difficult to describe because of the lack of detail in the recorded information. Certain databases, such as the Home Accidents Surveillance System (Consumer Safety Unit, 1996), exist but do not take into account all the potential injuries presenting to the A&E department.

The issue of whether to collect broad or in-depth information about the accident is also very important in the design of accident surveillance studies. McClure and Burnside (1995) discussed this problem in relation to accident surveillance in Australia. They concluded that it is the goals of the surveillance that should direct the method adopted. Replacing a system that collects detailed accident information with one that ensures complete case identification would lead to less information about the causation of accidents being collected, thus giving a weaker theoretical base on which to build accident prevention strategies.

Although studies of accident surveillance have been carried out in both hospital and primary care environments, the difficulty in building up a complete picture of accident occurrence arises as the result of the number of injuries not being reported to health care professionals. This means that researchers need to choose their target populations in relation to the utilisation of the data they produce. As the aim of this study is to reduce the number of accidents presenting to an A&E department, data will be collected about children attending the department. This study will in the future expand to consider children who attend their GP following an accident and those who do not seek medical attention.

Although many epidemiological studies of accidents exist, there is a large gap in terms of the evaluative research of accident prevention activities. Criticisms of accident prevention studies include the fact that they are poorly conceived and concentrate on the delivery or reception of the health message rather than actual health gain (Roberts *et al.*, 1993). This emphasises the need for sound data on the actual circumstances of accidents to be collected in order to identify the need for preventative action. In order to discover risk factors and successful interventions for a population such as that of Wolverhampton, it is essential that the relevant information for this area is used to underpin the work.

Definition of an accident

A specific definition of 'an accident' is difficult to determine because of its complex nature. One of the only common components of accident definitions in the literature is the use of the *International Classification of Diseases* (WHO, 1992) to code accidents and injuries. Therefore, for the purposes of this study, an accident was defined as:

An external occurrence causing any unintentional injury or potential injury, which may be coded by the *International Classification of Diseases* (10th Revision, WHO, 1992) by S and T codes. Assaults and intentional injury are excluded.

Intentional injury and assault were not addressed because of the large differences in cause and possible prevention strategies that exist. This definition does not assume that accidents are unpredictable or impossible to prevent and implies that the cause of the injury involved an event external to the individual involved, for example a fall, the ingestion of medication, a burn, an animal bite and so on. In addition, as this study was based in an A&E department, it was assumed that an injury or potential injury was sustained for which medical advice had been sought.

Aims of the research

The overall research question for this study was:

What are the target groups and priorities for accident prevention for children and young adults who attend the A&E department at New Cross Hospital, Wolverhampton?

In order to answer this question, the objectives for this study were developed as follows:

- To determine the most common injuries sustained by those under 18 years of age who attend the A&E department at New Cross Hospital following an accident
- To identify the most common circumstances in which specific injuries occur for children and young adults who attend the A&E department
- To differentiate between risk factors for accidents in this age group according to various demographic factors, for example gender, ethnic group, social status and housing
- To identify target groups for accident prevention strategies
- To identify priorities for accident prevention action in the Wolverhampton area, with reference to attendance at the local A&E department.

Methodology

Data collection tool

A structured questionnaire was designed using a series of closed questions, from which answers were categorised. The questionnaire was administered as a structured interview to maintain consistency in the coding of the data. Three main areas of information were collected by the questionnaire:

1. *Demographic details*, for example age, gender, education, housing, social status, family structure and ethnic group
2. *Accident details*, for example the date and time of the accident, the exact place of the accident, who was present at the time of the accident, the activity at the time of the accident, the mechanism of the accident, the weather at the time of the accident, and protective clothing worn and footwear
3. *Injury and treatment information*, for example the region of the body injured, the treatment and investigations in the department, whether the child was admitted and follow-up details.

The questionnaire was designed using a computer package, FormPro for the Macintosh, which enabled data to be read electronically using an optical scanner.

Sample details and data collection procedure

The target population for this study was all the attendees of the A&E department at New Cross Hospital aged less than 18 years old. Only those children and young adults presenting to the department with an injury that had not previously been treated in an A&E department were eligible for inclusion. Any child or young adult who was unconscious, very distressed or unable to consent to take part in the study was excluded.

The order of patient contact with the research nurse was determined by the order of booking at the reception desk. The actual size of the sample varied according to a variety of issues, for example the number of people attending the department, seasonal variations, the time of day, holiday periods and so on. Each interview lasted approximately 10–15 minutes.

The data collection period for this study was 1 year, during which all times of day, days of the week and seasons of the year were equally represented. This allowed cyclical patterns in accidents to be identified as well as seasonal variations. Partial data collection has been validated in the past (McClure and Burnside, 1995) and, although it may under-represent some aspects of data, a comprehensive picture of the pattern of events can still be obtained. To gain detailed information about accident circumstances, sensitivity of the data, rather than broadness of collection, is required.

The most important factor for an individual attending the A&E department was the treatment of his or her injury. The interview for this study did not interfere with this treatment in any way and occurred prior to treatment, unless this was not possible or the injured person preferred to be interviewed following treatment.

Ethical considerations

Because of the potential vulnerability of the participants in this study, it is important that ethical issues such as informed consent, confidentiality, anonymity and the rights of the individual are considered. Obtaining consent for vulnerable groups such as children is a widely debated issue. Koren *et al.* (1993) describe the age of assent for children as being as low as 7 years old. These children should, therefore, be given the opportunity to participate in giving consent, justifying obtaining both verbal and written consent from the child and the parent or guardian. If the child was unable to write because of injury or age, verbal consent was obtained. Where there was no accompanying person and the child was not deemed able to give valid consent by the research nurse, that child was not included in the sampled population. Consent was considered to be 'informed consent' because of the opportunity given to all participants, including the parent or guardian, to read a project information sheet and/or discuss the project with the research nurse prior to signing the consent form.

At all stages of contact with participants and their guardians, confidentiality and anonymity were assured. Also, the right to refuse to participate and to withdraw at any time was emphasised. Permission to conduct the study was obtained form the Wolverhampton Local District Ethics Committee.

Results

Analysis

The results presented in this chapter are the preliminary analysis of data collected during the first month of the study, March 1997, in the A&E department in Wolverhampton. Analysis was performed using descriptive and summary statistics. Tests of association using the Chi-squared statistic (χ^2) are presented at a significance level of 0.05.

During the month of March 1997, 63 children and young adults were surveyed in the A&E department. Two of these participants were excluded from the analysis as their casualty cards could not be located post-study. All the results are thus based on the remaining 61 children and young adults.

Demographic and social information

Figure 8.1 illustrates the age groups of the study participants.

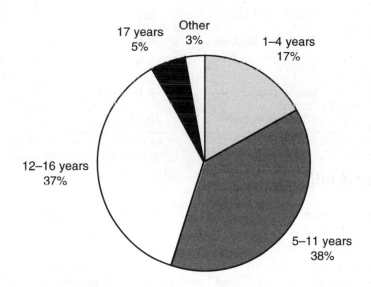

Figure 8.1   Age groups of survey participants

The sample was 47.6 per cent female and 52.4 per cent male. No significant association was found between gender and age. The majority of participants lived in owner-occupied homes (54 per cent), while 34.9 per cent were from Council-owned properties and 7.9 per cent lived in privately rented properties. Almost all the children and young adults lived in houses (93.7 per cent). The Standard Occupational Classification (OPCS, 1991) was used to describe both the male and female head of the family (if applicable). Of those male heads of households in full-time employment, 62.1 per cent were classified as groups III, IV and V. However, 22.2 per cent of the total sample had no male head of household, while only 1.6 per cent had no female head of household. The ethnic origin of participants is illustrated in Table 8.1.

Table 8.1   Ethnic origin of the children and young adults surveyed

Ethnic group	Percentage of sample
Asian – Bangladeshi	1.6
Asian – Other	6.3
Black – Caribbean	4.8
Indian	3.2
Mixed parentage	4.8
White – UK born	79.4

Accident details

The most common day for an accident to occur in the sampled population was Thursday. In the month sampled, 60.3 per cent of accidents occurred on a school weekday. There was an even split between accidents occurring indoors (49.2 per cent) and outdoors (50.8 per cent). No association was found between age and gender in relation to indoor or outdoor accidents. Indoor accidents occurred at home (48.7 per cent of total indoor accidents) or at school/nursery (51.3 per cent of total indoor accidents). There was an association between age group and the location of an indoor accident ($\chi^2 = 25.14$ with 12 df). Younger children aged 1–4 years were more likely to be injured at home than were older children. Of the accidents that occurred in the home, 36.8 per cent occurred in the living room and 21 per cent in the kitchen. Figure 8.2 shows the most common area in the school where accidents occurred.

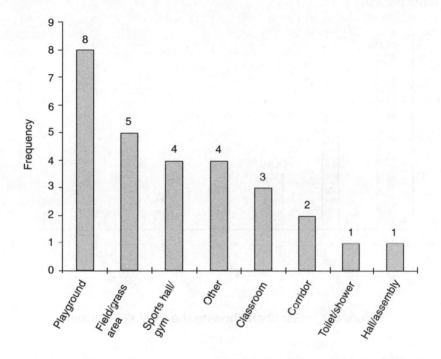

Figure 8.2   Bar chart to show area in school where accidents occurred

An association was found between the age group and the part of the school (χ^2 = 23.8 with 15 df). Children between the ages of 12 and 16 were more likely to have accidents during lessons than were those of any other age group.

Falls made up 39.7 per cent of the causes of accidents. Other causes included: struck a static object (14.3 per cent), a third party (11.1 per cent) and cutting and piercing (7.9 per cent). A closer analysis of falls showed that 68 per cent of all falls occurred on the same level and 32 per cent were from one level to another. Only 16 per cent of falls involved stairs or immovable steps.

At the time of the accident, only 11.1 per cent of participants had been wearing any protective clothing. There was an association between gender and the wearing of protective clothing (χ^2 = 7.2 with 1 df). No females reported the use of any while 21.2 per cent of males did wear some type of protective clothing. When footwear at the time of the accident was analysed, the most common type of footwear worn was sports shoes (42.9 per cent).

Figure 8.3 shows the most serious injury with which each participant presented.

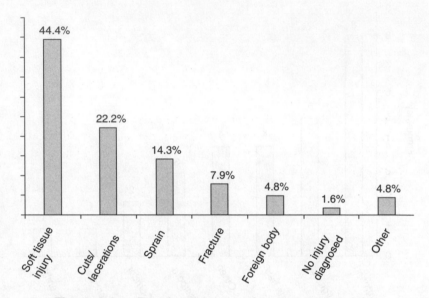

Figure 8.3   Bar chart showing the most serious injury

Discussion

These results were presented as an example of how the information collected by this study may be analysed. It is not the intention of the authors to make generalisations from the results to the whole population of children in the UK. However, the results do illustrate how the information could be used to further accident prevention strategies in the local area.

Limitations and methodological issues

A consideration of the methodological issues provides an opportunity to reflect on the research process and its application to evidence-based practice. This enables nurses to consider the appropriateness and validity of applying findings from a particular research study to their practice. One of the main limitations of this study is the actual sampling technique used, that is, a partial sample. However, as previously discussed, this is essential in order to gain the depth of information required for this study. In the past, many studies have used questionnaires to collect accident surveillance data; see, for example, Sahlin *et al.* (1990) and McClure and Burnside (1995). This technique, however, introduces its own bias, such as discriminating against those that cannot read or write. The use of a self-completed questionnaire for this study would be very time-consuming for the participants and require a high level of concentration. This may not be appropriate in an anxiety-provoking environment such as the A&E department or for the age-related reading and comprehension ability of the child involved.

The use of a structured interview maintains standardisation and comparability, enabling the responses to be easily quantified and coded, and thus increasing the reliability of the results. In addition, as the questionnaire is completed by the interviewer, the number of participants whose questionnaires are not fully completed is reduced. The use of an interview allows participants to expand on their answers so that additional detail can be written on the questionnaires and used to qualify the answers at a later stage.

The minimisation of interviewer bias is achieved by adhering to the order of registration in the department. This means that the interviewer cannot 'pick and choose' whom to approach. This also enhances the random element in the study. It will not be possible to interview all eligible people in the department because of the vast number that sometimes register within a short time period. If a potential participant is not interviewed, the reason will be recorded, for example: went home before being interviewed, did not answer when their name was called, was missed while interviewing another participant or refused to participate.

Conducting an interview requires the interviewer to have a high level of self-awareness in order to prevent the introduction of bias. Care must be taken not to pre-empt answers and not to appear judgemental. For this study, a rapport between the interviewer and interviewee needed to be achieved within a short space of time in order to allow a trusting relationship to develop in such an emotional environment. If the interviewer was not comfortable asking questions to clarify any points, the quality and reliability of the data collected might be questionable.

Another potential source of bias could also be the reliance on children, especially the very young, describing the actual accident and the circumstances involved. A dependence on children's recall of a stressful event such as an accident may be considered unreliable because of the stress and anxiety involved. However, children's memo ries of traumatic events and distress do not appear adversely to affect this process. Peterson and Bell (1996) found that there was no rela tionship between stress and memory for children aged between 2 and 13 years, apart from the actual event of being treated by the doctor if the child was very distressed. This study was also based on the actual experiences of children attending an emergency room following an accident rather than a laboratory situation, which is where most previous research was focused. Therefore, the actual involvement of all ages of child in this survey, especially prior to seeing a doctor, could be considered a strength rather than a weakness.

Developing accident prevention strategies

The broad aim of this study is to provide evidence on which to base health promotion strategies. The question 'why is this important to nurses?' can easily be asked. Its importance lies in the ability of nurses to contextualise the environment in which they work. This information can be used in a variety of ways, for example as a rein forcement of present practice, to provide insight into typical risk factors, to increase knowledge of common accident variables, thus enabling the identification of prevention strategies, to raise aware ness of the problem of childhood accidents presenting to A&E and so on. Hopefully, this will contribute towards high-quality care in any situation. An example of using accident surveillance information to inform accident prevention work could be the identification of the age group 12–16 as being at risk of injury during school lessons. This could be used as an area in which school nurses could work with teachers in order to raise the awareness of the problem. The analysis of school accident data alongside those from the A&E department would allow for this issue to be considered more fully. This would enable a strategy to be developed specifically to reduce this risk factor in the local area.

The prevention of accidents is a highly complex issue. Although many models of health promotion exist, deciding which actual approach is most successful in reducing accidents is highly controver sial. Educational approaches are frequently adopted, but these can be criticised as being passive, control being firmly left with the health professionals. Although education may be used in an attempt to reduce accidents, it may be more effective when used in conjunction with other approaches, for example environmental or legislation (NHS Centre for Reviews and Dissemination, 1996).

The identification of target groups for accident prevention work from the surveillance study can occur in a number of ways. As illustrated in this chapter, the data collected can be analysed in terms of age, gender, social class, type of accident, place of accident and many factors more. This enables detailed analysis to generate specific problem areas. For example, the most common place for outdoor accidents to occur during March 1997 was the school playground. If this were repeated in the full study, all accidents that occurred in school playgrounds could be analysed to discover whether a particular age group, gender, type of accident, set of weather conditions and so on were most frequently involved. This information could be related to age, developmental stage and theories of play. Health promoters, whether nurses, teachers or other professionals, would then have detailed information with which to plan appropriate accident prevention strategies, thus illustrating the importance of this type of study to provide the evidence with which to underpin further developmental and evaluative research.

The data collected in the full, year-long study could also be used as a baseline against which to compare attendance at the A&E department following particular prevention strategies. This approach is important as it allows an in-depth analysis of the pattern of accidents following prevention intervention. Although Sahlin and Lereim (1990) adopted a similar approach in children aged 0–6 years over a 2-year period in Norway, they found a change in accident occurrence only for very small children. This emphasises the need for very detailed surveillance rather than a broad scope of surveillance, as used in Sahlin and Lereim's (1990) study, to observe comprehensively the pattern of accidents in a specific area. This is the approach adopted in our accident surveillance study.

The ability to identify particular problems for certain age groups and gender will enable highly specific accident prevention strategies to be determined. Rather than purely focusing on the education of parents, actually involving children in age- and gender-specific prevention strategies would help to contextualise the problem. In Oxford, an Injury Minimisation Programme aimed at 10–11-year-olds was designed to give children a positive attitude towards accident prevention and to support their knowledge through the acquisition of skills (Orzel, 1996). This approach utilises the relevant cognitive and physical skills of children in this age group, thus making the prevention work highly specific and evidence based. Although Orzel's (1996) work was not based on accident surveillance data, the use of such data would have enabled specific topics to be identified as being especially relevant to the age group involved. This would also have allowed the ongoing surveillance of accidents to be utilised in the evaluation of the prevention strategy's impact.

The use of a structured interview to collect data for this accident surveillance study gives participants and accompanying adults the opportunity to express their feelings about the accident and how it might have been prevented. Although, for the purposes of this study, these data have not been formally recorded or analysed, this is an important issue that will be addressed in the later development of this study. Rice *et al.* (1994) suggest that people living in a particular community are ideally located in terms of recognising specific dangers in their own environment and suggesting ways of reducing these dangers. It can, therefore, be argued that it is essential to involve the community in the design of accident prevention projects and that a trusting relationship should be developed between the researchers and the community under study. High-quality, realistic and specific accident prevention targets require the detail collected in local accident surveillance studies to be considered alongside the views, perceptions and attitudes of the community local to that area. This approach moves the emphasis away from the health professional and places it on those who have the higher risk of being involved in a specific type of accident. By adopting this approach, the social as well as environmental, behavioural and educational aspects of accidents are taken into consideration.

The implications of accident surveillance data for nursing practice

The results of an accident surveillance study such as this have wide implications for all nurses working with children and their families. This research will enable local nurses to incorporate highly specific local data into their practice. For the purposes of this discussion, three groups of nurses who are involved in A&E work will be considered: health visitors, paediatric nurses and general nurses working in A&E. This is not intended to exclude the work of other nurses involved in accident prevention with children, for example school nurses, but reflects the basis from which this study originates.

In Wolverhampton, all children aged less than 16 years who attend the A&E department are referred to a liaison health visitor, although not all of these children are routinely visited at home. Liaison health visitors are in an ideal position to use, in their everyday practice, the data collected by local accident surveillance studies. This may involve the identification of people who have attended A&E and are from high-risk groups in terms of the type of accident or injury. For example, if the majority of accidents in children aged under 5 years occur in the home, the living room being the most common location, health visitors should incorporate this knowledge into their everyday practice. The liaison health visitors can then use this knowledge in a variety of ways, for example at an educational level, providing details of access to safety equipment, or looking at changing some aspect of the child's environment or behaviour. Although health visitors may not be able to carry out these activities themselves, they can act as a resource for people in the community, thus emphasising the importance of a multiagency approach to accident prevention.

However, account must be taken of the context in which post-accident visits by health visitors occur. Reynolds (1996) identified how post-accident support visits by health visitors may provoke guilt in parents, although health visitors are in an ideal situation to observe the safety of the home environment. This observation can then be integrated with health visitors' knowledge of child development to promote safety, although limitations to the help possible, for example the finance available, may be frustrating. However, a knowledge of accidents derived from accident surveillance data can provide a basis on which health visitors can work towards specific goals with at-risk groups prior to accidents occurring. In this context, basing health visitors' accident prevention practice on locally derived accident surveillance is of extreme importance.

Paediatric nurses have specialist knowledge in all aspects of caring for children, including communication and teaching. Therefore, in terms of interpreting the importance of accident surveillance data, they appear to be vital components of the A&E team. However, the need for registered children's nurses (RSCNs or RNs (Child)) in many A&E departments is not accepted, and they are sometimes viewed as a token presence, often not having special responsibility for children (Bentley, 1996). Thus, as many of the children attending A&E will be cared for by general nurses, the need for these nurses to be aware of the implications of accidents, including their causes and outcomes should be stressed. By integrating accident surveillance data such as age, gender and the social context of the child into their assessment of children, A&E nurses will be basing their practice on locally determined research findings.

The use of local accident surveillance data also has implications for the quality of care of children in the A&E department. Communication and information are two areas that have been shown to be lacking when considering parental perceptions of the quality of care of children in the A&E department (Davis, 1995). However, if nurses working in this environment have an adequate knowledge of local

problems in terms of accident occurrence and risk factors, they will
be able confidently to undertake accident prevention activities within
their everyday practice.

Actual accident prevention work in the A&E department often has
an educational emphasis. Ferguson (1994) conducted a small survey
of A&E departments in one region of London to clarify A&E nurses'
perceptions of their role in accident prevention. All departments who
responded gave health promotion advice on request, but only 3 out
of 14 departments had specific accident prevention material available
in their child examination rooms. The information that is contained
in such types of educational material needs to be based on locally
collected accident data in order to address important local accident
patterns and risk factors. For example, the national trend for boys to
have significantly more accidents than girls was not upheld in the
analysis of accident surveillance data for March 1997 in Wolverhampton. Only a slight increase in the ratio of boys to girls reporting
accidents to the A&E department was seen. The equality in gender
seen in the A&E department in this area should, therefore, be
reflected in the local accident prevention material if this trend is
found over the whole year.

Nurses can expand their roles to include a more proactive
approach to accident prevention by participating in local action
groups or accident prevention groups, which allow multiagency co-
operation at both a professional and a community level. Again, in
order to derive most benefit from such an approach, the use of accident surveillance data from the local area provides the base of
evidence on which to build. An expansion of the A&E nurse's role
in terms of accident prevention is suggested in Figure 8.4.

There are potentially many reasons why nurses do not routinely
become involved in accident prevention work within an A&E
department. Attendance at the A&E department can involve great
stress and anxiety for both children and the people accompanying
them. It may, therefore, be insensitive actually to discuss prevention
strategies at this time as a feeling of attaching blame may arise and
thus generate more tension. Each situation must thus be individually assessed. Sbaih (1997) identified one area of the nurses' work
in A&E to be taking risks. In A&E, this may occur as seemingly
more important issues may require the nurse's immediate attention,
so accident prevention work is not seen as being important.
However, taking into account the large amount of A&E department
work that is generated by childhood accidents, this role cannot be
over-emphasised. In this respect, the involvement of nurses in activities such as accident surveillance studies will enable a nursing

focus to assume importance in the design of future accident prevention strategies.

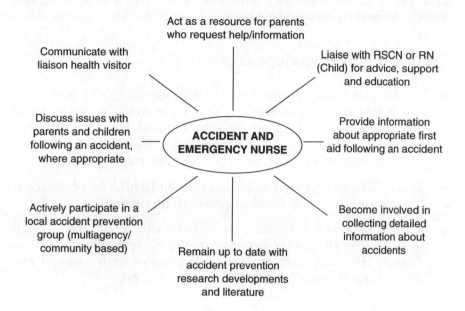

Act as a resource for parents
who request help/information

Communicate with
liaison health visitor

Liaise with RSCN or RN
(Child) for advice, support
and education

Discuss issues with
parents and children
following an accident,
where appropriate

ACCIDENT AND
EMERGENCY NURSE

Provide information
about appropriate first
aid following an accident

Actively participate in a
local accident prevention
group (multiagency/
community based)

Become involved in
collecting detailed
information about
accidents

Remain up to date with
accident prevention
research developments
and literature

Figure 8.4   Suggested strategies for A&E nurses to
become involved in accident prevention work

Conclusion

Providing evidence of the problem of childhood accidents is a vital step towards the development of accident prevention strategies. After their comprehensive review of accidents in children and adolescents, the NHS Centre for Reviews and Dissemination (1996, p. 12) recommended that:

> Community-based programmes should be based upon data derived from surveillance systems, they should target specific injuries and age groups and use these data systems to monitor the impact of the programme.

This recommendation reflects the ethos of this study. Being able to determine the details of accidents, their circumstances, causes and consequences from a variety of perspectives, for example behavioural, environmental and social, enables a specific, localised profile of children's accidents to be developed. Nurses working with children and their families in a variety of settings can then utilise this information to inform their work in terms of accident prevention and health promotion. Clinical practice will thus be underpinned by relevant, locally derived research evidence.

Proposed future developments

- To design a health promotion initiative involving different agencies working at various levels, that is, primary, secondary and tertiary, which is focused on issues raised from the original surveillance study. This will be developed within the framework of accident prevention projects already underway in the area.

- To explore the awareness of parents and children of accident prevention issues and accident prevention practices.

- To compare the accident surveillance and health promotion initiatives with similar projects in the West Midlands and in Europe. This will enable the consideration of both national and cross-cultural issues in accident prevention work.

References

Bentley J. (1996) 'Child-related services in general accident and emergency departments', *Journal of Advanced Nursing* **24**: 1184–93.

Child Accident Prevention Trust (1992) *The NHS and Social Costs of Children's Accidents: A Pilot Study*, London, CAPT.

Consumer Safety Unit (1996) *Report on 1994 Accident Data and Safety Research. Home Accident Surveillance System*, London, DTI.

Davis J. E. (1995) 'Children in accident and emergency: parental perceptions of the quality of care. Part 1', *Accident and Emergency Nursing* **3**: 14–18.

Department of Health (1992) *The Health of the Nation*, London, HMSO.

Department of Health (1995) *The Health of the Nation Key Area Handbook: Accidents*, London, HMSO.

Ferguson A. (1994) 'Child accident prevention as a health promotion issue – how extensive is the problem and how far have A&E departments responded to the recommendations made?', *Accident and Emergency Nursing* **2**: 193–9.

Hutchby P. (1996) *Report on the Public Health of Wolverhampton*, Wolverhampton, Department of Public Health.

Koren G., Carmeli D. B., Carmeli Y. S. and Haslam R. (1993) 'Maturity of children to consent to medical research: the baby-sitter test', *Journal of Medical Ethics* **19**(3): 142–7.

McClure R. J. and Burnside J. (1995) The Australian Capital Territory Injury Surveillance and Prevention Project', *Academic and Emergency Medicine* **2**(6): 529–34.

NHS Centre for Reviews and Dissemination (1996) 'Prevention of unintentional injuries in children and young adolescents', *Effective Health Care* 2(5): 1–16.

Office for Population Census and Surveys (1991) *Standard Occupational Classification*, London, HMSO.

Orzel M.-N. (1996) 'Injury minimisation programme for schools', *Accident and Emergency Nursing* 4: 139–44.

Peterson C. and Bell M. (1996) 'Children's memory for traumatic injury', *Child Development* 67: 3045–70.

Pless I. B. (1991) 'Accident prevention', *British Medical Journal* 303: 462–4.

Reynolds L. (1996) 'A qualitative evaluation of the post accident notification system to health visitors', *Journal of Advanced Nursing* 23: 97–105.

Rice C., Roberts H., Smith S. J. and Bryce C. (1994) 'Lay voices and professional research on child accidents'. In Popay J. and Williams G. (eds.) *Researching the People's Health*, New York, Routledge.

Roberts H., Smith S. and Bryce C. (1993) 'Prevention is better…' *Sociology of Health and Illness* 15(4): 447–63.

Roberts I. and Power C. (1996) 'Does the decline in child injury mortality vary by social class? A comparison of class specific mortality in 1981 and 1991', *British Medical Journal* 313: 784–6.

Sahlin Y. and Lereim I. (1990) 'Accidents among children below school age. Changes of incidence after intervention', *Acta Paediatrica Scandinavica* 79: 691–7.

Sahlin Y., Stene T. M., Lereim I. and Balstad P. (1990) 'Occurrence of injuries in a defined population', *Injury* 21: 155–7.

Sbaih L. C. (1997) 'The work of accident and emergency nurses. Part 1: An introduction to the rules', *Accident and Emergency Nursing* 5: 28–33.

Stilwell P. and Stilwell J. (1995) 'A locality focus on health for Wolverhampton', *Health and Social Care in the Community* 3: 181–90.

World Health Organization (1992) *International Statistical Classification of Diseases and Related Health Problems*, 10th Revision, Geneva, WHO.

Further reading

Dolan K. (1997) 'Children in accident and emergency', *Accident and Emergency Nursing* 5: 88–91.

Harker P. and Moore L. (1996) 'Primary health care action to reduce child home accidents: a review', *Health Education Journal* 53: 322–31.

Kendrick D., Marsh P. and Williams E. I. (1995) 'General practitioners: child accident prevention and *The Health of the Nation*', *Health Education Research* 10(3): 345–53.

Roberts I., Kramer M. S. and Suissa S. (1996) 'Does home visiting prevent childhood injury? A systematic review of randomised controlled trials', *British Medical Journal* 312: 29–33.

Towner E., Dowswell T., Simpson G. and Jarvis S. (1996) *Health Promotion in Childhood and Young Adolescence for the Prevention of Unintentional Injuries*, London, HEA.

9 Children's knowledge of their internal anatomy

Claire Gaudion

Introduction

Paediatric nurses have an essential role to play in the health education of sick and healthy children. Health teaching is inseparable from both family advocacy and children's rights. The Gillick judgement (Barnes, 1985) clarified the principle that parents have responsibility for their children rather than rights over them, and highlighted the concept of 'sufficient understanding' – that the child's knowledge of what is happening and of the consequence of their choices is critical if children are to be involved in decisions and consent to treatment.

An understanding of children's cognitive development, and how children perceive their internal anatomy, is of benefit when communicating with and teaching children of different ages (Eiser, 1984). Appropriate health education has the ability to allay anxiety and empower children and their families in an otherwise threatening and intrusive environment. For this to happen effectively, the explanations that are delivered must be understood by the listener, otherwise they are pointless. Paediatric nurses deal with a diversity of ages and cognitive abilities, so their approach to teaching and the provision of information must be individually tailored to meet the child's, or family's, educational needs. Developmental psychologists have discussed the use of guidance and prompting to enhance the level of knowledge that children can demonstrate (Vygotsky, 1978); however, limited nursing research has addressed this area. This study aims to gain an appreciation of children's knowledge of their internal anatomy and to explore methods of eliciting information from children.

Literature review

An extensive review of the literature regarding children's knowledge of internal anatomy led to three main discoveries. First, the published literature appears to extend over a wide period of time from Schilder

148

and Wechsler's (1935) study of internal anatomy to Badger and Jones' (1990) study of deaf and hearing children's conceptions of body interior, a minority of these studies having been published recently. Second, the actual number of studies concerned with children's knowledge of their internal body is limited. Finally, the literature provides evidence for the relationship between children's knowledge of internal anatomy, cognitive development and effective communication. This literature review aims to demonstrate these relationships and the need for this study, before briefly examining previous studies.

Much literature reflects the increasing concern of children's rights and suggests that true advocacy can only occur in an atmosphere of good communication. The Children Act 1989 (DoH, 1990) endorses the importance of obtaining children's views, and The Children's Charter (DoH, 1996) strongly reaffirms the responsibility of the children's nurse to provide appropriate explanations to children regarding health care. However, children's views and how they think and conceptualise remain ignored by some professionals (Pithers, 1994). Nurses may be too presumptuous in judging children's level of understanding before making an assessment, and consequently communication may occur at an inappropriate level (Eiser, 1984). Nurse–patient communication is notoriously difficult, the potential for misconceptions and inaccuracies being vastly increased when the patient is a child.

For nurses, an appreciation of how children think and conceptualise is an imperative aid to effective communication. Childhood cognition has received increased attention from developmental psychologists, notably Piaget and Inhelder (1969) and Vygotsky (1978). Numerous disparities between these developmental theories have been presented; pivotal to this study are their perceptions of childhood cognitive progression.

Piaget devised sequential stages through which he believed children progressed before attaining adult intelligence; although he insists that development is continuous, he does allow for the existence of these stages. Each stage leads progressively to the next so the order of the stages is the same for all children. The speed of movement is, however, definitely individual. Piaget rightly recognised that, irrespective of age or stage, children develop at an individual pace, a concept with which Vygotsky agrees. Piaget's views of 'learning' are, however, significantly less optimistic. He does not eliminate the possibility that specific attempts to teach children may make a difference, yet he believes that this process of maturation cannot be readily accelerated. More correctly, Vygotsky places more emphasis on the child's potential to improve given 'some slight assistance', the teacher maintaining the responsibility for determining what help is needed. This point is pivotal as each nurse's teaching role will be determined by which perspective influences his or her practice.

A limited number of studies have investigated what children know about their anatomy, with similar results. Unfortunately, many of the earlier writings were largely speculative and primarily reflected adults' beliefs about how children viewed their bodies rather than children's actual conceptions. Children's perceptions of anatomy and physiology were generally considered collectively, and most studies made comparisons between children of varying ages. This literature search revealed one study involving intervention strategies that compared two teaching modalities used in the instruction of internal body parts (Vessey, 1988) and literature that reviewed teaching children about their internal bodies (Vessey *et al.*, 1990). The main impetus for Vessey's study and discussion was the consideration of appropriate methodologies, language and timing, congruent with children's cognitive level and understanding. This pivotal study explored the use of a multisensory teaching method employing anatomical dolls, and a cognitive perceptual teaching approach using two-dimensional drawings. Post-testing using recall and recognition memory approaches was carried out 1–6 weeks after the intervention, the multisensory approach being shown to be significantly more effective.

A general consensus exists within the findings that children's knowledge of anatomy is greater with increasing age (Gellert, 1962; Kotchabhadaki, 1985). Investigations have suggested that children initially perceive their bodies to be composed of the heart, brain and bones (Porter, 1974; Brumback, 1977; Gibbons, 1985), especially regional structures such as the hips, arms and legs (Brumback, 1977). Any knowledge of the respiratory, gastrointestinal, reproductive or immune systems was less frequently indicated. Children were, however, familiar with the stomach and the lungs (Porter, 1974; Denehey, 1984).

Schilder and Wechsler's (1935) results suggested that children with a mental age of less than 11 years believed the inside of their bodies to contain food, Nagy's (1953) results agreeing with this. Children often believe that the body has inside it what we put inside it, demonstrating the concrete nature of children's thought. The studies that incorporated a drawing technique noted that despite being requested to mention internal parts of the body, a number of subjects also made reference to external features (Badger and Jones, 1990).

Contrary to earlier studies (Tait and Ascher, 1955), Gellert (1962) and Porter (1974) discovered that boys knew more body parts than girls. Porter, however, maintains that because the differences between each sex were slight, illogical or not maintained at every age level, the evaluation of these findings presents difficulties. McEwing (1996) also noticed distinct sex differences, boys always exceeding girls in their knowledge.

Although most studies reached some general agreements about children's knowledge, both Quiggin (1977) and Smith (1977) noted a wide variability in the level of knowledge that children displayed. They reported that this pervasive finding proves how explanations for children must be individualised to suit their understanding of their bodies.

Various methodological designs have been used in this field of study, yet they have been predominantly quantitative, the most popular methods being interviews and a projective drawing technique in which children were issued with an outline of a human figure and requested to draw in it what they perceived the body to contain. An earlier study describes a similar projective method but with the omission of a pre-drawn body outline (Tait and Ascher, 1955), although no rationale is given for the preference for either technique. A problematic feature of this method in terms of comparison with other studies, or an analysis of results, is the variation in size of the drawings when a standard body outline is not used. A further limitation of all existing studies is the absence of standardised scoring procedures. Researchers have failed to document exactly how all aspects of the drawings were objectively analysed (Porter, 1974; Quiggin, 1977). Porter (1974) observed that 'children were remarkably able to visualise and draw the internal parts of the body. Structures were drawn with accuracy and relatively proportionate.' Unfortunately, no description of how this conclusion was drawn is offered.

Eiser and Patterson (1983) attempted to resolve this dilemma of reliability, both authors independently coding the children's drawings. This method does not completely assure objectivity as there was a 94 per cent agreement rate between them and the remaining discrepancies needed to be resolved by discussion. This is of great significance to the present study.

A pertinent feature of Quiggin's (1977) study was the combined method used to enable a comparison to be made between the results of unprompted children (using the inside of the body drawing test) and the results obtained when knowledge was probed more deeply (using the inside of the body drawing test and a questionnaire). Unfortunately, no discussion of developmental theories is given to support the hypothesis, and it is not apparent why this dual method was chosen. The results fail to conclude whether one test was more productive than the other to elicit information; instead, Quiggin (1977) reported that the amount of information gained from one child using both methods together was greater than that obtained using one part alone. Perhaps no significant difference between the methods was discovered.

Methodology

A research statement, 'to investigate children's (aged 7–8) knowledge of internal anatomy and to demonstrate whether their knowledge differs between each sex', and a research question, 'can the use of prompting positively affect children's ability to demonstrate knowledge about their internal anatomy?', were proposed. The overall aim was to validate an instrument with which to measure children's knowledge of their anatomy – a standardised scoring procedure.

The sample comprised 20 healthy school children, aged 7–8 years old. Those excluded from the study were children outside this age group, children who did not have a written or spoken knowledge of the English language, children with learning difficulties and disabled children. This particular age group of children was chosen for two reasons. First, the children had not yet undergone any formal school teaching on internal anatomy, which would have interfered with results from differing schools. Second, children of this age are capable of expressing themselves verbally for the interview component of the study; Dale *et al.* (1980) and Piaget (1953) provide evidence to demonstrate that articulation skills are suitably developed as a vehicle for transmitting verbal messages when children reach approximately 7–8 years of age.

A randomised sample was thought to represent most closely the total population. Random stratification meant that schools could be chosen from differing geographical locations and an equal number of each sex could be incorporated. To select appropriate schools from varying socio-economic areas, a list of eligible primary schools was divided into two areas according to their rural–urban geographical location and to the resources available within the surrounding area. Four schools were selected. Within each school, the subjects were divided according to their sex, so that an equal number of each sex would participate in the study. The researcher then selected every xth boy and then every xth girl to obtain five subjects from each school.

Although the number of subjects was small ($n = 20$), Polit and Hungler (1991) suggest that when the researcher has reason to believe that the independent and dependent variables are strongly interrelated, a relatively small sample is generally adequate to demonstrate the relationship statistically.

Informed consent was obtained from the parents and assent from the children. The local research ethics committee and head teachers of each school granted ethical approval.

Two research tools were used for collecting the data. First was the unprompted technique, which incorporated a 'projective' drawing method. The second technique was the prompted technique, conducted as individual interviews and using a life-size anatomical rag doll created by the researcher (Figure 9.1). Both methods consider evidence from the literature, stating that 7- and 8-year-olds can begin to make sense of internal body systems only if physical models and pictures allow them to 'see' inside the body (Lieberman *et al.*, 1992).

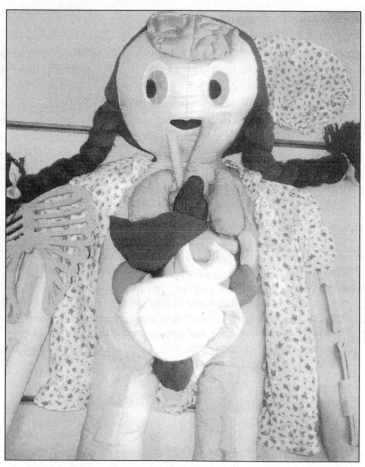

Figure 9.1   Anatomical rag doll (photograph by author)

The unprompted technique

A body outline was issued to each child, and they were asked to draw and label 'everything they could think of that was inside their bodies'. The data were collected in a classroom environment, and the children were allowed 15 minutes to complete the task. This projective drawing technique is a simple method for measuring psychological attributes and is particularly useful when investigating children. The technique takes advantage of children's creative ability, imaginary nature and desire to draw. Most importantly, this technique was used to obtain information from children who were entirely unprompted.

The prompted technique

The rag doll was used in combination with individual interviews. All the organs were removed from the rag doll prior to the interview. The child was asked a series of questions (Figure 9.2) and, in response to each question, was expected to name internal body parts. These parts were then handed to the child to position on the rag doll. Following each interview, the rag doll was photographed. The photograph was than enlarged so that the results from both techniques could be scored using the same standardised method. The questions were devised to represent each of the main physiological systems of the body.

What pumps your blood to every part of your body?
When you breathe in, where does the air go?
Where does your food go when you have swallowed it?
Which parts of your body help you to break down and mix food?
Where do you store your 'wee' before you go to the toilet?
What allows your body to move and stops you from being 'wobbly'?
Where are your memories and where do you do your thinking?
Are there any other parts of the body that you have not mentioned
that you can think of?

Figure 9.2   Interview schedule

The rag doll was made by the researcher to serve as a representation of the human figure, similar to the body outline. The rag doll needed to be unique enough to capture the child's interest, and realistic to avoid creating false impressions, but not so much so that it frightened the child. The internal parts were created out of different coloured fabrics to distinguish easily between them. In addition, the rag doll reached a height of approximately 125 cm and was therefore large enough for the children to compare the parts with their own bodies.

A repeated measure design, in which each subject participated in both parts of the study, enabled a more auditable comparison to be made. There were two main reasons for altering the data collection instruments used within each part of the study. First, the subjects might have become bored, and second, if a drawing technique had been used for both parts, the children might have been tempted to redraw the same organs for the second part of the study.

Grid scoring system

The researcher, in order to ensure that the measuring process was consistent in every instance, devised a standardised grid scoring system. A standard-sized grid was maintained for each internal part, with different scores in each compartment of the grid for each organ. The allocated scores referred to the position of the body parts, each organ scoring a maximum of 5 points for correct positioning. A higher score thus represents a more accurate response. Because each internal part occupies an individual place in the body, separate scoring grids were created for each one.

Accurate positions of internal organs were confirmed using anatomical textbooks. Transparencies were prepared for each internal part named by the subjects to superimpose upon each drawing or photograph. The photographs representing the completed versions of the rag doll were enlarged, and the scoring grid was accurately scaled to match.

The position of an organ was scored according to the location of the most central point; should the centre fall on a compartment margin, a half score was awarded. The subjects were supposed to label every item they drew, and consequently any unlabelled items were ignored. Paired organs, for example the lungs and kidneys, were considered separately. However, when only one of the paired organs was represented, it was assumed that it was positioned on the correct side; if two were positioned on the same side, one was presumed to be correct and the other, accordingly, scored lower.

The criteria used in this study to decide whether an item such as a joint should be considered as internal or external was that any label that only reached the body margin was considered to be external; if the label pointer extended into the body outline, the item was considered to be internal.

Internal parts that are not confined to a specific location but are distributed throughout the body, for example the veins and muscles, were automatically scored 5 points. Additionally, accessory organs (such as the teeth, tongue and tonsils) were awarded 5 points if they were shown within the region of the head and neck. Bones were scored slightly differently. When the correct number of bones was positioned within a region (for example, the upper and lower arm or leg), the maximum score was allocated, crediting the child for his or her knowledge of the limb joints.

Data analysis and results

Following the transformation of the raw data into numerical form using the grid scoring system, the findings were analysed in two parts. Part 1 addressed the research statement, and Part 2 presented a comparison of the prompted and unprompted techniques used. A mean of 7.4 parts was known by the respondents (Table 9.1), a slight difference being demonstrated between the knowledge of girls and of boys (mean 7.9 for girls and 6.9 for boys). This difference was not, however, significant. A total of 26 different internal parts were referred to overall, but the maximum number that was mentioned by any individual subject was 13, the minimum being 2.

Table 9.1   Number of internal parts mentioned

	Girls	Boys	All	Unprompted	Prompted
Mean number of internal parts	7.9	6.9	7.4	5.8	9.1
Maximum	13	11	13	11	13
Minimum	2	4	2	2	4

The most commonly named internal parts were the heart (100 per cent), the brain (82.5 per cent), the arm bones (82.5 per cent) and the leg bones (85 per cent). However, the lungs (60, left, and 57.5 per cent, right), stomach (60 per cent), oesophagus (37.5 per cent) and rib bones (42.5 per cent) were also mentioned quite frequently.

The children's knowledge of the position of internal parts was analysed from two different aspects. First, their knowledge of position was evaluated for each internal part. Second, the researcher focused on the children's knowledge of position for all the internal parts collectively, producing an overall score for each child.

The internal parts positioned correctly the most frequently were the heart (94.5 per cent), the brain (82.5 per cent), the arm bones (60.5 per cent), the leg bones (63 per cent) and the lungs (52.5 per cent). However, the stomach (39 per cent) and the oesophagus (31 per cent) also obtained relatively high position scores. From the overall scores for each child, a comparison could be made of boys' and girls' knowledge. The descriptive statistics were subjected to statistical analysis using t-tests and confirmed the results to be insignificant.

Mean position scores for the unprompted (26.0) and prompted (38.5) groups (scored according to the grid scoring system) produced descriptive statistics. The differences between groups were confirmed using paired t-tests and showed the results to be extremely significant, demonstrating a confidence interval of 99 per cent. The mean number of internal parts was also clearly higher when children were prompted (9.1 compared with 5.8 unprompted; see Table 9.1 above) so the original research question was clearly 'supported'.

To summarise, the findings of this study were:

- The children appear to have demonstrated a standard of knowledge that is congruent with previous research.
- The children's knowledge appears to be extremely varied and individual, even within a limited age range.
- The children demonstrate a higher standard of knowledge when prompted.

Discussion

Congruent with these earlier studies, children appear to be most knowledgeable about the heart, brain and limb bones (Porter, 1974; Brumback, 1977; Gibbons, 1985). The lungs, stomach, oesophagus and rib bones were also well represented. The internal parts that scored most positively may reflect children's appreciation of the importance of these parts to body functioning, although this was not investigated. Children may develop an understanding of these internal parts first reflecting their sensorimotor and then their concrete thinking, as described by Piaget and Inhelder (1969). For example, children develop an awareness of their hearts because of the sensory stimulation of their hearts beating, and a knowledge of their bones through touch and self-exploration.

Many children acknowledged that their bodies contained a stomach (60 per cent) but were unable accurately to position it (39 per cent); they knew that food must be contained somewhere but were unsure of the exact location. Schilder and Weschler (1935) suggested that children believe their bodies to contain what they put inside them and what they know comes out. These simplistic views represent their concrete thought; moreover, the ability of some children to discuss more complex aspects of internal phenomena reflects the beginnings of abstract thinking (Lieberman *et al.*, 1992).

There was considerable variation in the accuracy of the responses obtained from each child, affirming the concept of individuality recognised by developmental theorists. The researcher speculates that these variations in children's knowledge may be influenced by the environmental sources from which children develop their perceptions. This finding may be attributed to the availability of educational literature, reading books and general children's television programmes; cartoons especially have a tendency to use skeletons, reinforcing children's knowledge of their bones, as demonstrated by the results of this study. Quiggin's (1977) study also acknowledged a substantial variation between the standard of answers obtained from the individual children.

In response to the research question, the mean number of internal parts was clearly higher when the children were prompted (9.1) than unprompted (5.8), despite the range being equal. A dramatic increase in the frequency with which individual organs were mentioned, between the unprompted and prompted techniques, was apparent: internal parts such as the penis and rectum were only noted in the unprompted responses, possibly because of the intimate nature of these parts. Although the penis protrudes externally from the body, it is referred to as an internal organ because its associated anatomy extends internally. Perhaps the children were more likely to mention these organs 'privately' on the drawing than verbally during the interview, which may have caused embarrassment. Other parts, such as the teeth and tongue, which were not referred to during the prompted technique, could be explained by the presence of the facial features on the rag doll, so the children did not feel it necessary to mention them again. The intestines and kidneys were only named by the respondents when they were prompted, which demonstrates that children already possess the knowledge but are better able to elicit it with further guidance.

Children whose knowledge was prompted were capable of scoring substantially higher than when they completed the projective drawing technique. The findings of this study vindicate Vygotsky's concept that 'able instruction' has the potential to enhance children's understanding. Indeed, this notion is pivotal to the nurse's role as an educator: our ability to elicit knowledge from children will determine the quality of each child's experience.

Limitations of the study

The study encompassed some limitations within each methodological component. The sample studied was unfortunately small as the amount of time needed to collect the data was considerable and a smaller sample prevented extensive classroom disruption. A few schools denied access because of their busy calendars, further reducing the sample size. Problems have been identified with fully disclosing the nature of the study when requesting informed consent as this can distort and misdirect the results of a study, either consciously or subconsciously. However, the extent to which this influenced these findings cannot easily be determined.

The data collection method used in this study may be heavily criticised as the use of two research tools introduces an additional variable and subsequently eliminates experimental control. Nevertheless, the use of a single method may have produced invalid results, as previously discussed. The researcher is also aware that the results in the prompted technique may have been affected by the child's previous experience of undertaking the unprompted test. However, both tests were carried out during the same morning for each school, thus minimising the time for conferring and questioning.

The accuracy of the projective drawing method has been debated. It has been suggested that children's inborn artistic abilities vary greatly, which would affect their ability to demonstrate their understanding. This study followed guidance provided by Cratty (1977), who demonstrated that drawing is a valid and accurate means of obtaining data from children aged 7–8 years.

The scoring grid used to interpret the children's responses was accurately reduced to suit the size of the photographs of the rag doll, but the data collection tools (the drawings and the rag doll) were actually different sizes. The larger surface area of the rag doll provided an increased opportunity for error when positioning the organs. This was not a problem as the results demonstrated more positive scores for the prompted technique; hence the increased chance of error indicates that children displayed an even better knowledge when prompted. The size of the rag doll may have also positively affected the results. The 'life-size' appearance may have encouraged a more accurate perception of internal anatomy on the part of the children as they were able to relate the rag doll to their own bodies. The close proximity of the desks meant that some discussion and copying was inevitable, despite close supervision and requesting the children to 'hide' their work and work in silence. Within each class, additional instructions contributed by the teachers varied so some children were unfairly advantaged.

Conclusions and recommendations

The limitations of this study reduce the substantive and statistical significance of the findings, and restrict the potential for generalisation of the findings. Nevertheless, this pilot study can offer significant and practical recommendations regarding the nursing care of children. Importantly, the advantages of prompting children are advocated. Until we have gained an accurate appreciation of what children know, education cannot be delivered effectively. Not only is it essential to educate children about health in a correct manner, but also the way in which knowledge is obtained from children (or how we assess their knowledge) can have a huge impact on the results. The methods employed in this study could be adapted for use in clinical practice in order to gain an insight into children's conceptions of their internal anatomy.

The wide range of responses obtained from such a limited age group demonstrates that the knowledge that individuals possess can vary immensely, emphasising the importance of individual assessments of knowledge and tailored teaching strategies based on the children's experience, age and ability.

The contribution of a reliable tool for measuring children's knowledge of their internal anatomy will hopefully benefit further studies, and the study overall may be valuable in generating further research. Clearly, the importance of communicating information and emphasising the need to probe children's knowledge accurately to assess that knowledge must not be underestimated. Paediatric nurses have an essential role as children's advocates, and as information giving has been suggested to be the key to empowerment (Campbell and Glasper, 1995), this study should assist paediatric nurses in their pursuit of children's advocacy.

References

Badger T. A. and Jones E. (1990) 'Deaf and hearing children's conceptions of the body interior', *Pediatric Nursing* 16(2): 201–5.

Barnes A. (1985) 'After Gillick – the implications for nursing', *Professional Nurse* 1(3): 79.

Brumback R. A. (1977) 'Characteristics of the inside-of-the-body test drawings performed by normal school children', *Perceptual and Motor Skills* 44: 703–8.

Campbell S. and Glasper E. A. (1995) *Whaley and Wong's Children's Nursing*, London, C. V. Mosby.

Cratty B. (1977) *Perceptual and Motor Development in Infants and Children*, New York, Macmillan.

Dale S., Nader P. R. and Hymovich D. P. (1980) 'Middle childhood'. In Hymovich D. P. and Chamberlin R. W. (eds) *Child and Family Development: Implications for Primary Health Care*, New York, McGraw-Hill.

Denehey J. (1984) 'What do school-age children know about their bodies?', *Pediatric Nursing* 10(4): 290–2.

Department of Health (1991) *An Introductory Guide for the Children Act, 1989*, Lancashire, DoH.

Department of Health (1996) *The Patient's Charter: Services for Children and Young People*, London, HMSO.

Eiser C. (1984) 'Communicating with sick and hospitalised children', *Journal of Child Psychology and Psychiatry* 25(2): 181–9.

Eiser C. and Patterson D. (1983) '"Slugs and snails and puppy-dog tails" – children's ideas about the inside of their bodies'. *Child: Care, Health and Development* 9: 233–40.

Gellert E. (1962) 'Children's conceptions of the content and functions of the human body', *Genetic Psychological Monographs* 65: 293–411.

Gibbons C. L. (1985) 'Deaf children's perceptions of internal body parts', *Maternal-Child Nursing Journal* 14(4): 37–46.

Kotchabhdaki P. (1985) 'School-age children's conceptions of the heart and its functions' (Monograph 15), *Maternal Child Nursing Journal* 14: 203–69.

Lieberman L. D., Clark N. M., Krone K. V., Orlandi M. A. and Wynder E. L. (1992) 'The relationship between cognitive maturity and information about health problems among school age children', *Health Education Research* 7(3): 391–401.

McEwing G. (1996) 'Children's understanding of their internal body parts', *British Journal of Nursing* 5(7): 423–9.

Nagy M. H. (1953) 'Children's conceptions of some bodily function', *Journal of Genetic Psychology* 83: 199–216.

Piaget J. (1953) *The Origins of Intelligence in Children*, London, Routledge & Kegan Paul.

Piaget J. and Inhelder B. (1969) *The Psychology of the Child*, New York, Basic Books.

Pithers D. (1994) 'Acting fair (Children Act, Advocacy)', *Nursing Times* 90(8): 32.

Polit D. F. and Hungler B. P. (1991) *Nursing Research: Principles and Methods* (4th edn), Philadelphia, J. B. Lippincott.

Porter C. S. (1974) 'Grade school children's perceptions of their internal body parts', *Nursing Research* 23(5): 384–91.

Quiggin V. (1977) 'Children's knowledge of their internal body parts', *Nursing Times* 28: 1146–51.

Schilder P. and Wechsler D. (1935) 'What do children know about the interior of the body?', *International Journal of Psychoanalysis* 6: 355–60.

Smith E. C. (1977) 'Are you really communicating?' *American Journal of Nursing* Dec.: 1966–68.

Tait C. D. Jr. and Ascher R. C. (1955) 'Inside-the-body-test', *Psychosomatic Medicine* 17(2): 139–48.

Vessey J. A. (1988) 'A comparison of two teaching methods on children's knowledge of their internal bodies', *Nursing Research* 37(5): 262–7.

Vessey J. A., Braithwaite K. B. and Wiedermann M. (1990) 'Teaching children about their internal bodies', *Paediatric Nursing* 16(1): 29–33.

Vygotsky L. S. (1978) *Mind in Society*, Cambridge, MA, Harvard University Press.

Further reading

Eiser C., Patterson D. and Eiser J. R. (1983) 'Children's knowledge of health and illness: implications for health education', *Child: Care, Health and Development* 9: 285–92.

Hall D. (1991) *Health for All Children: Report of the Third Working Party on Child Health Surveillance*, Oxford, Oxford University Press.

Thompson S. W. (1991) 'Communication techniques for allaying anxiety and providing support for hospitalised children', *Journal of Child and Adolescent Psychiatry* 4(3): 119–22.

Webber I. (1995) 'Reaction of the family and child to illness and hospitalisation'. In Campbell S. and Glasper A. (eds) *Whaley and Wong's Children's Nursing*, London, C. V. Mosby.

10 Can information leaflets assist parents in preparing their children for hospital admission?

Karen J. Stone

Introduction

This chapter discusses the findings and implications of a small undergraduate study designed to investigate the perceived usefulness of an information leaflet entitled 'Preparing your child for hospital: a parents' guide'. The study was carried out in a combined child and adult ear, nose and throat (ENT) unit to which children are admitted for elective surgery. A leaflet was developed and appropriately field-tested before being mailed to a group of parents for evaluation. Data were subsequently collected, an analysis of which demonstrated considerable parental satisfaction with the information contained in the leaflet. The results of this small study indicate that a well-designed information leaflet showing the importance of pre-admission preparation for children will assist and encourage parents to prepare their child for hospitalisation.

Background

The Patient's Charter: Services for Children and Young People (DoH, 1996a) highlights the importance of information giving to families with children in hospital. The focus of this study was to develop and evaluate the usefulness of an information leaflet designed for parents that was related to the psychological preparation of children prior to admission for elective surgery.

At the time of this study, children were admitted for ENT surgery to a combined unit catering for adults as well as children, with no provision of pre-admission preparation. The advantages of pre-admission preparation to a child's psychological wellbeing were investigated by reviewing the available literature and attending a pre-admission programme developed in the child health directorate of the same hospital. It was felt that children who were to be admitted for ENT surgery should also be provided with the opportunity to experience the benefits of pre-admission preparation. With the limited resources available, the most appropriate and realistic way of offering pre-admission preparation appeared to be by means of a family information leaflet.

Many hospitals send out leaflets to patients undergoing an elective admission. It has been repeatedly demonstrated, however, that these leaflets lack adequate advice for parents about preparing their child for hospital (Stewart, 1984; Muller *et al.*, 1992). For this reason, there was a need to develop a leaflet with the specific intention of informing parents about the psychological preparation of their child for hospital admission and elective surgery.

Review of the literature

The literature was reviewed in three distinct domains, which were believed to be central to the proposed area of study:

- Information giving to children and their families
- The preparation of children for hospital admission
- The design and production of family information leaflets.

The giving of information to children and their families

Giving information to children and their families has become an integral part of the philosophy of paediatric nursing. The sharing of relevant knowledge and information is now accepted as a fundamental right and valued as good caring practice (Robertson, 1995). This philosophy, among others, is reflected in, for example, the Department of Health (DoH) publications *The Welfare of Children and Young People in Hospital* (1991), *The Patient's Charter: Services for Children and Young People* (1996a) and *Child Health in the Community: A Guide to Good Practice* (1996b).

A number of authors describe the provision of information as being central to family empowerment (Coombes, 1995; Swanwick, 1995; Browne *et al.*, 1996). Empowerment in a broad sense can be described as a process of helping people to assert control over the factors that affect their lives and thus Gann (1990) states that information giving is the key to empowerment. If this is true, empowerment cannot occur in ignorance, so nurses should attempt to provide families with the relevant and appropriate information. Being in possession of information will assist parents and children to understand fully the care they receive, enabling them to achieve a sense of control. Information can help parents and children to feel like equal partners in care provision. However, partnership in care is only possible when parents and children are fully informed and their needs recognised.

The provision of information plays a key role in family-centred care. The sharing of unbiased and complete information with parents about their child's care on an ongoing basis in an appropriate and supportive manner is one element of family-centred care described by Shelton *et al.* (1987). Birch (1993) emphasises that the need for effective communication between health professionals, children and their families is vital to the success of family-centred care and ultimately the welfare of the child. It can, therefore, be suggested that readable and comprehensible information leaflets, as an effective way of communicating, have a role to play in promoting family-centred care.

Parental dissatisfaction with information provision

Although giving information is viewed as commendable, Bradford and Singer (1991) have shown that parental dissatisfaction is often associated with a perceived lack of information and emotional support.

Ball *et al.* (1988) carried out a small study in Southampton in which 35 parents were questioned about their views of their children's nursing care using a questionnaire, the results of which showed that parents were overall generally satisfied with the care that they and their children had received. However, these authors reported that one area of care with which parents were not fully satisfied was that of information giving, several questions included in the questionnaire being specifically targeted to this subject. The results showed that some parents did not understand what doctors had told them and felt uncomfortable asking questions. In addition, some parents found that the information given to them was not always consistent. The authors state that comments to open-ended questions also reflected a need for more information, and in light of this, nurses should be encouraged to give parents more information, both formally and informally.

While and Crawford (1992) conducted a small study to investigate
the experiences of 10 children admitted for day surgery. The main
results indicated that the provision of more information needed to be
addressed in order to improve standards of care. Although the study
was of a small scale, it demonstrates the need for effective and reassuring information giving to parents.

Collectively, the studies by Ball *et al.* (1988), Bradford and Singer
(1991) and While and Crawford (1992) highlight the fact that
increased consumer satisfaction with care can be achieved by the
improved provision of information to both parents and children.
Information leaflets are one medium that can be used to package
such information. In the child health domain, information leaflets
have an important role to play in achieving the goal of improved
information provision for parents.

One particular area in which parents are requesting information is
in relation to how they can best prepare their child for hospital admission. Shelley (1992) analysed 82 telephone calls and letters received
from parents at the Action for Sick Children's national office. The
results of this audit showed that 28 per cent of these parents wanted
information on preparing their child for hospital admission.

Preparing children for hospital admission

The pioneering work of psychologists James Robertson (1958) and
John Bowlby (1960) first led to the recognition that children might
suffer psychological trauma during a stay in hospital. The importance of the psychological preparation of children for hospitalisation
and surgical intervention is now well recognised within child health
nursing and is considered a vital element of care (Eiser, 1990; Bailey,
1992; While, 1992).

Visintanier and Wolfer (1975), in testing variations of psychological preparation and supportive care designed to increase the adjustment of children (and their parents) hospitalised for elective surgery
($N = 84$), showed that children who had received psychological
preparation were significantly less upset and more co-operative. In
addition, their parents reported significantly greater satisfaction and
less anxiety than did children or parents in the control groups.

Other more recent studies confirm these results. Bielby (1984)
describes the work of the Royal National Throat, Nose and Ear
Hospital, which developed and evaluated the film *Marc Goes to
Hospital* as a method of preparing children for ENT surgery. The
results showed that children who had received some form of prepara-

tion achieved lower scores on fear-related variables and required less post-operative analgesia than did those children in the control group who had received no preparation. Post-hospitalisation, children who had undergone preparation were less behaviourally disturbed, made an earlier physical recovery and returned to school sooner than the children in the control group. The mothers of children in the preparation group were more satisfied with hospitalisation than were those in the control group.

A similar study was carried out by Adams *et al.* (1991) in Birmingham. In response to the results of a parental questionnaire, which showed dissatisfaction with the routine admission procedure, a booklet was developed that parents could use to help to explain hospital procedures to their child. Twenty children were allocated to a control group, receiving routine verbal information, and 20 children to an experimental group, being given the booklet. The results of the study showed that children who had been prepared for surgery using the booklet showed less anxiety overall than did the children who had not received the booklet, these children also showing significantly less anxiety while in theatre. Children who received the booklet had fewer problems when they returned home, and their parents were significantly more satisfied with the care provided by the hospital.

Both of these studies were carried out in specific hospitals evaluating specific preparation procedures, and the fact that both sets of results support the idea that 'pre-admission preparation enables a child to cope more positively with hospital exhibiting less anxiety and fewer behavioural problems after discharge' suggests that this theory can be applied generally to paediatric nursing. This argument is supported by other papers describing interventions in practice to provide pre-admission preparation, for example Glasper and Stradling (1989).

Children's concepts of hospital and illness

One major argument put forward to support pre-admission preparation is that it allows the opportunity to correct children's misconceptions about hospital and illness.

Perrin and Gerrity (1981) asked 128 healthy children attending kindergarten up to eighth grade standardised questions about illness. The responses that the children gave were recorded and scored according to Piaget's theoretical framework of cognitive development. The results showed that although the response varied widely at all ages, there was a systematic progression in the children's under standing of illness-related concepts with age. The findings of Perrin and Gerrity (1981) have been replicated by numerous other studies, for example Brewster (1982) and Bibace and Walsh (1980). All of these studies showed that children below the age of 5 frequently believe that illness may be attributed to disobedience and be a form of punishment.

Internal mechanisms are hard for children to imagine. Eiser and Patterson (1983) asked 26 children at each of four age levels (6, 8, 10 and 12 years) to draw the insides of their bodies and answer some questions on body organisation and function. The results showed that knowledge increased with age. The children's responses to questions about how their bodies worked revealed some basic misunderstanding and errors. Explanations of function tended to focus on the external, visible aspects, with considerable confusion over what took place inside.

Swanwick (1995) states that children perceive the body in a global way and as a surface entity; for example, the cause of illness is where the pain presents on the surface of the child's body. Sharman (1985) suggests that children below the age of 8 describe body parts as simply being necessary for life, with a high proportion of 4-year-olds believing that they cannot live without their tonsils.

It is important for nurses to have an understanding of children's concepts of health, illness and the insides of their bodies in order to inform the content of pre-admission preparation. Explanations can be given to the child based on concepts with which they are familiar and able to understand. The misconceptions that children hold, for example that illness is a punishment and that children cannot live without their tonsils, can be corrected.

Children's concepts of hospitals, what doctors do and what medical treatment involves have been shown to be based on quite distorted views. Brewster (1982) studied a group of 50 chronically ill hospitalised children aged between 5 and 12 years. Their results showed that children below the age of 10 may believe that doctors and nurses deliberately hurt them, and below 7 years of age medical procedures are viewed as a punishment. Numerous other studies have investigated children's thoughts about hospital; Eiser (1990), for example, states that children under 5 years of age may think that hospitals are a place where people go to become ill rather than to get better. Children can also believe that admission to hospital can last for years rather than days or weeks (Eiser, 1987).

Pre-admission preparation provides the opportunity for children to explore their beliefs about hospitals and medical procedures with an adult who can correct the child's misconceptions by providing information. As a result, the child can feel reassured about the intent and purpose of hospital admission.

Who should prepare children for hospital admission?

A review of the pertinent literature reveals that parents are the most suitable people to tell children about hospitals (Rodin, 1983; Stewart, 1984). Parents have a unique knowledge of their child's individuality. While accurate information can be provided by hospital staff, parents have the ability to interpret this information and to tailor it to suit each individual child. This view formed the reasoning behind this particular study, which aimed to design a pre-admission leaflet for parents.

Preparing children for hospital admission using information leaflets

Pre-admission leaflets are mailed out by many hospitals and have become a recognised tool in preparing children for hospitalisation. The adequacy and effectiveness of some of these leaflets may, however, be questioned. Many leaflets are not specifically written for child patients and their parents, and few give information that can help parents to prepare their child for hospital (Muller *et al.*, 1992; Glasper and Thompson, 1993). An evaluation by Stewart (1984) of 22 pre-admission leaflets identified that only one contained a section for parents related to preparing their child for hospital admission.

Methodology

The aim of the study

The primary aim of this small study was to design and evaluate an information leaflet to help parents to prepare their child for elective admission to hospital and surgical intervention.

The design and production of information leaflets

The design of a leaflet is of major importance if the intended objectives are to be met. Information leaflets have been shown to fail in their intended purpose because of inappropriate or missing content, the degree of readability and poor layout and presentation (Albert and Chadwick, 1992; Sturmey, 1993; Robertson, 1995). The effectiveness of writing does not end with the words put on paper, but also depends on how attractively the words are packaged (Cox, 1989).

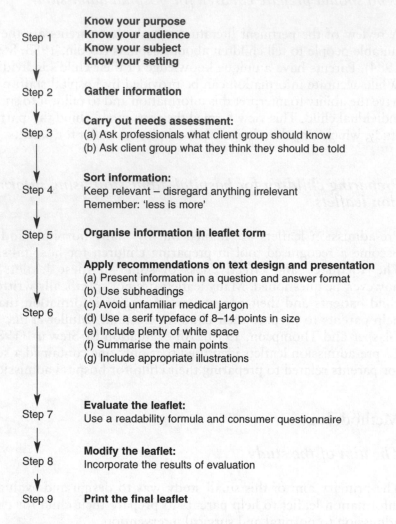

Step 1   **Know your purpose**
          Know your audience
          Know your subject
          Know your setting

Step 2   **Gather information**

Step 3   **Carry out needs assessment:**
          (a) Ask professionals what client group should know
          (b) Ask client group what they think they should be told

Step 4   **Sort information:**
          Keep relevant – disregard anything irrelevant
          Remember: 'less is more'

Step 5   **Organise information in leaflet form**

Step 6   **Apply recommendations on text design and presentation**
          (a) Present information in a question and answer format
          (b) Use subheadings
          (c) Avoid unfamiliar medical jargon
          (d) Use a serif typeface of 8–14 points in size
          (e) Include plenty of white space
          (f) Summarise the main points
          (g) Include appropriate illustrations

Step 7   **Evaluate the leaflet:**
          Use a readability formula and consumer questionnaire

Step 8   **Modify the leaflet:**
          Incorporate the results of evaluation

Step 9   **Print the final leaflet**

Figure 10.1   Flow chart to summarise the recommended
steps for designing a family information leaflet

There are many papers that discuss techniques for the effective writing of patient information materials (Wong, 1989; Glasper and

Burge, 1992; Nancekivell, 1995). These papers were utilised in order to create a step-by-step approach for the design of information leaflets (Figure 10.1).

The content of a leaflet

Before putting pen to paper, would-be leaflet designers must consider the message that is to be conveyed to the reader (Nancekievell, 1995). It is recommended that all the information required should be gathered from an appropriate source. Glasper and Burge (1992) suggest that a prudent exercise to undertake is a needs assessment, which involves finding out what the experts think the client group should know, followed by finding out what the client group think they should be told. The material gathered must then be organised into a logical order and a rough draft of the final product created. The content must be current and up to date and written material should contain only essential relevant information, interesting but irrelevant details being omitted (Wong, 1989). The reader should be informed adequately but not overloaded with a lot of 'nice to know' as opposed to 'need to know' facts. The key to memorability is simplicity, the operating principle being 'less is more'.

Text design and presentation

Many authors make practical suggestions for text design and presentation; these are summarised in step 6 of Figure 10.1.

Readability of information leaflets

Readability formulae have been advocated by a number of authors for assessing and evaluating the readability of family information leaflets (Deller and Walker, 1994; Arthur, 1995). Readability formulae were originally designed as 'predicative averages' to rank the reading difficulty of books used in a specific grade at school (Pichert and Elam, 1985). These formulae generally involve counting the length of sentences, the number of polysyllabic words and/or the number of words considered to be unfamiliar to a standard population (Pichert and Elam, 1985). Examples of readability formulae are the Spache grade level score, FLESH, FOG and SMOG (Spadero, 1983).

Several limitations of readability formulae have been documented. They fail to take into account all the variables influencing reading difficulty, including content presentation, organisation and sentence complexity, the reader's background knowledge and reader interest (Wong, 1989). For these reasons, a readability formula should not be the sole medium of assessment to indicate the readability of an information leaflet.

Piloting a leaflet

Piloting a leaflet is an important part of its production. Authors advocate that a leaflet should be piloted using the client group for whom it is intended and modified accordingly (see, for example, Glasper and Burge, 1992). Discrepancy has been documented between the professional's view of the family's needs for information and their actual needs (Campbell *et al.*, 1993; Coulter and Koester, 1985). Piloting a leaflet can help to guard against this. It is essential that material is reviewed by the families for whom it is intended in order to ensure it has fulfilled their needs and is presented in an appropriate form (Campbell *et al.*, 1993).

Evaluating a leaflet

Having designed a family information leaflet, the final stage of its production is evaluation. Arthur (1995) refers to the *Patient's Charter*, which indicates that patient information should be clear and comprehensible. Furthermore, unless written information is evaluated, health professionals are not fulfilling the obligations of the *Patient's Charter*. In reality, patient education material is often not evaluated. If this is the situation, it cannot be determined whether the education material designed has met the needs of the patient group for whom it was intended.

Designing the parent information leaflet

The leaflet 'Preparing your child for hospital: a parents' guide' (Figure 10.2) was designed by following the steps outlined in Figure 10.1 above. A review of the literature relating to the psychological effects of hospitalisation on a child, children's thoughts about health and illness, and preparation techniques informed the content of the

Figure 10.2 A copy of the leaflet used in the main study, 'Preparing your child for hospital. A parent's guide'

Why should I prepare my child?

-To help your child cope with their stay in hospital.

-To help your child feel less frightened.

-To help your child to understand why they are going to hospital.

-To correct any wrong ideas your child may have about hospital.

NAME: _____ WARD: _____

Nameband

What common fears do children have about hospitals?

-Fear of being in a strange place.

-Fear of separation from family.

-Believe that doctors and nurses may hurt them

-That a stay in hospital is a punishment for being naughty

How can I prepare my child?

-Tell your child a few days before or when you feel it is appropriate, that they are going to hospital to have an operation.

-In a simple way explain what the operation is for, that it will make something better.

-Tell your child that they will have a 'special hospital sleep' while they have their operation.

-Tell your child they may have pain after their operation which can be made to go away by medicine.

-Always tell your child the truth, do not lie to them, e.g. that something will not hurt when it might.

-Encourage your child to express their feelings.

-Only tell your child that you will stay with them while in hospital if this is what you are going to do.

-Involve brothers and sisters so they know what is happening

-Do not let your child see your own anxieties as this may make them more frightened.

What activities may help me to prepare my child?

Drawing and painting.
This can help your child to show many of their feelings.

Books.
Reading a book about 'going to hospital' with your child can help them to feel more confident.

Games.
Playing 'hospital games' using toys and dressing up clothes can help your child to act out their fears and concerns.

Talking.
Listen to your child and be alert for any wrong ideas they may have.

These activities can help your child to ask questions about their visit to hospital. Answer them in a truthful and simple way.

Figure 10.2 (cont'd)

Preparing Your Child For Hospital.
A Parent's Guide.

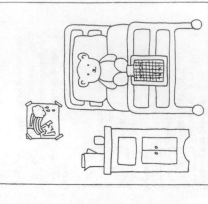

This leaflet aims to answer the questions you may have about preparing your child for a stay in hospital.

Try to arrange a visit to the ward a few days before your child's operation if you feel this will help your child. This can make you and your child feel happier about their admission to hospital.

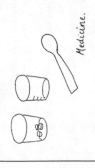

Medicine.

Remember,

-**Prepare** your child as much as you can, the best way is by giving them **information.**

-In a simple and **truthful way tell** your child what is **happening.**

-Try to be involved in **your child's care** as much as possible.

If you have any questions please contact the ward where your child is going to stay.

Ward:

Tel:

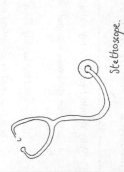

Stethoscope.

leaflet. A preliminary draft of the leaflet was formatted incorporating the information acquired through the literature review.

In addition to the literature review, a needs assessment was conducted to ascertain what information professionals thought parents should be given. Informal, unstructured interviews were carried out with four nurses and the Director of Education, who worked in a local school. Each professional was asked to comment on the draft leaflet and give ideas for how it could be improved. Responses were recorded and the leaflet changed to incorporate the comments given.

Attention was next paid to text design and presentation, implementing the advice presented in the literature. Further modifications were made to the leaflet (Stone, 1994/95).

Subjecting the leaflet to SMOG testing

The leaflet 'Preparing your child for hospital: a parents' guide' (Figure 10.2) was subjected to SMOG testing to give an indication to the author of the reading ability that was required to read and understand the leaflet. This formula was selected as it was suggested by the literature reviewed to be the easiest and most accurate method (Wong, 1989), one based on 100 per cent comprehension (Spadero, 1983). Table 10.1 outlines the steps to be taken when subjecting literature to SMOG testing.

Table 10.1   Steps taken when subjecting literature to SMOG testing

Step 1	Count 10 consecutive sentences at the beginning, middle and end of the material (total = 30). A sentence is any list of words ending in a full stop, a question or an exclamation mark
Step 2	Count every word of three or more syllables in the 30 sentences. If a word is repeated, count the repetition too
Step 3	Obtain the nearest square root of the number of three or more syllable words
Step 4	Add three to the square root. This gives you the SMOG grade, that is the reading age expressed as a school grade

Adapted from McLaughlin (1969).

The results showed that the reading ability required to read the leaflet mirrors that of a ninth grade student, which is the equivalent of 12 years of age. To ensure that the highest percentage possible of the intended target group of readers can read and understand an information leaflet, it is best to make it as simple as possible. Couchman and Dawson (1992) suggest, however, that the average reading age in the UK might be as low as 9 years of age.

A survey of parent views of an information leaflet designed to assist parents in preparing their child for hospital

The study took place in an ENT unit in a general hospital over a period of 3 months. The study was descriptive, comprising a small-scale survey. A parental questionnaire was the chosen method of data collection, which ensured that the leaflet was evaluated from the consumers' point of view. A discrepancy has been documented between the professional's views of the family's need for information and their actual needs (Campbell et al., 1993, Coulter and Koester, 1985). It is essential that information material is reviewed by the families for whom it is intended in order to ensure that it has fulfilled their needs in an appropriate form (Campbell et al., 1993). This gives further support to the use of a parental questionnaire as a data collection tool.

An initial pilot study was carried out to determine that the questionnaire designed was clearly worded, that all possible answers had been catered for and to see whether it generated the type of information envisaged. The pilot study also provided an opportunity to pre-test the leaflet and identify any necessary alterations. Six parents on the ENT ward where the main study was to be carried out were given a copy of the leaflet during the post-operative period and asked to complete a questionnaire.

For the main study, 40 copies of the leaflet were sent to parents with the initial letter informing the parent of the date for their child's ENT surgery. During the child's post-operative period, parents who had received the leaflet were asked whether they would be willing to complete a questionnaire. The final sample size consisted of only 16 parents, attributable to cancelled operations and parents not being resident on the ward during the times of data collection.

Results of the parental survey

Sample characteristics

The children of the parents included in the study were aged between 3 and 13 years, eight being boys and eight girls. Seven of the children had previously been admitted to hospital.

Leaflet design

Parents were asked several questions relating to the overall design of the leaflet. The responses are summarised in Table 10.2.

These results suggest that, overall, parents liked the way in which the leaflet was designed, being easy to read and understand. This concurs with advice given within the literature reviewed relating to leaflet design.

Table 10.2 Parental responses to questions relating to the design of the leaflet

	Number		Percentage	
Question	Yes	No	Yes	No
Did you find the leaflet easy to understand?	16	0	100	0
Is the leaflet set out in a way that makes it easy to read?	16	0	100	0
Would it be better to present the information using cartoons?	4	12	25	75
Do the pictures go with the text?	13	1	*	*
Would you prefer more pictures?	3	13	*	*
Is the typing big enough?	15	1	94	6

* Percentages were not calculated as two respondents did not answer these questions.

Content of the leaflet

The main content of the leaflet was organised as a question and answer format into four sections:

- Why should I prepare my child?
- What common fears do children have about hospitals?
- How can I prepare my child?
- What activities may help me to prepare my child?

A Likert-type scale containing both positively and negatively worded statements was constructed to examine parental opinion about the value of each section within the leaflet. The results are presented in Table 10.3.

Table 10.3   Parental opinion of the value of each section within the leaflet

Statement	Response*			
	SA	A	D	SD
The information contained within the leaflet about why I should prepare my child for hospital was not helpful (–ve)	0	1	10	5
It was helpful to have a list of common fears children have about hospitals (+ve)	6	9	1	0
I did not find the advice relating to specific ways in which I could prepare my child for hospital admission valuable (–ve)	0	0	14	2
The suggestions within the leaflet concerning activities that parents can use to prepare their child, such as the use of games and books, were generally helpful (+ve)	3	12	1	0

* SA, strongly agree; A, agree; D, disagree; SD, strongly disagree.
(–ve) = negatively worded statement, (+ve) = positively worded statement.

It can be said of the above results that parents generally agreed that each of the four sections was necessary and satisfactorily written, being of help and value in assisting them to prepare their child for admission to hospital.

Preparation methods used by parents

The majority of parents (15) felt that the leaflet gave them an informed choice to decide how to prepare their child for hospital admission. All the parents stated that they had prepared their child. The age of the child influenced the method of preparation used by the parents, the most popular methods being talking and using books (Table 10.4). Younger children preferred talking, drawing and painting, school-age children books and role play, and teenagers talking. These results fit with the recommendations made within the literature that the method of preparation must be age appropriate.

Table 10.4   Preparation methods used by parents

Methods of preparation	Times used	
	Number	Percentage
Talking	8	50
Talking and books	4	25
Talking and games	1	6
Talking, drawing and painting	1	6
Talking, books, games, drawing and painting	1	6
Talking, books, games and role play	1	6

The age groups for whom the parents believed the leaflet was most suitable

Parents were asked to comment on which age group of children they felt the leaflet could particularly benefit. Their comments suggested that the leaflet would be of most benefit to parents whose children were aged between 3 and 12 years. In practice, it would be more feasible to distribute a leaflet routinely to all parents regardless of their child's age, making the administration process simpler.

Discussion of the results of the parental survey

Parents were asked to comment on how beneficial they felt the leaflet was for themselves and their children. Results showed that all parents felt that the leaflet was either beneficial or very beneficial. The aim of the leaflet was to educate parents on how they could prepare their child for hospital. With the knowledge obtained by reading the leaflet, the majority of parents (15) felt that they were in a position to be able to choose and decide how to prepare their child. In light of this, it can be said that the leaflet assisted in the empowerment of parents. All parents stated that the leaflet should continue to be distributed before the child's admission to hospital. This reflects the need identified within the literature reviewed of parents wanting to receive more information on preparing their child for hospital admission (Shelley, 1992; Coombes, 1995).

Parents were asked to indicate discrepancies in the leaflet and whether there were ways in which it could be improved. Their answers gave concrete suggestions for additional content and for improvements of the overall presentation. It was suggested that information should be included about parental involvement in care and facilities on the ward for parents, for example that parents could accompany their child to the anaesthetic room and that fold-up beds were provided, enabling parents to sleep next to their child.

Collectively, the results of the parental questionnaire illustrated that the leaflet did help parents to prepare their child for elective admission to hospital; it can thus be said that the aims of the study had been met.

Limitations of this study

Several limitations to this study have been identified. The success of the leaflet in preparing the child for hospital requires much interaction between the parent and the child, the quality of which will clearly always be variable. The availability of resources to the parents, for example time and materials such as books and drawing and painting equipment, as well as the parent–child relationship, will influence the quality of the interaction. Future research could probe and explore more deeply the way in which parents prepare their children.

Developing an additional leaflet aimed directly at the child may help to decrease this dependency on the interaction between parent and child. However, the cognitive abilities of children differ in accordance with their age. Therefore, several leaflets would have to be developed pitched at different age levels. Despite this, the addition of such a leaflet may assist parents in preparing their child by providing a focal point from which to begin the preparation process.

The non-experimental design of this study does not allow inferences to be made regarding the significance of these findings, but it is recognised that non-statistically significant results can have practical implications within the field of nursing (Burns and Grove, 1993). In the case of this study, it was the parents' views of a leaflet that were being investigated. Views can not always be expressed as quantitative data, but this does not mean that they hold no value. The views of the sample of parents included in this study have indicated that a leaflet has been designed that helps parents to prepare their child for hospital admission. All the parents included in this study stated that they felt that distribution of the leaflet should continue.

Implications and recommendations for clinical practice

1. *A thorough investigation into the presentation of information and effective writing skills resulted in the production of a leaflet that all parents included in this study found easy to understand.*
    The steps followed in designing the leaflet have been seen to be effective. They can provide a useful protocol for developing future family information leaflets and will help to guard against poor design. SMOG testing provides a useful indication of how difficult a leaflet is to read. A questionnaire for consumers ensures that the leaflet has fulfilled their needs in an appropriate form, helping to prevent any discrepancy between the professional's view of the family's need for information and their actual needs.

2. *The content of the leaflet 'Preparing your child for hospital: a parents' guide' was helpful and valuable in assisting parents to prepare their child for hospital admission*
    Having received and read the leaflet, parents were placed in a position to choose and decide how to prepare their child. It can be said that the leaflet did meet a parental need for advice

related to preparing a child for hospital, as identified by Stewart (1984), Shelley (1992) and Coombes (1995).

3. *The leaflet 'Preparing your child for hospital: a parents' guide' has been shown to be a useful pre-admission tool*
   In practice, such leaflets are easy to administer and relatively cheap to produce. It must, however, be remembered that although leaflets can be supplied, a nurse cannot 'make' a parent read or carry out the suggestions within it. A leaflet can only attempt to improve the pre-admission preparation that a child receives.

4. *The visual appeal of the leaflet 'Preparing your child for hospital: a parent's guide' could be improved by high-quality printing*
   The printing of the leaflet on high-quality paper, and the addition of coloured illustrations, would make the leaflet more visually appealing. In practice, however, restrictions on the print quality that can be achieved result from limited financial resources.

Creating and developing an information leaflet that meets an identified need within a clinical setting is an intervention that can lead to improved satisfaction with care and family empowerment. The methodology used in this study can provide helpful guidance for nurses working within different clinical settings so that they can develop and create family information leaflets that reflect the identified information needs of children and their families.

Conclusion

The results of this small study have indicated that a well-designed leaflet can help parents to prepare their child for elective admission to hospital. The step-by-step approach used in the design of this leaflet is an effective protocol that can be followed for future documents. The use of a parental questionnaire for data collection ensured that the leaflet met the needs of the parents for whom it was intended, enabling them to prepare their children for hospital admission.

References

Adams J., Gill, S. and McDonald M. (1991) 'Reducing fears in hospital', *Nursing Times* 87(1): 62–4.
Albert T. and Chadwick S. (1992) 'How readable are practice leaflets?', *British Medical Journal* 305(6864): 1266–8.

Arthur V. A. M. (1995) 'Written patient information: a review of the literature', *Journal of Advanced Nursing* 21(6): 1081–6.

Bailey R. C. (1992) 'Children in theatre: meeting their needs', *British Journal of Theatre Nursing* 2(3): 4–8.

Ball M., Glasper A. and Yerrell P. (1988) 'How well do we perform? Parents' perception of paediatric care', *Professional Nurse* 4(3): 115–18.

Bibace R. and Walsh M. (1980) 'Development of children's concepts of illness', *Pediatrics* 66(6): 912–17.

Bielby E. (1984) 'A childish concept', *Nursing Mirror* 159(18): 26–8.

Birch E. (1993) 'The key to real partnership. The importance of parent information', *Child Health* 1: 25–6.

Bowlby J. (1960) 'Separation anxiety', *International Journal of Psychoanalysis* 41: 89–113.

Bradford R. and Singer J. (1991) 'Support and information for parents', *Paediatric Nursing* 2(4): 18–20.

Brewster A. B. (1982) 'Chronically ill hospitalised children's concepts of their illness', *Pediatrics* 69(3): 355–62.

Browne D., Campbell S., Glasper E. A. and Glasper J. (1996) 'Pursuing strategies of patient empowerment – a preliminary evaluation of CD-ROM generated health promoting information system', *Southampton Health Journal* 12(1): 38–43.

Burns N. and Grove S. K. (1993) *The Practice of Nursing Research, Conduct, Critique and Utilization* (2nd edn), Philadelphia, W. B. Saunders.

Campbell S., Kelly P. and Summersgill P. (1993) 'Putting the family first', *Child Health* 1(2): 59–63.

Coombes R. (1995) 'From parent to expert', *Child Health* 2(6): 237–40.

Couchman W. and Dawson J. (1992) *Nursing and Health Care Research*, London, Scutari Press.

Coulter D. L. and Koester B. S. (1985) 'Information needs of parents of children with epilepsy', *Journal of Development and Behaviour of Pediatrics* 6(6): 334–8.

Cox B. G. (1989) 'The art of writing patient education materials', *American Medical Association* 4: 11–14.

Deller R. and Walker J. (1994) 'Evaluating advice booklets for parents', *Health Visitor* 67(12): 421–3.

Department of Health (1991) *The Welfare of Children and Young People in Hospital*, London, HMSO.

Department of Health (1996a) NHS: *The Patient's Charter: Services for Children and Young People*, London, DoH.

Department of Health (1996b) *Child Health in the Community: A Guide to Good Practice*, London, DoH.

Eiser C. (1987) 'What children think about hospitals and illness', *Professional Nurse* 3(2): 53–4.

Eiser C. (1990) *Chronic Childhood Disease. An Introduction to Psychological Theory and Research*, Cambridge, Cambridge University Press.

Eiser C. and Patterson D. (1983) 'Slugs and snails and puppy dogs tails: children's ideas about the insides of their bodies', *Child Care, Health and Development* 9: 233–40.

Gann R. (1990) 'Patient information', *Health Libraries Review* 7(4): 233–6.

Glasper E. A. and Burge D. (1992) 'Developing family information leaflets', *Nursing Standard* 6(25): 24–7.

Glasper E. A. and Shadling P. (1989) 'Preparing children for admission', *Paediatric Nursing* 1(5): 18–20.

Glasper E. A. and Thompson M. (1993) 'Preparing children for hospital'. In Glasper E. A. and Tucker A. (eds) *Advances in Child Health Nursing*, London, Scutari Press.

McLaughlin G. (1969) 'SMOG grading – a new readability formula', *Journal of Reading* 12: 639–46.

Muller D. J., Harris P. J., Wattley L. and Taylor J. D. (1992) *Nursing Children. Psychology, Research and Practice* (2nd edn), London, Chapman & Hall.

Nancekivell S. (1995) Guidelines for writing parent/patient materials. Unpublished internal document, Toronto, Editorial Services, Hospital for Sick Children.

Perrin E. C. and Gerrity P. S. (1981) 'There's a demon in your belly: children's understanding of illness', *Pediatrics* 67(6): 841–8.

Pichert J. W. and Elam P. (1985) 'Readability formulas may mislead you', *Patient Education and Counselling* 7: 181–91.

Robertson J. (1958) *Young Children in Hospitals*, New York, Basic Books.

Robertson L. (1995) 'The giving of information is the key to family empowerment', *British Journal of Nursing* 4(12): 692.

Rodin J. (1983) *Will this Hurt?*, London, RCN.

Shelley P. (1992) 'Finding out what parents want', *Action for Sick Children, Cascade* Jul.: 4–5.

Shelton T., Jepson E. and Johnsen B. (1987) *Family-centred Care for Children with Special Health Care Needs*, Washington, DC, Association for the Care of Children's Health.

Spadero D. C. (1983) 'Assessing readability of parent information materials', *Pediatric Nursing* 9(4): 272–8.

Stewart A. (1984) 'Prepared for parting', *Nursing Mirror* 159(17): 15–18.

Stone K. J. (1994/5) 'Preparing your child for hospital: a parent's guide', *Child Health* 2(4): 165.

Sturmey P. (1993) 'The readability and human interest of information leaflets from major British charities: an unintelligible boring replication', *Mental Handicap Research* 6(2): 174–83.

Swanwick M. (1995) 'Power where it belongs. Empowerment in child health', *Child Health* 2(6): 232–6.

Visintanier M. N. and Wolfer J. A. (1975) 'Psychological preparation for surgical pediatric patients. The effects on children's and parents' stress responses', *Pediatrics* 56(2): 187–201.

While A. (1992) 'Day case surgery', *Maternal and Child Health* 19(6): 184–6.

While A. and Crawford J. (1992) 'Paediatric day surgery', *Nursing Times* 19(6): 184–6.

Wong P.C. (1989) 'Write, right', *Canadian Nurse* 85(2): 28–30.

11 Promoting adolescent sexual health: enhancing professional knowledge and skills

Rachael L. Smith

Introduction

This chapter explores the role of health professionals in promoting sexual health and briefly reviews the literature examining aspects that influence young people's sexual knowledge, skills and behaviour, as well as the role of the nurse as a sexual health promoter. A small-scale research study is described that utilised a qualitative approach to explore further the development of young people's sexual health by interviewing a sample of student nurses. Findings and possible implications for a number of health professionals are discussed.

Health promotion and education are viewed as important areas related to the health of children; as such, they are an integral part of the role of health professionals. Children and young people should have a right to be cared for holistically as unique individuals. These are belief statements with which few health professionals would disagree, particularly as adult health status is likely to be greatly influenced by the healthy, or unhealthy, habits and lifestyles laid down in childhood and adolescence. However, providing holistic care for this client group should include the important area of sexual health. Health professionals who work with young people have a responsibility and role in the promotion of sexual health and the provision of health education.

The reality for many health professionals is that opportunities to engage in sexual health promotion or education may not happen every day. Thus, developing and maintaining skills and competence in this domain may not be easy. Recognising opportunities when they do occur may be a necessary first step. Developing the ability and skills to meet such challenges is also vital. Not to do so could be considered to be professional negligence.

This chapter explores some of the issues related to the promotion of adolescent sexual health. It gives an overview of a small research study undertaken in partial fulfilment of a MA in Education (Smith, 1995) and draws upon the extensive literature in this area, as well as on the tentative conclusions from this small study, in order to discuss possible implications for clinical and educational practice. The partnership between clinical practitioners and educational colleagues in developing expertise and skills in this important aspect of professional practice is endorsed in all the implications discussed.

It is important to highlight that the study was undertaken in partial fulfilment of a Master's programme. As such, certain boundaries were applied, not least in ensuring it was a manageable research project completed in the given time limit. The author acknowledges that the focus of heterosexuality and the consideration of the female perspective may be limiting to the breadth of understanding required.

The need for sexual health promotion

It is well recognised that rewarding personal and sexual relationships promote health and wellbeing but that sexual activity can also have undesired consequences, such as unwanted pregnancy and the transmission of human immuno-deficiency virus (HIV) and other sexually transmitted diseases (STDs) (DoH, 1993a). HIV infection presented perhaps the greatest new public health challenge of the twentieth century. Preventing its transmission depends upon lifestyle behaviour, which for some may require sustained changes. First sexual intercourse, at whatever age, has health implications by marking the initiation into sexual activity, which, if unprotected, carries the risks identified. Furthermore, cervical carcinoma is known to be associated with age at first intercourse as well as with the number of sexual partners, the incidence now increasing, with presentation at a younger age (Curtis *et al.*, 1988). The possible sequelae associated with STD infection, such as ectopic pregnancy and infertility, are also well documented (Svenson *et al.*, 1992).

Scally (1993) suggests a national objective in order to ensure that when young people reach maturity, they possess the knowledge and skills to enable them to deal confidently with their sexuality and to avoid the undesirable consequences of sexual intercourse. Kasen *et al.* (1992) assert that the goal should be to empower young people with the tools necessary to exercise control over risk-related behaviours and to build self-confidence that these tools can be used effectively, even in difficult situations.

Literature review

There is extensive literature related to adolescent sexual health, the following being a brief highlight of some key sources. Readers wishing to explore the literature more fully may find the review and analysis undertaken by Smith (1997a, b) a helpful starting point.

Acquiring sexual health knowledge and skills

The importance of school sex education is stressed by Green and Delaney (1994) and Scally (1993). Studies have demonstrated marked variations in sex education, and young people have often expressed disappointment with its content and delivery (Curtis *et al.*, 1988; Woodcock *et al.*, 1992a). The minimal success in changing behaviour as a result of traditional sex education in British schools is highlighted by Mellanby *et al.* (1995). The relationship of parents and significant others to the development of sexual knowledge, skills and attitudes has been the focus of a number of studies (Allen, 1987; Curtis *et al.*, 1988; Woodcock *et al.*, 1988b; Prendergast, 1992), which highlight the difficulties for parents and the influence of peers and siblings.

The British National Survey has recently reported data on sexual activity and age of first sexual activity (Wellings *et al.*, 1994). The importance of young people being able confidently to access contraceptive advice and/or contraceptives has been stressed (Allen, 1991; RCOG, 1991; Peckham, 1992; Scally, 1993). An important aspect to be explored in considering young people's ability to access advice and manage their own sexual health is decision making linked to self-efficacy.

Rational decision making versus self-efficacy

Are decisions concerning sexual behaviour always based on a rational decision-making process? The notion of rationality in relation to sexual behaviour has been discussed by a number of authors (Fishbein and Ajzen, 1975; Loewenstein and Furstenberg, 1991; Petosa and Jackson, 1991; Ingram *et al.*, 1992; Ingram, 1993). The consensus of opinion is that theories of rational decision making alone have little to offer to our understanding of adolescent sexuality.

A key concept in Bandura's (1989) social learning theory is self-efficacy. This central and pervasive personal mechanism concerns people's beliefs regarding their capability in exercising control over events affecting their lives. Studies have applied and explored the theory in relation to adolescent sexuality (Breakwell *et al.*, 1991; Rosenthal *et al.*, 1991; Basen-Engquist and Parcel, 1992; Kasen *et al.*, 1992). Kasen *et al.* call for the link between self-efficacy and behaviour to be exploited in programmes related to sex education rather than offering just the more traditional knowledge-only approaches. Building confidence in mastering skills and appraising confidence with each new situation or role that arises is seen as crucial to exploiting this link.

A feminist analysis exploring the differential power base inherent in heterosexual relationships has been explored (Ingram *et al.*, 1991; Holland *et al.*, 1991, 1992; Aggleton and Kapila, 1992). The authors claim that it is males who call the tune and take the lead role in determining outcomes, women adopting a subordinate sexual role. They raise questions on how safer sexual practices can be promoted within a gendered relationship and how young women can be helped to develop assertiveness and negotiation skills.

Professional role

Nurses, midwives and health visitors have a mandate to be involved with sexual health education and promotion (DoH, 1993b). The evidence suggests, however, that there are perceived difficulties in undertaking this role (Webb, 1985; Akinsanya and Rouse, 1991; Russell, 1992; McHaffie, 1993). Several writers emphasise that nurses, as representative individuals of the general population, are also learning about their own sexuality and coming to terms with this (Savage, 1987; Holly, 1989; Davidson, 1990; Russell, 1992).

The research study

As noted in the introduction, a brief overview of the research study undertaken by the author is offered. My interest in the topic area stemmed from the professional need as a lecturer in child health to include adolescent sexual health in the curriculum, as well as an awareness that many nursing recruits have not long passed through their adolescent years. Furthermore, developing sexual health/identity can be viewed as a lifelong process.

The aims of the study were therefore two-fold. The first was to explore possible factors that influence the development of a select sample of young people's sexual health (the select sample being a group of young recruits into nursing). The second was to develop an understanding of young nurses' feelings with respect to a professional sexual health promotion role.

The subjects of the study were young adults (18–20 years of age) from one cohort of students within the first 3 months of a pre-registration Diploma in Nursing Sciences 3-year programme. Within the age range specified, there were a possible 48 subjects, five of whom were male, reflecting the female domination of such courses. The intention was to have a stratified sample, all five males being invited to participate and 20 females being randomly selected.

Approval to approach eligible students was gained from the Head of School, and the whole cohort was seen by the researcher to give a brief introduction to the study and to herself as the researcher. Contact with the subjects was made through a personal letter with a return slip to indicate consent. Only one male consented, and it was thus deemed necessary to withdraw the male from the main study. Eighteen female subjects agreed to participate. These subjects were contacted by telephone to arrange an interview time at an acceptable venue where privacy could be assured. Recognising the potential sensitivity of the study, the occupational health department was contacted to act as a referral source.

The study adopted a qualitative approach, the data being collected by semi-structured individual interviews, the questions of which arose from a theoretical framework derived from the literature. The research design needed to find ways of collecting descriptions while preserving the spontaneity of the subjects' lived experiences (Oiler, 1982). It was recognised that the researcher's own set of preconceptions and experiences could influence the way in which the subjects described their experiences and the way in which the data were used, interpreted and analysed. The ability to 'bracket', enabling the researcher to 'intuit' from the data, was seen as a key skill (Oiler, 1982; Beck, 1992) . This involves:

> Looking at the experience with wide open eyes, with knowledge, facts, theories held at bay; concentrating on the experience is absolutely necessary. (Oiler, 1992, p. 180)

The aim of the study was to elicit not personal sexual histories from the subjects but instead the experiences of developing sexual health knowledge and skills. The interview schedule thus consisted mainly of a set of open-ended questions, with a proposed sequence and identified prompts, to allow flexibility to probe for more depth, remove any misunderstandings and to encourage co-operation and rapport between the interviewer and participant (Cohen and Manion, 1989). A 'conversation with a purpose' style was adopted, requiring the facilitating skills of the interviewer (Baker, 1991) while eliminating cues that would lead the participant to respond in a particular way (Robson, 1993).

A pilot study, consisting of the first four conducted interviews, was undertaken to validate the interview questions and to evaluate the researcher's performance as an interviewer. As with the main study, the audiotaped interviews were transcribed verbatim. An analysis of the transcripts indicated that the tool was reliable. However, some changes in the wording of the questions and more explicit prompts were made to ensure that the subjects were questioned on the same key areas, thus as much as possible eliminating researcher bias. The interview technique and the questions were re-examined to ensure that, as far as possible, neither would direct respondents towards socially desirable responses, thus reducing the potential for subject bias.

The main study was conducted with 14 subjects. The interview consisted of three main question areas. The first asked subjects to reflect on their formative years to consider how they learnt about sexual matters. The prompts referred to school sex education, home life and other people or agencies who were significant in their learning.

The second question area asked about relationship skills, with the aim of exploring some of the complex issues related to sexual self-efficacy and the empowerment of young women within heterosexual relationships. The potentially more sensitive nature of this was recognised, and thus a form, derived and adapted from a sexual self-efficacy scale cited by Rosenthal *et al.* (1991), was used. The items on the form were preceded by the statement 'Young people need to be able to...', in order to allow the subjects to answer generally about young people as a whole. The items related to buying condoms and/or contraceptives; discussing their use with a potential partner; carrying a condom around with them 'just in case'; discussing with a partner the use of a condom for AIDS protection when other means of contraception were being used; and refusing a sexual advance by their partner.

The final question area focused on the subject's perceived role as a nurse. The script introducing the question acknowledged that nurses probably spend more time than any other health care worker with patients, and it could, therefore, be suggested that nurses should have a role in helping patients with their sexual health needs. The subjects were asked whether they had considered this aspect of the nurse's role before starting their course and what they felt about having such a role, particularly with young clients.

The transcribed audiotapes were replayed several times in order for the researcher to become immersed and 'extraordinarily familiar' with the data (Field and Morse, 1985). Robson (1993) argues that, unlike quantitative data, there is no clear and accepted set of conventions for the analysis of qualitative data; they must, however, be dealt with systematically. The content was analysed to connect themes to the literature wherever possible.

The findings are briefly discussed under three headings.

Reflection on the learning process

Overall, the findings of how the subjects remembered learning about sexual matters supported the literature (Curtis *et al.*, 1998; Woodcock *et al.*, 1992b). All 14 subjects were able to cite some memories of sex education in their secondary schooling. While the amount and content were variable, it was generally considered to be limited, with a predominant biological focus, some inclusion of contraception and contraceptives and a small amount of discussion related to contemporary and moral issues.

The 1993 Education Act removed work on AIDS, HIV, STDs and aspects of human behaviour other than the biological from the Statutory Orders for Science (Green and Delaney, 1994). For the subjects in this study, who were in secondary education before the Act became mandate, it would appear that the small amount of sex education was indeed biological, to the exclusion of other important aspects associated with the development of sexuality and health.

For these subjects, the teaching methods used in school sex education were mainly didactic and teacher centred. The use of videos was poorly evaluated, and the descriptions gave evidence of their inappropriate content and use as a teaching tool. The teacher's skill of facilitation was questioned as a result of a perceived embarrassment about the topic area. This was directly linked to disruptive classroom behaviour, which was viewed as a hindrance to learning. The few subjects who spoke more positively of their sex education identified the teacher's ability as being crucial to a satisfactory programme. This included an ability to be open about sexual matters, treating pupils like adults and always answering questions. The need to start sex education earlier was supported by the majority of subjects.

The part played by the subjects' home life in learning about sexual matters supports that where parents play an active part, it is predominantly the mother who undertakes the teaching of daughters. Just under half of the subjects spoke very positively of their mother's role. An equal number were less positive, two being adamant that their mothers played no part. These two subjects were from families in which the parents were separated or divorced, which the subjects felt was an important factor. Just as teachers who were embarrassed were rated low in their ability, parents similarly viewed as such were not considered able to cope with this part of the parental role. In this study, fathers appeared to take no part or a significantly lesser role. How the relationship between the mother and daughter influenced the daughter's sexuality and the weak correlation of fathers' sexual attitudes to their daughters' sexual development was noted by Yaber and Greer (1986).

The role of friends in learning about sexual health issues was stated as discussing and chatting about sexual matters, learning thus being seen as more informal. Half of the subjects were unsure that this informal talking could be equated to actual learning. This possibly refutes Allen's (1987) belief that friends are considered to be a main source of sex education for teenagers, and supports Curtis *et al.* (1988), who state that friends discuss relationships rather than actually gaining knowledge from each other.

Thirteen out of the 14 subjects had not consulted, while at school, a general practitioner (GP) or family planning clinic (FPC) for advice or help to do with sexual matters. The reasons given for not consulting a GP were male gender and older age as well as a perceived potential lack of confidentiality. The main reason for not consulting an FPC was a lack of awareness of the services available.

Relationship skills

The data revealed considerable consensus from the subjects regarding the skills that young people need to develop, particularly the importance of learning to talk, communicate and discuss issues with the opposite sex. These were seen as fundamental to building a relationship. There was a link between learning to relate to the opposite sex in terms of asserting one's individual rights, and the notion of trusting one's partner. The complex nature of building relationships was explored by some of the subjects.

The findings from the items on the form, aimed at exploring perceptions related to sexual self-efficacy, demonstrated the complexity of developing relationship skills. Four out of the five items evoked predominantly positive responses from the subjects. It was agreed that young people need to be able to purchase contraceptives, although the difficulty of actually buying condoms and the possible labelling of a girl if she did were seen as deterrents. There was a perception on the part of some subjects that this was easier for boys, who might be considered to be acting responsibly by buying them. Curtis *et al.* (1988) and Small *et al.* (1993) highlight the potential for dual standards between the expected behaviour of girls and that of boys.

The need to discuss the use of contraceptives with a potential partner was recognised as a necessity, as was the need to discuss the use of condoms when other contraceptives were being used. However, the difficulty for a female in raising the issue of condom use, particularly if she were on the 'pill', was not dismissed lightly. It was also agreed that a young person should be able to refuse a sexual advance by a partner, but this was again qualified by perceived difficulties. The findings support the literature (Holland *et al.*, 1992; Ingram *et al.*, 1992) that young women can potentially find negotiating sexual safety difficult, which may be indicative of the differential power base inherent in heterosexual relationships, as discussed by Ingram *et al.* (1991), Aggleton and Kapila (1992) and Holland *et al.* (1991, 1992).

The item on the form evoking the most varied response was that young people should be able to carry condoms around with them 'just in case'. The range from full agreement to definite disagreement was indicated. However, a frequent comment referred to what this would say about the girl's willingness to have sex and the reputation she would get. The findings suggest that, even knowing that sexual intercourse may and can take place when it has not been planned, the negative response to a female who is prepared with a condom 'just in case' outweighs the likelihood of her taking such action.

There is a suggestion in the findings that young people perceive that they cannot be helped to develop relationship skills and that learning can only really occur through 'trial and error'. This expressed belief was accompanied by the acknowledgement that a 'trial and error' approach to learning can lead to serious mistakes. In addition, young people need to develop self-confidence and assertion skills, and there is a need for cultural change, leading to a more open climate in terms of being able to talk about and discuss sexual matters.

The role of the nurse

The majority of the subjects had not considered that helping patients with their sexual health needs was part of a nurse's role. Only two subjects stated they had thought about this aspect before starting their course and gave examples relating to the sexual health needs of clients with learning disabilities.

The findings also indicate some perceived uncertainty over whether the nurse does have a role in helping patients with their sexual health needs or what such a role would entail. Some subjects acknowledged that it is probably part of the role of the nurse but stated that their current knowledge and skills would be inadequate to fulfil such a role. The subjects' perceptions of a professional sexual health role with young people revealed that well over half of them believed that this might not be as difficult as with older people, the similarity in age being seen to be an advantage. Some subjects identified that young people may favour asking young nurses and target them for advice because of the similarity of age.

A few subjects explored the possible difficulties of this role and that undertaking it, particularly with young patients, required the development of professional skills as well as the meeting of personal needs. This was expressed in a variety of ways, such as exploring personal perceptions and possible hang-ups, developing an understanding of other people's lifestyles and not allowing personal opinions to cloud one's professional judgements. One subject also spoke of the potential sexual factor in the nurse–patient relationship, which she recognised as implicit and needing professional skills to handle.

The majority of the subjects spoke of the need to ensure that their knowledge was sound and accurate, mainly expressed in terms of factual, biological knowledge. Some subjects felt that there should be a compulsory part of the course that revisited the basic biological knowledge that might have been missed in their initial education. A few spoke of the need to go beyond the basic facts and develop knowledge related to wider concepts such as sexual practices, homosexuality and sexuality in general. The importance of developing communication skills in order to undertake a sexual health role was raised by a large number of subjects.

Just under half of the subjects spoke of the need to have awareness of their own sexuality in order to help others. Many, whether in relation to the development of communication skills or the need to explore sexuality, identified the need for small groups to facilitate this type of learning.

Discussion and implications for practice

The learning process

The findings of this study regarding how young people gain sexual health knowledge and skills appear to support much of the literature. School sex education, which has the potential to be an important avenue for young people to learn and master sexual skills, fell short of this goal for the majority of subjects. The findings suggest that, for these young people, the opportunity for school sex education to play a significant part was missed or at least not fully exploited.

The RCOG report (1991) states that health authorities should provide separate and comprehensive sexual health services for young people. The findings of this study may suggest that, even if such services were available, these young people were unaware of them or how to access them. One subject stated that even in the school of nursing and midwifery, information related to the nearest FPC was not readily available. For many, starting a nursing course may be the first occasion of living away from home, allowing newfound freedom. Providing information, within the school of nursing and midwifery, on contraception services and the way in which to access them would appear to be very important.

There are several implications for health professionals in relation to these findings and the literature reviewed. There is the definite need to develop professional expertise and actively seek opportunities to influence sex education programmes. This may be in terms of strengthening and widening the sex education beyond a purely biological focus. Few *et al.* (1996) explored the partnership between school nurses and teachers in sexual health education. The A PAUSE project (Mellanby *et al.*, 1995; see Chapter 12) is an excellent example of partnership between health and teaching professionals incorporating peer teaching, which is demonstrating significant results. Evidence of best practice, on the part of school nurses or others, must be shared with all professionals working with children and young people in order to develop our own expertise.

In addition, there may be an important role in enabling parents and significant caregivers to be able to help their children develop positive sexual health knowledge and skills. The challenge facing parents in this role should not be lightly dismissed. The perception that some parents may abdicate this role to the school may be related to their own upbringing and a lack of guidance and support in undertaking this role, as well as to the real difficulties of knowing how to give answers and information to their children. How often have we told parents, or heard others say, 'Just answer your child's questions as honestly as possible and take your cues from them.' Finding a balance between honesty, truthfulness and giving information at the child's level of maturity without causing undue anxiety and discomfort is no easy task. Understanding and interpreting cues from children is not always straightforward, at times requiring great insight and skill.

Sexual self-efficacy

The findings of this study revealed that these young people believed the development of relationship skills to be important for looking after one's own, and any potential partner's, sexual health. The importance of sexual self-efficacy, developing confidence in one's own ability to control and negotiate sexual activity, while being recognised by these subjects, does not appear to have been facilitated. The experience of these young people in not having addressed the acquisition of such skills in a 'taught' way may have influenced some in their belief that it is not possible to facilitate this development.

There are implications for further developing programmes that explore these important relationship skills for young people, both building on and benchmarking good practice. The work of Mellanby *et al.* (1995) is one example of the involvement of the School Nursing Service working in partnership with colleagues in education, which also capitalises on peer teaching. Health professionals need to consider the health education models they employ in their professional practice. An essentially information-giving approach, often used in the delivery of health education and commonly known as the medical model, has been shown to be flawed in relation to sexual health education and promotion for young people (Petosa and Jackson, 1991; Ingram *et al.*, 1992; Rosenthal *et al.*, 1992).

More appropriate and creative methods need to be developed and employed to enable young people to master these skills. Skills-based models, such as Bandura's (1989) 'mastery experience', need to be explored and adopted into practice. Again, the dissemination and sharing of best practice is vital in order to enhance effective professional and clinical practice.

There are implications here for nurse teachers. A comparison of the findings of this study and the literature reviewed would suggest that recruits into nursing, in relation to the study area, are not significantly different from other young people. They appear to have a variety of life experiences to draw upon and are at different stages of their own sexuality, yet the profession they are entering has a sexual health promotion/education role implicit in its claimed holistic approach. This must emphatically underline the need for a full and well-informed curriculum in relation to sexuality and sexual health needs, both in terms of one's personal needs and in enabling others in this important aspect of living. Professionals may need to challenge their own personal beliefs and perceptions, which may affect their professional practice. The ENB's (1994) Open Learning Pack is an excellent resource in designing and delivering just such a component of the curriculum. The recent moves towards developing reflective practice skills and engaging in clinical supervision can only strengthen this aspect of nursing's professional practice, if utilised to their fullest potential.

Nurses starting their career

The finding in the study that the majority of recruits into nursing had not considered a sexual health role as being part of the nurse's role may not be surprising. Hogan, back in 1980, stated that the traditional, stereotypical role of nurses was very slow to change. Indeed, some literature suggests that qualified nurses themselves pay little attention to this role and certainly demonstrate difficulty in situations in which sexuality impinges on health care (Bond *et al.*, 1989; Akinsanya and Rouse, 1991; McHaffie, 1993).

While the findings of the study showed some uncertainty with regard to whether the nurse has a sexual health role and what that may entail, it is also encouraging that some subjects had an awareness that their current knowledge and skills would be inadequate to fulfil this role.

The findings regarding how the subjects felt about helping other young people with their sexual health needs raise some discussion points. Having found that the idea of the role *per se* was met with some uncertainty and concern, the response that a similarity in age (that is, young patient and young nurse) would be an advantage may be somewhat surprising. The findings relating to the first two question areas of the study highlighted quite significant deficits with respect to the development of the subjects' own sexual health knowledge and skills. Russell (1992) noted that nurses are likely to be affected by their culture and upbringing, which will impact on their ability to discuss sexuality issues with relative strangers. The subjects' own experience of being able to relate to younger people in this area will no doubt have influenced their beliefs and may give a true reflection that young patients may indeed target young nurses for advice and help.

The suggestion in the findings that pre-registration curricula should revisit basic biological aspects relating to sexual health knowledge is probably a reflection of the subjects' own biologically focused school sex education. Educationalists must ensure a sound knowledge but in ways that take into account individual students' varying levels of knowledge. The mandate of the DoH (1993b) is that nurses, midwives and health visitors are to be involved in sexual health education and promotion. If this is to be fulfilled, there is a need for educationalists to explore creative teaching and learning methods to take the purely factual knowledge into the domain of attitudes and skills acquisition. Both pre- and post-registration education requires critical analysis and an evaluation of the current contribution. A partnership between clinical and educational colleagues is called for in order to develop appropriate education and training for the sexual health role of nurses. Assessing need and providing care in relation to sexual health is a new area of concern for many practitioners (ENB, 1994).

Webb (1985) believes that nurses are part of society as a whole, with the same queries, doubts and emotions as their patients. It could be suggested that it is unrealistic to expect young nurses to have come to terms with their own sexuality, a notion explored by Savage (1987). To enable nursing students to progress along the continuum related to their own sexuality, there is a need for teachers who are both self-aware and adept in the domain of affective skill development. Furthermore, an appropriate expertise in the field of sexual health is an additional requirement. Practitioners in clinical and practice areas also need to be self-aware and able to support other practitioners in developing skills related to sexual health promotion and/or education. The findings of the study support the need for clearly articulated curriculum aims, philosophy, content, teaching methods and evaluation strategies for the facilitation of sexual health knowledge, skills and attitudes.

Conclusion

The literature reviewed and the tentative findings from this small-scale study raise many important issues for health professionals working with children and young people, and for nurse educationalists. The study sample of student nurses is unrepresentative of the total young population, but the subjects were key informants with insider knowledge (Mackenize, 1994) who shared an essential characteristic with the young population as a whole (Robson, 1993), that of having recently progressed through adolescence and experienced the area of human development under scrutiny. An important aim of the study was to explore the feelings of young nurses in relation to their chosen career and the promotion of the sexual health of young people. It is acknowledged that because of the limitations already noted and the small sample size, no generalisations can be drawn from the findings of this study. A replication of this study is needed in order to be able to generalise more widely.

Returning to the introduction of this chapter, children and young people have the right to have their sexual health needs met; aspects of their future health and wellbeing rest on this. This calls for health professionals who can rise to the challenges implicit in this part of their role and who are willing to develop the necessary expertise. It also calls for pre-registration and continuing professional education that can enable practitioners to fulfil their responsibility and role.

References

Aggleton P. and Kapila M. (1992) 'Young people, HIV/AIDS and the promotion of sexual health', *Health Promotion International* 7(1): 45–51.

Akinsanya J. A. and Rouse P. (1991) *Who will Care? A Survey of the Knowledge and Attitudes of Hospital Nurses to People with HIV/AIDS*, Norwich, Anglia Polytechnic University, Faculty of Health and Social Work.

Allen I. (1987) *Education in Sex and Personal Relationships*, London, Policy Studies Institute/Blackmore Press.

Allen I. (1991) *Family Planning and Pregnancy Counselling Projects for Young People*, London, Policy Studies Institute.

Baker P. (1991) 'Interview'. In Cormack D. F. S. (ed.) *The Research Process in Nursing*, Oxford, Blackwell.

Bandura A. (1989) 'Perceived self-efficacy in the exercise of personal agency', *Psychologist* 2(10): 411–24.

Basen-Engquist K. and Parcel G. S. (1992) 'Attitudes, norms and self-efficacy: a model of adolescents' HIV-related sexual risk behaviour', *Health Education Quarterly* 19(2): 263–77.

Beck C. T. (1992) 'The lived experience of post partum depression: a phenomenological study', *Nursing Research* 41(3): 166–70.

Bond S., Rhodes T. J., Philips P. R. *et al.* (1989) *A National Survey of HIV Infection. AIDS and Community Nursing Staff in England: A Summary Report*, Newcastle, University of Newcastle-upon-Tyne, Healthcare Research Unit.

Breakwell G. M., Fife-Schaw C. and Clayden K. (1991) 'Risk-taking, control over partner choice and intended use of condoms by virgins', *Journal of Community and Applied Social Psychology* 1: 173–87.

Cohen L. and Manion L. (1989) *Research Methods in Education* (3rd edn), London, Routledge.

Curtis H. A., Tripp J. H., Lawrence C. and Clarke W. L. (1988) 'The influence of teenage relationships and sex education', *Archives of Diseases in Childhood* 63: 935–41.

Davidson N. (1990) *Boys will be...? Sex Education and Young Men*, London, Bedford Square Press.

Department of Health (1993a) *The Health of the Nation. Key Area Handbook: HIV/AIDS and Sexual Health*, London, HMSO.

Department of Health (1993b) *Targeting Practice: The Contribution of Nurses, Midwives and Health Visitors*, London, DoH.

English National Board (1994) *Caring for People with Sexually Transmitted Diseases, Including HIV Disease*. Open Learning Pack, London, ENB.

Few C., Hicken I. and Butterworth T. (1996) *Partnerships in Sexual Health and Sex Education*, Manchester, University of Manchester.

Field P. A. and Morse J. M. (1985) *Nursing Research: The Application of Qualitative Approaches*, London, Croom Helm.

Fishbein M. and Ajzen I. (1975) *Belief, Attitude, Intention and Behaviour: An Introduction to Theory and Research*, Reading, MA, Addison-Wesley.

Green J. and Delaney F. (1994) 'Beyond the bike-sheds', *Health Service Journal* 9 June, p. 10.

Hogan R. (1980) *Human Sexuality. A Nursing Perspective*, New York, Appleton-Century-Crofts.

Holland J., Ramazonoglu C., Scott S., Sharpe S. and Thomson R. (1991) 'Between embarrassment and trust: young woman and the diversity of condom use'. In Aggleton P., Hart G. and Davies P. (eds) *AIDS: Responses, Interventions and Care*, London, Falmer Press.

Holland J., Ramazonoglu C., Sharpe S. and Thomson R. (1992) 'Pleasure, pressure and power: some contradictions of gendered sexuality', *Sociological Review* 40(4): 646–73.

Holly L. (ed.) (1989) *Sexuality: Teaching and Learning*, Milton Keynes, Open University Press.

Ingram R. (1993) *Can we have a Policy on Sex? Setting Targets for Teenage Pregnancies*, Occasional Paper, IHPS, Southampton, University of Southampton.

Ingram R., Woodcock A. and Stenner K. (1991) 'Getting to know you... young people's knowledge of their partners at first intercourse', *Journal of Community and Applied Social Psychology* 1: 117–32.

Ingram R., Woodcock A. and Stenner K. (1992) 'The limitations of rational decision-making models as applied to young people's sexual behaviour'. In Aggleton P., Davies P. and Hart G. (eds) *AIDS, Rights Risk and Reason*, London, Falmer Press.

Kasen S., Vaughan R. D. and Walter H. J. (1992) 'Self-efficacy for aids preventive behaviors among tenth grade students', *Health Education Quarterly* 19(2): 187–202.

Loewenstein G. and Furstenberg F. (1991) 'Is teenage sexual behaviour rational?', *Journal of Applied Social Psychology* 21(12): 957–86.

McHaffie H. (1993) *The Care of Patients with HIV and AIDS: A Survey of Nurse Education in the UK, A Report*, Edinburgh, University of Edinburgh, Institute of Medical Ethics.

Mackenize A. (1994) 'Evaluating ethnography: considerations for analysis', *Journal of Advanced Nursing* 19: 774–81.

Mellanby A. R., Phelps F. A., Crichton N. J. and Tripp J. H. (1995) 'School sex education: an experimental programme with educational and medical benefit', *British Medical Journal* 311: 414–17.

Oiler C. (1982) 'The phenomenological approach in nursing research', *Nursing Research* 31(3): 178–81.

Peckham S. (1992) *Unplanned Pregnancy and Teenage Pregnancy. A Review*, Southampton, Wessex Research Consortium IHPS, University of Southampton.

Petosa R. and Jackson K. (1991) 'Using the health belief model to predict safer sex intentions among adolescents', *Health Education Quarterly* 18(4): 463–76.

Prendergast S. (1992) *This Is the Time to Grow Up: Girls' Experiences of Menstruation in School*, Cambridge, Health Promotion Trust.

Robson C. (1993) *Real World Research*, Oxford, Blackwell.

Rosenthal D., Moore S. and Flynn I. (1991) 'Adolescent self-efficacy, self-esteem and sexual risk taking', *Journal of Community and Applied Social Psychology* 1: 77–88.

Rosenthal D., Hall C. and Moore S. (1992) 'AIDS, adolescents and sexual risk taking: a test of the health belief model', *Australian Psychologist* 27(3): 166–71.

Royal College of Obstetricians and Gynaecologists (1991) *Report of the Working Party on Unplanned Pregnancy*, London, RCOG.

Russell P. (1992) Sex and the student nurse. Student nurses' perceptions of their preparation and role in promoting the sexual health of patients. Implications for education. Unpublished dissertation, Southampton University.

Savage J. (1987) *Nurses, Gender and Sexuality*, London, Heinemann.

Scally G. (1993) 'Teenage pregnancies – the challenge of prevention', *Midwives Chronicle*, Jul.: pp. 232–9.

Small S. A., Silverberg S. and Kerns D. (1993) 'Adolescents' perceptions of the costs and benefits of engaging in health-compromising behaviours', *Journal of Youth and Adolescence* 22(1): 73–87.

Smith R. (1995) Engaging young people – the promotion of sexual health. Unpublished dissertation, University of Southampton.

Smith R (1997a) 'Promoting the sexual health of young people. Part 1', *Paediatric Nursing* 9(2): 24–7.

Smith R (1997b) 'Promoting the sexual health of young people. Part 2', *Paediatric Nursing* 9(3): 24–7.

Svenson L. W., Varnhagen C. K., Godin A. M. and Salmon T. L.(1992) 'Rural high school students' knowledge, attitudes and behaviours related to sexually transmitted disease', *Canadian Journal of Public Health* 83(4): 260–3.

Webb C. (1985) *Sexuality, Nursing and Health*, Chichester, John Wiley & Sons.

Wellings K., Field J., Johnson A. and Wadsworth J. (1994) *Sexual Behaviour in Britain. The National Survey of Sexual Attitudes and Lifestyles*, London, Penguin.

202   *Rachael L. Smith*

Woodcock A., Stenner K. and Ingram R. (1992a) 'Young people talking about HIV and AIDS: interpretation of personal risk of infection', *Health Education Research* 7(?), 229–17.
Woodcock A., Stenner K. and Ingram R. (1992b) 'All those contraceptives, videos and that...: young people talking about sex education', *Health Education Research* 7(40): 517–31.
Yaber W. and Greer J. (1986) 'The relationships between sexual attitudes of parents and their college daughters' or sons' sexual attitudes and sexual behaviour', *Journal of School Health*, 56(2): 68–72.

Further reading

Readers may find the following papers helpful. They were identified from the NHS CRD Systematic Review 1998 database.

Kim N., Stanton B., Li X., Dickersin K., and Galbraith J. (1997) 'Effectiveness of the 40 adolescent aids-risk reduction interventions', *Journal of Adolescent Health* 20(3): 204–15.
Kirby D., Short L., Collins J. *et al.* (1994) 'School-based programs to reduce sexual risk behaviour: a review of effectiveness', *Public Health Reports* 109(3): 339–60.
Oakley A., Fullerton D, Holland J. *et al.* (1995) 'Sexual health education interventions for young people: a methodological review', *British Medical Journal* 310: 158–62.

12 Added Power and Understanding in Sex Education (A PAUSE): a sex education intervention staffed predominantly by school nurses

John Rees, Alex Mellanby, Jenny White and John Tripp

Introduction

'Life is rather like a tin of sardines – we're all of us looking for the key'. (Alan Bennett)

The National Health Service (NHS) Centre for Reviews and Dissemination (Dickson *et al.*, 1997) has suggested that despite the best efforts of education and medicine, school-based sex education programmes that result in behaviour change continue to be rare. Indeed, there is a growing body of evidence to suggest that traditional approaches to sex education are failing to meet the needs of young people. Added Power and Understanding in Sex Education (A PAUSE), reported by Mellanby *et al.* (1995a), is a programme now staffed predominantly by school nurses, which has shown positive medical and educational benefits that are, we believe, unique in Europe (Mellanby *et al.*, 1995b).

The original research project has been developed as a service provision to secondary schools in and around the programme's 'home town'. A PAUSE is also being developed in consultation with schools and health authorities in different parts of the UK. This chapter outlines the background, the theoretical perspectives, the transitions, the potential future and some recommendations from this work.

203

Background

Beyond human immuno-deficiency virus and acquired immune deficiency syndrome

During the 1980s, the threat of human immuno-deficiency virus/acquired immune deficiency syndrome (HIV/AIDS) focused initially on homosexuals and identified, albeit inappropriately, 'high-risk' groups. Holland *et al.* (1990a) note that the public fear of the spread of HIV/AIDS to heterosexual groups is cited as being responsible for the increasing concern for (young) people's sexual conduct, health and wellbeing. Despite the international picture, the HIV/AIDS pandemic anticipated for the UK has been, as a public health issue, less devastating than was initially predicted. It may, however, be argued that an increased awareness of HIV/AIDS has provided funding and an increasing willingness to address sexual health issues. This has reinforced the desire for effective educational strategies.

Long before the advent of HIV/AIDS, health professionals, educationalists, parents and young people were concerned with the undesirable consequences of sexual activity, especially for younger teenagers (Bell, 1966). Most adults, either in their professional capacity or as the parents of teenagers, have, at some stage, worried about adolescents' sexual health, that is, becoming pregnant or causing pregnancy, contracting a sexually transmitted disease or suffering the emotional upset that can follow an unsatisfactory relationship or inappropriate physical contact. 'Inappropriate' is pejorative only in as much as it includes any physical contact that the recipient would have preferred, either at the time or retrospectively, not to have happened. While Holland *et al.* (1990b) note that the reasons for sexual activity may vary, Curtis *et al.* (1988) found, and Ingham (1997) confirmed, that the majority of women report immediate and/or subsequent regret with respect to their first sexual encounter.

Physical and societal changes

Over the past 100 years, the average age of menarche appears to have been falling and, until the mid-1970s, showed little sign of levelling off (Roche, 1979). This pattern has been inversely mirrored by the increase in the school-leaving age, resulting in physically mature individuals who are treated like children in school. At the same time, the average age of marriage has risen, leaving an ever-widening 'window of fertility'.

The latter part of the twentieth century has been characterised by social changes of unprecedented rapidity. Many of the effects of childhood ailments have been eradicated and controlled, the majority enjoy a better standard of living, and the population is generally less prone to disease. Young people are, however, now presented with challenges, opportunities and media perspectives that were unimaginable to our forebears. Such changes include real and perceived issues: new perspectives on the role of women and changing patterns of employment; marital breakdown and divorce statistics that would have previously been unthinkable; legal and interpretative changes concerning homosexuality and abortion; the availability of effective contraception; popular culture; and improved global communication.

Such circumstances present us with exciting times in which to live but are attended by concerns regarding the rapidity of some of those changes. Take this fast-ageing joke: *Two four-year olds in the play-ground; one said 'I found a condom on the patio!' The other asked 'What's a patio?'*, reflecting a social and linguistic revolution in the UK, particularly as it was told to one of the authors by his septuagenarian mother!

Teenage sexual activity

Adolescent sexual activity is clearly not, and never has been, without risk. Watney (1987) notes that risks of intercourse have changed somewhat and that these risks have come into sharp focus for an increasing number of (young) people during recent years. Adolescence is, for many, characterised by the initiation of intimate physical relationships and a variety of other behaviours that might result in harm to themselves and others. Many of these behaviours are essential in the process of 'growing up' and developing independence. However, adolescents' bodies and social expectations change with what must seem to be bewildering rapidity. Young people now have perhaps less chance than their predecessors of knowing what societal 'goalposts' exist, and we need to recognise that the majority of sex education is simply not meeting their needs. In England in 1995, there were more than 27,000 terminations carried out on teenage women (Chief Medical Officer, 1996). Genuis and Genuis (1995) suggest that this figure has not changed much in recent years, and Hadley (1997) explains that young adults have the highest prevalence of sexually transmitted disease, and that such rates of infection are increasing, which has been confirmed most recently by Nicholl *et al.* (1999).

It would be easy to assume from the media that we are in the midst of a teenage pregnancy explosion, but the reverse is, in fact, true: teenagers are far less likely to get pregnant today than they were 25 years ago. In 1970, 82.4 per 1000 women (aged 15–19) conceived; this figure has now dropped to 58.6 per 1000, and the rate of teenage motherhood has fallen from 71.4 to 38.0 in the same period (Johnson *et al.*, 1994; Office of National Statistics, 1996), although these figures tell us little about how many of these pregnancies are planned. Despite the increase in teenage sexual activity in the UK, the general decline in conception rate may be an indication that more young people are successfully avoiding unwanted pregnancy. As the age of first intercourse falls (Johnson *et al.*, 1994), the conception rate of sexually active teenagers may also be declining.

Sexual health strategies, including sex education

There is, however, no cause for complacency as the teenage pregnancy rate in the UK is the highest in Europe. Despite international support for an improved health promotion policy (WHO, 1986), there is strong evidence to suggest that the *Health of the Nation* (sexual health) strategy is doomed to failure. In 1989, the Department of Health (DoH) determined a national average conception rate for young women, aged 13–15 years, to be 9.5 per 1000. This figure determined one of the *Health of the Nation* targets (DoH, 1992). By 1993, this national rate had dropped to 8 per 1000, although the latest figures (for 1994; Office of National Statistics, 1996) show an increase, and Adler (1997) rightly suggests that it is difficult to imagine how the target of 4.8 will be reached by the year 2000. The subsequent *Our Healthier Nation* (DoH, 1998) failed to include sexual health targets, an omission that is, at the time of writing, only slightly ameliorated by the promise of a national sexual health strategy.

Sex and relationships education in secondary schools is identified as a means of addressing sexual health issues (DES, 1986; RCOG, 1991; DoH, 1992). Although many fear that there may be conflicting values and societal attitudes surrounding sex education, there is clearly a need for high-quality, age-appropriate sex education in schools (BMA, 1997). This should complement that provided by parents in preparation for healthy relationships (Sex Education Forum, 1997) and be part of a wider personal, social, health and citizenship education curriculum (QCA/DfEE, 1999). Unfortunately, there is all too frequently a marked gender difference in the way in which boys and girls are taught sex education by their parents and in many schools (Holland *et al.*, 1996). Sex education has traditionally been biologically factual and all too often taught in a knowledge-based, didactic manner (Hirst, 1994). It was frequently aimed at young women, particularly regarding menstruation and types of contraception – most of which were, and remain, inappropriate for teenagers (Lenderyou and Rey, 1997). All too often, the 'tampon lady' talked exclusively to girls while the boys were kept busy until their female peers returned from their rite of passage, perpetuating and reinforcing the stereotype that such topics were not part of boys' understanding or vocabulary. Young gay men have also reported that the fear of prejudice and violence has led them to deny their sexuality (Mason and Palmer, 1996). Such exclusion also perpetuates many gender stereotypes that may make intimate or contraceptive negotiation more difficult for young women later in life (Holland *et al.*, 1998).

There is a growing realisation that while we are not meeting the needs of young people generally, we are specifically failing our young men (Walker and Kushner, 1997). Sex education that focuses on the reproductive aspects of intercourse may engage girls but frequently leaves boys bored, disruptive and hostile (Measor *et al.*, 1996). Reinforcing the notion that sexual health is not an issue for boys has serious implications for their sexual and mental health (Sex Education Forum, 1997).

Regis (1996, p. 1) describes a 'consensus view' that 'School's health education should be about promoting informed choice, perhaps even valuing the quality of decision over its content.' He quotes Kolbe (1981), who suggested that 'turning a shallow, conformist non-smoker into an independent, rational and self-aware person who decides to smoke, may even be seen as a health education success' (p. 25). This paper argues that sex and relationships education should be seen as part of a health initiative and cannot be value free. As recommended by the World Health Organization (WHO, 1998), this must have a clear focus for young people to promote their own sexual and emotional wellbeing as part of their wider health needs. Such a philosophy also demands that they must protect their own physical and emotional health and that of their (potential) partner(s), but expects us all to accept responsibility to reduce ill-health and medical risk.

Challenges for the future

The challenge for society, educators and especially health professionals is to invoke the 'Heineken principle': 'How can we reach those parts which conventional education cannot reach?' Health and education professionals with parents, working with and for young people, must ensure that as many young people as possible receive a sexual health education that is appropriate to their needs, those of their community and the wider society of which they are part. The National Curriculum requires that sex education be taught in all secondary schools but *effective* sex education that can be shown to have significant educational or medical advantages for young people is far less common (Wight, 1997). Improved school-based sex education, in which the vast majority of young people are present, is essential. This must be a skills-based curriculum founded on accurate knowledge that empowers young people to accept responsibility for their own wellbeing and that of others. This approach, emphasising the need for teenagers to develop skills in obtaining and negotiating contraception, rather than simple knowledge, has been recommended (Abraham *et al.*, 1991). The importance of linking school sex education programmes with improved contraceptive services has also been emphasised (Dickson *et al.*, 1997).

Theoretical perspective

Sex and relationships education, like any other health intervention, must be firmly based on effective theory. Schaalma *et al.* (1996), and more recently Jemmott *et al.* (1998), reported a greater belief and behavioural change as a result of participating in a programme based on the theories described below, compared with the outcome seen in students receiving more traditional approaches. If a programme is not soundly based on theory, it may simply slide into delivering factual information. An approach that focuses on, for example, attempting to teach *all* the methods of contraception, *all* the sexually transmitted diseases and *all* the ways in which to catch or avoid them has *not* been shown to result in young teenagers being less likely to conceive or contract disease. It may not even enable them to retain accurate knowledge since much of it is irrelevant to them.

Information alone does not empower teenagers to manage their emotions and relationships. Enhanced self-esteem and self-efficacy, improved assertiveness and a respect for and tolerance of others all need to be addressed as part not only of sex education, but also of the wider personal and social education that should be an educational entitlement for all. This is especially pertinent when considering one of the most powerful human drives (to reproduce), which is influenced by external pressures and unrealistic beliefs about the activities of others. It is unsurprising that cognitive-based, adult-derived health education is not associated with a reduction in some outcomes that are unwanted by teenagers or adults. Models that rely on information dissemination and/or attempting to improve services are often adult in their perspective, and it may be that adolescents do not find such approaches appropriate or useful.

Meta-analyses suggest that although some experiments may have been imperfect, it is currently apparent that only programmes based on theories such as social learning (Bandura, 1976), and associated theories such as social inoculation (McGuire, 1964) and social norms (Baric and Harrison, 1977), have demonstrated behavioural change (Fong, 1994; Kirby *et al.*, 1994; Oakley *et al.*, 1996). The main assumption of such approaches is that people's behaviour is best understood according to their perceptions of their social environment (Conner and Norman, 1996).

Such theories do not always sit comfortably with traditional approaches to teaching and learning in schools. These theories collectively posit that behavioural change may be effected when the 'learner' negotiates, in a collaborative style with the 'teacher', and has the opportunity to practise and gain confidence in, behaviours that are subsequently to be employed. In sex education, most of this is obviously applied to 'proxy' behaviour since, despite requests from students (usually male) for 'practicals', this approach would not be acceptable! These theories can, however, be used to formulate approaches that seek to enhance relationships and reduce the susceptibility of young teenagers to unwelcome pressure.

If sex and relationships education is to be effective, and for some teenagers such efficacy will result in controlling the pace of their physical relationships and countering unwelcome sexual pressures, we need to do more than simply improve knowledge. Creating, developing and maintaining supportive environments and enhancing personal skills are central principles of social learning and its associated theories, and were major premises of the WHO Ottawa Charter (1986). Teenagers' behaviour is shaped not only by personal factors, but also by interactions with their environment and other individuals. Collaborative learning can take place through imitation but is enhanced by the opportunity to rehearse desired behaviours. These principles imply that effective sex education is based on improving self-efficacy and will result in a belief on the part of the individual that he or she can effectively use such skills or methods of protection (Bandura, 1995)

As children reach adolescence, many experience increased vulnerability, experiment with different lifestyles and increasingly seek independence from their families. Decisions to smoke tobacco, drink alcohol, take other illegal drugs or engage in higher-risk sexual activity are assumed to be partly dependent on their cognitive maturity (Stuart-Smith, 1996) and their ability to resist social pressure from others. A key component of social influence theory is therefore education on social pressures and how to deal with them. Theory translates into practice where a variety of classroom techniques are employed to allow students to identify and counteract social pressure in relationships. Students are encouraged to demonstrate communication skills in small group and whole class discussions and within role plays.

Adding Power and Understanding in Sex Education (A PAUSE): a research project and results

The A PAUSE project was established in 1990, following research (Curtis *et al.*, 1988) funded initially by the South Western Regional Health Authority and later by the Research and Development Directorate of the South and West NHS Executive. The research team of health and education professionals reflected a collaborative approach to sex and relationships education, employing the classroom management skills of a teacher and the medical credibility of a doctor, working together with young people. The team devised a curriculum and classroom process based on the theoretical constructs of effective programmes identified in a world literature review and using a collaborative learning, social influences model (Mellanby *et al.*, 1996).

The two original intervention schools were matched with local and distant populations – comprehensive schools – from similar urban/semi-rural cities in different parts of the UK. Students from these comparison or control schools reflected the socio-economic and academic profiles of the intervention schools. The theoretical basis of the evaluation, using quantitative methodologies, is described elsewhere (Mellanby *et al.*, 1995a) but comprises an individual, anonymised questionnaire to year 11 students (mean age 16 years) to determine their personal knowledge, beliefs and behaviour. Three successive cohorts of students in year 11 were required to complete a questionnaire under 'examination conditions', invigilated by the research team. The results of the programme were published

(Mellanby *et al.*, 1995a), showing that the intervention population ($n = 387$), when compared with the local ($n = 455$) and distant ($n = 2856$) controls, demonstrated significant differences both from controls and from previous data in the intervention schools. This included an increase in knowledge related to contraception, sexually transmitted diseases and prevalence of sexual activity (χ^2 for trend $p < 0.001$ for all three series). Questions asked, included for example, whether post-coital contraception was effective 2 days after sexual intercourse. The number of correct answers to this question increased in the programme populations from 33 per cent (1992) to 70 per cent (1994) and was 22 per cent higher than that of the control groups in 1994 (relative risk [RR] 1.47; 95 per cent confidence interval [CI] 1.37–1.59). Other questions asked teenagers about the prevalence of diseases and sexual activity. The percentage of programme students who incorrectly believed that 'more than half of all teenagers have had sex by the time they are 16' fell from 59 per cent (1992) to 46 per cent (1994) (χ^2 for trend $p < 0.001$) and was 14 per cent lower than that of the overall control population (RR 0.77; 95 per cent CI 0.69–0.86).

Students were asked for responses to six statements suggesting that sexual intercourse was beneficial to teenagers and their relationships. These included questions such as 'Teenagers who have sex feel more "grown up"' and 'Young teenage girls (and boys in a separate question) get a bad reputation if they've had sex.' In 1994, a greater proportion of students from the programme schools than from either of the control school groups disagreed with all the statements. In particular, 86 per cent of the programme group, compared with 71 per cent of the local controls, disagreed that sexual intercourse made young people's relationships last longer (RR 1.22; 95 per cent CI 1.13–1.31) and 49 per cent versus 39 per cent disagreed that girls get a bad reputation if they have sexual intercourse (RR 1.27; 95 per cent CI 1.09–1.48).

In successive years (1992–94), the percentage of students in the local control schools who had sexual intercourse increased. This did not happen in the programme schools, and overall there was a significant difference between the students receiving the intervention and those in both the local and the distant control schools. Increased educational aspirations, religiosity, fewer older siblings and rural residence are associated with a decreased likelihood of sexual activity at the age of 16 (Johnson *et al.*, 1994), and factors such as these had to be allowed for in a logistical regression analysis. These data indicated that the students in the control population were 1.45 times more likely to have had sexual intercourse than students who had received the A PAUSE programme (odds ratio 1.45; 95 per cent CI 1.13–1.87).

The programme and control schools were given prior access to the questionnaires and were given annual reports comparing their students' answers with those from other control schools. Within control populations, there was no annual increase in the number of correct answers, nor was there a difference in the control schools tested for more than 1 year compared with those newly recruited each year.

These results are, we believe, unique in Europe, consistently demonstrating that pupils aged 16 who have received the programme:

- increased their knowledge of sex, contraception and sexually transmitted diseases
- were less likely to believe that intercourse is important in relationships
- were more tolerant of the behaviour of others
- were less likely to be sexually active.

They were also nearly twice as likely to say that sex education was 'OK' than were students in the control groups.

A PAUSE: a service provision

The project has now secured funding from North and East Devon Health Authority for a service provision currently reaching eight high schools and agreed for seven more, but with plans to extend this to all the secondary schools in the health authority district. The programme currently serves nearly 7,000 young people aged 12–16. Pre- and post-session questionnaires are used as quality control measures, and evaluation is maintained through the year 11 questionnaire as both longitudinal and cross-sectional comparison data. Additional funding has been provided by the Wellcome Trust to maintain this evaluation and develop research as the technology has been adopted in other parts of the UK, specifically North Essex, North Tees and Sandwell health authorities.

Increasingly close collaboration with local schools and the communities that they serve is sought, and the programme now offers:

- curriculum support materials for year 7 or 8 (aged 11–13 years)
- three 1-hour sessions led by teachers and school nurses for year 9 (aged 13–14 years)

- four 'peer-led' sessions (recruited from sixth forms and the college of further education)
- three sessions in year 10 (aged 14–15 years)
- an annual report to each institution, based on data from the year 11 questionnaire, contributing to an audit of the schools' personal, social and health education curriculum.

Programmes based on appropriate theories and timed before the vast majority become sexually active (Baldo *et al.*, 1993) can be effective and can not only influence the knowledge, skills and attitudes of young people, but also empower them to manage their behaviour. The challenge is clear, as we move from research to service mode, to replicate these results on a wider scale.

As noted above, A PAUSE involves six adult-led sessions, co-facilitated by teachers and health professionals. A more detailed explanation of the session content, ethos and activities is beyond the scope of this chapter, but the purpose of the approach is to encourage young people to consider, discuss and reflect on aspects of sexual health. This relies on creating an atmosphere in which such issues may be negotiated by reducing the fear of personal comments and ridicule, concerns may be acknowledged and 'mythunderstandings' dispelled, and young people's perceptions of their social environment can be enhanced and effective relationships modelled.

The programme no longer employs a doctor in the classroom, although doctors from the Department of Child Health, in association with external agencies such as 'AIDSline', support the staff and peer training. Teachers have traditionally reported inadequate training for health education (Heathcote, 1989), a need that remains largely unmet. Teachers are, however, recruited and given additional training in the theory, methodology and ethos of the programme. The classroom medical credibility is now provided by health professionals (predominantly school nurses), who have a crucial role to play in the programme and develop their expertise through appropriate training and collaborative reflection with the teachers. The duality of this delivery is very important. The health professional provides medical credibility, is a source of accurate information and offers a realistic 'case study' that forms the basis of each session. The teacher provides classroom management skills and lends credibility in the eyes of the (sometimes sceptical) educationalists. Visiting teachers have been employed, but there are considerable benefits to be gained from training 'in-house' teachers as a contribution to their wider personal, social and health education and citizenship responsibilities.

To work collaboratively with pupils requires, almost by definition, those 'teaching' the session to lower their status in the classroom and raise that of the 'learners'. The inverted commas are apposite as titles such as 'teacher' and 'learners' are indicative of a didactic style (Brandes and Ginnis, 1986) and may consequently be less appropriate in a collaborative programme. This can be difficult for adults based in a school where the institutional ethos demands roles associated with control and discipline, and a government philosophy of education which appears to see students as empty vessels that need to be filled. This is exacerbated when external examinations, league tables and funding all collude to encourage teachers to fill as many vessels as quickly as possible.

Teachers (and doctors) are unaccustomed to diminishing their status (apparently relinquishing control) in the classroom, whereas health professionals such as school-based nurses are frequently better able to fulfil a supportive and collaborative role and are particularly adept at working in this manner. School nurses frequently have wide clinical experience yet are used to working with teachers and young people in the classroom environment (Few, 1995). Their additional qualifications lend them both knowledge and expertise with regard to health issues, and they are accustomed to working with a variety of external agencies. School nurses are often familiar adults within the school community, and their role in schools is seldom authoritarian or disciplinarian but sensitive to pupils' needs.

In most schools, there is a wide range of academic ability, socio-economic background and parental support. Such diverse populations need people who treat them with respect, listen to their needs and offer advice when required. Beyond the classroom, teachers, unlike school nurses, cannot offer confidentiality to pupils, and the school nurse is uniquely placed to offer access to medical services for young people (Brook Advisory Centres, 1996). Many teenagers will seek impartial, confidential advice, seldom needing complex or academic explanations; school nurses are well placed to offer all of this.

Although the A PAUSE health professionals are predominantly school nurses, the programme has had a policy of not utilising nurses in their 'home' institutions. This encourages young people to see the services represented as safe, confidential and accessible. This approach to school-based nursing is not one that all will find easy, although students' perceptions, to some extent, rely on the personality of the nurse and the role that the school encourages him or her to adopt. Recent financial constraints have, regrettably, threatened the essential services of school-based nurses in the UK (Norfolk Health Authority, 1995).

Groups of young people using this collaborative style of learning with teachers and nurses need to be allowed to explore their vocabulary, knowledge, social mores, norms and attitudes. Such discussion needs to have structure provided by a caring, non-judgemental, sensitive and experienced staff whose actions are part of their belief system and have a sound theoretical basis. They need to communicate to the young people, with and for whom they are working, that the young people are valued, respected and liked. For example, A PAUSE adults often suggest to the class: 'You are the experts here – you know what its like to be a teenager in the 1990s; I could tell you about the 'good old days' – but that might not be relevant to the twenty-first century!' There is a degree of factual information that is necessary for informed decision making, but it is the thoughts, feelings and self-efficacy of the young people that are crucial. If we are to empower teenagers to enjoy the benefits of mutually rewarding relationships, we need to work with them rather than make judgements or dictate their behaviour.

This process is not a 'value-free zone'. Kirby (1989) concludes that effective programmes also require focused objectives. One outcome measure of A PAUSE is to delay first sexual intercourse until after the age of 16, which is not an arbitrary figure that happens to coincide with the law: a study of pregnant teenage women (Curtis *et al.*, 1988) suggests that young people who have intercourse before they are 16 are usually in shorter-term relationships, are less effective contraceptive users and have more partners, with all the associated risks. These include a higher prevalence of sexually transmitted diseases, and of (or causing) pregnancy, with an increased long-term risk of infertility or cervical cancer. It is also the oldest age at which a collection of data for all young people is possible in school.

Although the A PAUSE school nurses are not specifically performing a medical service role in the classroom, they do inform and perhaps remind young people of the availability of local services. We are currently investigating the ease with which young people feel that they are able to access medical services. Many GPs make efforts to offer more teenage-friendly services, often supported by publications such as those from the Brook Advisory Service (1996). It may be more important to train young people to deal effectively with medical personnel by rehearsing the questions, strategies and assertiveness techniques required to meet their needs. We believe that this process is enhanced when, from the security of 'their own territory' (that is, the classroom), young people are able to meet, anticipate and rehearse effective strategies. These can be planned before venturing into the disproportionate power imbalance that many people feel when they contact a practice receptionist – even before entering the doctor's surgery.

It is particularly important, wherever possible, to maintain a gender balance in both the adult- and the peer-led sessions. Traditional, female-centred sex and relationships education implies a danger that sexual health, contraception and disease prevention are associated with the role of women. We need to allow *all* young people to recognise and understand that such issues are concerns that we *all* need to address, and that fulfilling relationships and effective parenting alter the life chances of children. If we are to encourage young men, who may not have a resident male role model, to accept their social, emotional and medical responsibilities, we must allow and encourage them to see that 'It's OK for blokes to talk about these things'.

Just as we cannot rely on effective sex and relationships education being delivered exclusively by one gender, so we must recognise that we cannot exclusively rely on adult-based delivery. Although Kirby (1995) noted the commonality of theoretical basis, he did not determine that a peer education component was an *essential* feature of effective interventions. Howard and McCabe's (1990) Postponing Sexual Involvement programme contains a peer-led component based on social learning and associated theories, which has been extensively used in North America and forms one, possibly essential, strand of A PAUSE.

Kirby *et al.* (1997) point out two methodological flaws of Howard and McCabe's (1990) study and suggest that the limitations of this particular programme may be partly the result of insufficient time allocation. Moreover, they note the difficulties of replicating a widespread dissemination of such technology, which are probably logistical rather than pertaining to the theoretical basis of the programme. A curriculum involving many institutions and personnel, while remaining true to theory, is potentially beset with many problems. Staff (and possibly peer) training – ensuring that those leading sessions do so with optimal clarity and skill, timetable negotiations and get the right staff at the right time, in front of the right students, all set in an educational and social context of other priorities – is a tall order.

The American cultural and teaching approach of Howard and McCabe's work required some adaptation for inclusion into British classrooms. In many ways, the sessions in the USA show an apparent formality in classroom structure, but the peer leaders were extremely extrovert, and the younger teenagers responded to a 'show business' approach. In A PAUSE, we have devised four sessions led by peer educators that revolve around distinct activities; these comprise 40 per cent of the programme.

Adults may be able to communicate facts, but teenagers are some-times suspicious when they start talking about behaviour. The peer-led sessions involve whole-class presentation and discussion, small group work and role plays. It is a collaborative approach, and from the peers' initial training, it is made very clear that peer leaders do not instruct younger teenagers on how to behave; nor do they impose their own experiences or values on younger students. The sessions are not free from value judgements because, as with the adult sessions, discussion will include values that the younger students consider important. For example, the peer leaders ask the students, in small groups, to write down all the reasons 'why *young* teenagers (13–14 years) might have sexual intercourse'. The students discuss these and are then asked to list the reasons 'why *young* teenagers might wish to wait before having intercourse'. The peer leaders then initiate a discussion that may acknowledge that 'being drunk', 'curiosity' or 'it's the next stage of their relationship' may be reasons why some people may have sex. They then ask the students to deter-mine which of the reasons are considered 'good enough' for them-selves or for a friend to start a sexual relationship. Virtually without exception, the younger teenagers denigrate and reject reasons related to undue pressure, or reasons that involve promoting the image of one partner at the expense of another. They also refute the idea that it is 'OK' for one partner to coerce the other into sexual activity. These are the main reasons year 9 students consider to be behind most sexual activity at their age. It is not surprising, therefore, that our unpublished data show that when the peer leaders discuss phys-ical expressions of affection, the vast majority of 13–14-year-olds believe that people of their age should stop short of sexual inter-course in their relationships. The only surprised individuals may be the observing adults who believed that this would not be the case.

As alluded to above, peer education programmes are increasingly popular and frequently thought to be 'a good thing', receiving appro-bation from many authors (Thomson, 1994). Despite their preva-lence, however, many peer-delivered programmes are criticised for their lack of a theoretical basis (Frankham, 1998), their efficacy is seldom questioned, and they are even more rarely evaluated with sufficient academic rigor (Milburn, 1995). We are currently evalu-ating the difference in knowledge, skills and attitudes, and behaviour between young teenagers who have received sessions led by their peers and those who have experienced similar, adult-led sessions. Early indications are that while adults may convey knowledge just as effectively, peer educators have a capacity to change social mythology and perceptions that outweighs that of adults. A number of authors acknowledge an international requirement to evaluate the potentials and research the effectiveness of such peer-led work.

A PAUSE does not rely entirely on either concerned adults or well-meaning youngsters but draws on a rigorous theoretical framework and best practice from around the world. Effective health education should not rely exclusively on either peers *or* adults but a combination of the two. It is also reasonable to suppose that the health of young people is best supported when they have easy and immediate access to high-quality advice and personnel. School-based nurses clearly have a crucial role here. Working together, adults and young people can capitalise on the advantages that sensitive experienced professionals can offer, augmenting this with the enthusiasm and realism of youth, and working for the best interests of the young people and the future of our communities.

Future developments and recommendations

Despite government's past initiatives (DoH, 1992; DfEE 1995), and assurances (Jowell, 1999; QCA/DfEE, 1999) from both health and education, traditional approaches to sex education endure and continue to fail to meet the needs of the first generation of the new millennium.

Strategic policy changes must be implemented to enhance existing good practice. Although secondary schools are required to provide sex education, neither content nor methodology is currently recommended. Parents have a unique right to withdraw their child from anything beyond the confines of the National Curriculum (science), and relationships, as part of personal and social education, are often poorly addressed, as well as being under increasing pressure from other areas of the curriculum. Section 28 of the Local Government Act 1988, which prohibits local authorities from a disproportionate 'promotion' of homosexuality or the advocacy of homosexuality as a better way of life, while not applying to schools, causes anxiety and misunderstanding. Primary schools may choose to omit sex education, and school-based nursing has been cut. All of these policies must be redressed.

Recent recommendations (BMA, 1997) indicate the need for additional research funding. This should involve a quantitative data analysis of outcomes and a qualitative investigation of process. There also remains a place for professional judgement and subjective participant evaluation from school pupils and their teachers; indeed, pupils' involvement in such a programme is strongly recommended.

If we are to reduce the longer-term costs of health care, we must promote good health. We can no longer be content with distributing leaflets and posters in an effort to improve the nation's health, or rely simply on a knowledge-based curriculum. There is an ever-increasing demand for research evidence of cost-effectiveness as well as a growing awareness that programmes must show not only subjective outcomes, but also positive, measurable, behavioural change. Programmes must be soundly based on theory and include rigorous evaluation. It is surely incumbent on heath authorities to promote and finance studies that are shown to be effective rather than continuing to fund unevaluated or methodologically inadequate projects.

From the A PAUSE perspective, we must continue to refine, enhance and develop the existing programme in Exeter, North Essex, Teesside and Sandwell schools. In common with many research departments, we must continue to innovate and to attract funding, which may include vigorously marketing the programme to other health authorities. In North Essex, A PAUSE, based on the same theory and methodology, employs a visiting health professional working with a regular class teacher. The teachers have been positively selected and trained, but such an approach clearly has a different per capita cost. We eagerly await the results of this approach. If the results are satisfactory, we will be in a position to support an *effective* school sex education programme, at a reduced cost, with methodology that sits comfortably with the philosophy and requirements of the educational community.

Colleagues with a background in drama and theatre in education (TIE) are pointing out the close similarities between well-documented approaches to theatre (such as socio-drama and forum theatre) and collaborative goals theory (Evans *et al.*, 1998). There is some fascinating and much-needed research to be undertaken here, considering approaches that have traditionally lain in the TIE domain but which need to be linked with a more rigorous assessment and evaluative process. TIE need not lose its intrinsic credibility nor deny its own innate worth but may continue to help young people to create their own meanings of the world. However, we may be able to evaluate such a process both in the usual terms and in ways that demonstrate behavioural change and have both medical and educational benefits.

Effective health education should rely not exclusively on either peers *or* adults but on a partnership of the two. There is currently a very strong movement in education, both in formal and youth/community settings, to adopt a variety of peer-led approaches.

Many schools, particularly given the reduction in support from external agencies, are eager to develop programmes surrounding a variety of health issues, including sexual health and anti-smoking, anti-bullying, anti-drinking and anti-drugs education. A skilled team of peers could also respond to local training needs from local schools. We have also considered the need for additional session(s), perhaps in year 11, which could be facilitated by year 13 (aged 17–18 years) peer leaders. We could recruit and train a small (12–15) team of peers who would be employed on a sessional basis but would have full-time availability throughout the year.

A PAUSE continues to be a successful intervention that will, we anticipate, provide positive health gain and measurable behavioural outcomes. This is by no means inevitable and, if we are to continue to refine this work, we must continue to innovate and develop the role that school-based nurses have to play in promoting and supporting the health of young people. As a society, we must develop the excellence of existing practice, drawing strength from the groundswell of education, medical and public opinion that supports the funding of more research into effective methodologies. To respond to the comment of Alan Bennett at the start of this chapter, we believe that through collaborative approaches to education, even if we do not hold the key to life, we have a plan to continue the search.

References

Abraham C., Sheeran P., Abrams D., Spears R. and Marks D. (1991) 'Young people learning about AIDS: a study of beliefs and information sources', *Health Education Research: Theory and Practice* 6: 19–29.

Adler M. W. (1997) 'Sexual health – a Health of the Nation failure'. *British Medical Journal* 314: 1743–7.

Baldo M., Aggleton P. and Slutkin G. (1993) 'Does sex education lead to earlier or increased sexual activity in youth?' *IXth International Conference on AIDS, Berlin.* Geneva, WHO, abstract PO-DO2-3444.

Bandura A. (1976) *Social Learning Theory*, Englewood Cliffs, NJ, Prentice Hall.

Bandura A. (1995) *Self-efficacy in Changing Societies*, New York, Cambridge Press.

Baric L. and Harrison A. (1977) 'Social pressure and health education', *Journal of the Institute of Health Education* 15(4): 12–18.

Bell R. R. (1966) 'Parent–child conflict in sexual values', *Journal of Social Issues* 22: 34–44.

Brandes D. and Ginnis P. (1986) *A Guide to Student Centred Learning*, Oxford, Blackwell.

British Medical Association (1997) *School Sex Education: Good Practice and Policy*, London, Board of Science and Education.

Brook Advisory Centres (1996) *What Should I Do? Guidance on Confidentiality and under 16s for Community Nurses, Social Workers, Teachers and Youth Workers*, London, Brook Advisory Centres.

Chief Medical Officer (1996) *On the State of the Public Health. The Annual Report of the Chief Medical Officer of the Department of Health for the Year 1995*, London, HMSO.

Conner M. and Norman P. (eds) (1996) *Predicting Health Behaviours*, Buckingham, Open University.

Curtis H., Lawrence C. and Tripp J. H. (1988) 'Social background and sexual experience of girls (pregnant before their 18th birthday)', *Archives of Disease in Childhood* 63: 373–9.

Department for Education and Employment (1995) *Science National Curriculum*, London, HMSO.

Department of Education and Science (1986) *Health Education from 5–16; Curriculum Matters 6*, London, HMSO.

Department of Health (1992) *The Health of the Nation: A Strategy for Health in England*, London, HMSO.

Department of Health (1998) *Our Healthier Nation*, London, HMSO.

Dickson R., Fullerton D., Eastwood A., Sheldon T., and Sharp F. (1997) *Effective Health Care: Preventing and Reducing the Adverse Effects of Unintended Teenage Pregnancies*, NHS Centre for Reviews and Dissemination, University of York, Churchill Livingstone.

Evans D., Rees J. B., Okagbue O. and Tripp J. H. (1998) 'Negotiating sexual intimacy: A PAUSE develops an approach using a peer-led, theatre-for-development model in the classroom', *Health Education* 6: 220–9.

Few C. (1995) 'Sensible sex education: a closer alliance between school nurses and the teaching profession at all levels will improve sex education in schools', *Nursing Times* 11 Oct: 59–60.

Fong S. (1994) *Youth to Youth Sexual Health Education Programmes: Summary Report*, Toronto, Toronto Department of Public Health.

Frankham J. (1998) 'Peer education: the unauthorised version', *British Educational Research Journal* 24(2): 179–93.

Genuis S. G. and Genuis S. K. (1995) 'Adolescent sexual involvement: time for primary prevention', *Lancet* 345: 240–1.

Hadley A. (1997) 'Teenage contraception', *British Journal of Sexual Medicine* Mar./Apr.: 13–16.

Heathcote G. (1989) 'Teachers, health education and in-service training', *Health Education Journal* 48: 172–5.

Hirst J. (1994) *Not in Front of the Grown-ups*, Sheffield's Health Research Institute, Sheffield Hallam University.

Holland J., Ramazanoglu C. and Scott S. (1990a) 'Managing risks and experiencing danger: tensions between government AIDS education policy and young women's sexuality', *Gender and Education* 2(2): 125–46.

Holland J., Ramazanoglu C. and Scott S. (1990b) *Sex, Risk and Danger: AIDS Education Policy and Young Women's Sexuality*, WRAP Paper 1, London, Tufnell Press.

Holland J., Mauthner M. and Sharpe S. (1996) *Family Matters: Communicating Health Messages in the Family*, London: HEA.

Holland J., Ramazanoglu C., Sharpe S. and Thomson R. (1998) *The Male in the Head: Young People, Hetrosexuality and Power*, London, Tufnell Press.

Howard M., and McCabe J. B. (1990) 'Helping teenagers postpone sexual involvement', *Family Planning Perspectives* 22(1): 21–6.

Ingham R. (1997) *The Development of an Integrated Model of Sexual Conduct Among Young People*, Southampton, University of Southampton.

Jemmott J. B., Jemmott L. S. and Fong G. T. (1998) 'Abstinence and safer sex: HIV risk-reduction interventions for African American adolescents', *Journal of the American Medical Association* 279(19): 1529–36.

Johnson A. M., Wadsworth J., Wellings K. and Field J. (1994) *Sexual Attitudes and Lifestyles*, Oxford, Blackwell.

Jowell T. (1999) *A Sexual Health Strategy for Britain*, Press Release at FPA Annual Conference, 23 March 1999.

Kirby D. (1989) 'Research on effectiveness of sex education programmes', *Theory into Practice* 28(3): 165–71.

Kirby D. (1995) Sex and HIV/AIDS education in schools have a modest but important impact on sexual behaviour. *British Medical Journal* 311(7207): 403.

Kirby D., Short L., Collins J. *et al.* (1994) 'School-based programmes to reduce sexual risk behaviours: a review of effectiveness', *Public Health Reports* 109(3): 339–60.

Kirby D., Korps M., Barth R. and Cagampang H. (1997) 'The impact of the postponing sexual involvement curriculum among youths in California', *Family Planning Perspectives* 29: 100–8.

Kolbe L. (1981) 'Propositions for an alternative and complimentary health education paradigm', *Health Education* May/Jun: pp. 24–30.

Lenderyou G. and Rey C. (1997) *Let's hear it for the boys!*, London, Sex Education Forum.

McGuire W. J. (1964) 'Inducing resistance to persuasion', *Advances in Experimental Social Psychology* 1(83): 191–229.

Mason A. and Palmer A. (1996) *Queer Bashing: A National Survey of Hate Crimes Against Lesbians and Gay Men*, London, Stonewall.

Measor L., Tiffin C. and Fry K. (1996) 'Gender and sex education: a study of adolescent responses', *Gender and Education* 8(3): 275–88.

Mellanby A. R., Phelps F. and Tripp J. H. (1995a) *Added Power and Understanding Sex Education – the Project and Results*, Exeter, University of Exeter.

Mellanby A. R., Phelps F. A., Curtis H. A., Tripp J. H. and Crichton N. J. (1995b) 'A sex education programme with medical and educational benefit', *British Medical Journal* 311: 453–77.

Mellanby A. R., Rees J. B. and Tripp J. H. (1996) *The Power To Be Me: The A PAUSE Sex Education Project in 'Sexual Awakening'*, London, MRC.

Milburn K. (1995) 'A critical review of peer education with young people with special reference to sexual health', *Health Education Research* 19(4): 407–20.

Nicholl A., Catchpole M., Cliffe, S., Hughes G., Simms I. and Thomas D. (1999) 'Sexual health of teenagers in England and Wales: analysis of national data', *British Medical Journal* 318: 1321–2.

Norfolk Health Authority (1995) *In a Class Apart: A Study of School Nursing*, Norwich Research Centre, Norfolk Health Authority.

Oakley A., Fullerton D., Holland J. *et al.* (1996) *Sexual Health Education Interventions for Young People: A Methodological Review*, London, Science Research Unit, London University Institute of Education.

Office of National Statistics (1996) *Conceptions in England and Wales 1994*, Birth Statistics, Series FM1 (96/2), London, HMSO.

Qualification Curriculum Authority/Department for Education and Employment (1999) *The Review of the National Curriculum in England – the Secretary of State's Proposals*, London, HMSO.

Regis D. (1996) 'Peer tutoring seems to work – but why?', *Education and Health* 13(5): 75–8.

Roche A. F. (1979) 'Secular trends in stature, weight and maturation', *Monograph of Social Research of Child Development* 44: 3–27.

Royal College of Obstetricians and Gynaecologists (1991) *Report of the RCOG Working Party on Unplanned Pregnancy*, London, RCOG.

Schaalma H. P., Kok G., Bosker R. J. *et al.* (1996) 'Planned development and evaluation of AIDS/STD education for secondary-school students in the Netherlands', *Health Education Quarterly* 23: 469–87.

Sex Education Forum (1997) *Supporting the Needs of Boys and Young Men in Sex and Relationships Education*, Sex Education Factsheet 11, London, Sex Education Forum.

Stuart-Smith S. (1996) 'Teenage sex: cognitive immaturity increases the risks', *British Medical Journal* 312: 390–1.

Thomson R. (1994) 'Moral rhetoric and public health pragmatism: the contemporary politics of sex education', *Feminist Review* 48: 40–61.

Walker B. and Kushner S. (1997) *Understanding Boys' Sexual Health Education and its Implications for Attitude Change*, Norwich, Centre for Applied Research in Education.

Watney S. (1987) *Policing Desire: Politics, Pornography and AIDS*, London, Methuen.

Wight D. (1997) 'Does sex education make a difference?', *Health Education* 2: 52–6.

World Health Organization (1986) *Ottawa Charter for Health Promotion. An International Conference on Health Promotion*, Copenhagen, WHO/EURO.

World Health Organization (1998) *Sexual and Reproductive Health Research Priorities for WHO 1998–2003*, Geneva, WHO.

Further reading

Jackson P. and Plant Z. (1997) 'Youngsters get an introduction to sexual health clinics', *Nursing Times* 92(21): 34–6.

Mellanby A. R., Pearson V. A. H. and Tripp J. H. (1997) 'Preventing teenage pregnancy', *Archives of Disease in Childhood* 77: 459–62.

Tripp J. H. and Mellanby A. R. (1995) 'Sex education – whose baby?', *Current Paediatrics* 5: 272–6.

13 The critically ill children study: a prospective study of the provision and outcome of paediatric intensive care in the South West

Siobhan Warne, Lynn Garland, Linda Bailey, Susan Edees, Patricia Weir and John Henderson

Introduction

There has in recent years been an increased focus, on the part of both professional bodies and the media, on the needs of critically ill children in the UK. The British Paediatric Association (BPA) survey published in 1993 identified a lack of paediatric intensive care beds in the UK and recommended that all critically ill children should be cared for in paediatric intensive care units (PICUs). The publication of *Paediatric Intensive Care: A Framework for the Future*, and its companion publication *A Bridge to the Future*, by the National Health Service (NHS) Executive (1997) reiterated these recommendations, although the impact of this has yet to be evaluated. The recommendations are based upon evidence from Australia and the USA demonstrating that critically ill children have an improved outcome if cared for in tertiary centres. A tertiary centre has been defined as a regional children's hospital with a dedicated PICU fulfilling set criteria of standards for medical staff, nursing staff and the facilities available (Pollack *et al.*, 1991).

There are, however, many differences in health care facilities, the case mix of patients admitted and intensive care resources and organisation when comparing the USA or Australia with the UK. No large-scale studies have been published identifying facilities for critically ill children and comparing the outcome with severity of illness in the UK.

Other reports have been written since the BPA published its survey, most recently *A Framework for the Future* (NHS Executive, 1997),

outlining the levels of staffing, training, equipment, services and facilities recommended for units caring for critically ill children.

The need for a large-scale regional UK study has been identified,
one that would identify the facilities available for critically ill children and use recognised severity of illness scoring tools and measurements of outcome on these children. It was felt that those children
requiring high-dependency care should also be identified and
included, especially those transferred directly from the ward to the
tertiary PICU. These children could be identified as being critically ill
in the ward area and should be included in any study attempting to
identify all critically ill children, despite their not being cared for on
an adult intensive care unit (AICU).

Having identified the need for such research, a pilot study using
the population, tools and measurements described was conducted in
the Exeter region, funding being received from the South West
Regional Health Authority NHS Executive, Research and Development grant scheme.

Literature review: structure and organisation of paediatric intensive care

A PICU has been defined as 'a facility designed, staffed and equipped
for the treatment and management of critically ill children from early
infancy to adolescence' (BPA, 1993, p. 4). The BPA working party on
intensive care documented that 20.5 per cent of children requiring
intensive care in 1991 were cared for in an AICU, 51 per cent in a
PICU and 28.6 per cent on a children's ward (Table 13.1).

Table 13.1   Identified areas of care for critically ill children

Area in which care was provided for critically ill children	Percentage of critically ill children cared for in each area
Adult intensive care unit	20
Paediatric intensive care unit	51
Paediatric ward	28

The working party consisted of representatives of the BPA, the Association of Paediatric Anaesthetists, the Association of Paediatric Surgery and the Royal College of Nursing. The report was based on a survey of all PICUs, AICUs, wards and units admitting children in the UK in 1991 (Table 13.2). There was an 84 per cent response rate. This did not include any PICU beds closed because of staff shortages. There were too few Registered Sick Children's nurses in all areas.

Table 13.2   Number of children requiring intensive care

Number of children admitted to hospital	600,000
Number of children requiring intensive care services	12,800
Number of beds available to provide at least high-dependency unit care	175

The National Health Service (NHS) Executive, in its critical appraisal of the report (1994), stated that although it was a useful source of information, there were a number of concerns:

- The response rate was only 84 per cent
- It was unclear what was meant by dependency levels 1, 2 and 3
- It did not state whether all high-dependency unit (HDU) admissions had been included
- There was a lack of UK evidence to support the recommendations put forward.

What was needed was a national audit of critically ill children, including those children requiring high-dependency care, looking at outcome adjusted for severity of illness.

Evidence from other countries, predominantly the USA and Australia, suggests that there is an improved outcome for children requiring paediatric intensive care when it is carried out in tertiary care paediatric units, particularly for those most severely ill (Pollack *et al.*, 1991; Shann, 1993a.) There have been few UK studies of the effectiveness of paediatric intensive care in tertiary or non-tertiary centres (Balakrishnan *et al.*, 1992), nor of the identification of patients who would benefit from transfer to a PICU from another hospital environment.

The BPA working party, in its 1993 report *The Care of Critically Ill Children*, recommended that paediatric intensive care in the UK should be carried out in a PICU if the child reaches dependency level 2 or 3 (Appendix 13.1). The level of provision of paediatric intensive care beds at that time was inadequate to meet these recommendations, the requirement being approximately 1 bed per 30,000–80,000 children (Paediatric Intensive Care Society, 1993; Yeh, 1992; Shann, 1993b; Barry and Hocking, 1994). Using an estimate of 1:48,000 (based on a childhood population of 13.5 million and the 1991 survey by the BPA of Intensive Care for Children in the UK), the BPA identified a UK shortfall of 72 beds.

The major evidence to support an improved outcome in tertiary care centres is from a study by Pollack *et al.* (1991) from Oregon, USA. A scoring system – the Pediatric Risk of Mortality (PRISM) – was used to predict mortality risk in critically ill children. This compared actual mortality with predicted mortality in tertiary and non-tertiary centres. It demonstrated an increased risk of mortality, adjusted for initial mortality risk, of up to seven times greater in non-tertiary centres. The mortality scores, which include some limited information on pre-morbidity, are based on physiological variables and their ranges in addition to diagnostic and other risk variables giving a risk of mortality score.

Non-tertiary centres in the USA cannot, however, be assumed to be equivalent to a district general hospital (DGH) in the UK. The case mix and staffing are considerably different so the results may not be directly applicable to the UK population. A more recently developed model – the Pediatric Index of Mortality (PIM) – based on eight variables measured at the time of first patient contact with intensive care, has been evaluated in a UK population (Pearson *et al.*, 1997) but has not been compared directly with PRISM.

The findings of the recent BPA survey (1993) did not demonstrate a significant difference in crude mortality, that is, in the number of children who died as a proportion of all children admitted to a unit without adjustment for initial severity of illness, between PICUs and AICUs. This observation may reflect differences in the case mix and illness severity of the populations treated, and it is important that mortality data are adjusted for these potentially confounding variables.

.dvantages and disadvantages of tertiary care

There are potential advantages associated with the care of children in tertiary care PICUs. It has been suggested that quality of care improves with a greater throughput of patients in larger units (Farley and Ozminkowski, 1992; this has been demonstrated in neonatal intensive care units in the UK (Field *et al.*, 1991). There is, however, one study of adult intensive care that refutes this (Rowan, 1994). In addition to this, families may benefit from child-orientated facilities and the counselling that may be available centrally, although the relationships between such facilities and patient morbidity have not been well evaluated. Combined with this, the centralisation of care may carry some cost advantages, because of a more efficient use of resources. Family-centred care is, however, more difficult to provide when services are centralised. When care is provided locally, the family retain their established support mechanisms.

In addition, the transport of critically ill children is difficult and carries an inherent risk of morbidity (Kanter and Tomkins, 1989). The risk of transferring a child is significantly reduced when the transfer is undertaken by a dedicated intensive care team, usually provided by the receiving PICU (Britto *et al.*, 1995). It may be advisable to arrange for the transfer of critically ill children at an early stage of a potentially progressive illness as increasing physiological instability is likely to increase the risk of transfer-related morbidity. The difficulty lies in selecting at an early stage those most likely to deteriorate, thus preventing an excess of children being transferred who do not necessarily require paediatric intensive care in a tertiary unit, with the consequent impact on the availability of beds and resources.

Methodology

Methods of evaluating outcome

The availability of suitable methods for evaluating the outcome of paediatric intensive care is controversial, there being a lack of standardised measurements that can be used for this purpose. Crude mortality data may not reflect differences in case mix in that tertiary centres are likely to care for 'sicker' children. Several systems have been developed to compare the outcome of intensive care, some using physiological variables based on the concept that physiological instability directly reflects the risk of mortality (Pollack *et al.*,

1988), others using therapeutic variables (Cullen *et al.*, 1974; Malstam and Lind, 1992). These scores may be artificially influenced by physician practices.

One of the most widely used scoring systems is PRISM, which is based on 14 physiological variables and indicates disease severity independent of diagnosis (Pollack *et al.*, 1988). The score was developed from the much larger Physiological Stability Index in order to reduce the number of physiological variables required to be measured, thus simplifying data collection.

The PRISM score (Table 13.3) was developed and validated in the USA. It has only been validated in a small UK population of 270 subjects in Glasgow (Balakrishnan *et al.*, 1992; Goddard, 1992), but it is currently the most accurate tool available for comparing outcomes between centres for a given severity of illness.

Table 13.3 PRISM Score (Pollack *et al.*, 1988)

Variables measured	
Systolic blood pressure	(mmHg)
Diastolic blood pressure	(mmHg)
Heart rate	(beats/min.)
Respiratory rate	(breaths/min.)
Arterial oxygen tension/	(PaO_2)
fractional inspired oxygen ratio	(FiO_2)
Arterial carbon dioxide tension	($PaCO_2$)
Glasgow coma score	
Pupillary reactions	
Prothrombin time/partial	
thromboplastin time ratio	
Total bilirubin time	(μmol/l)
Potassium	(mmol/l)
Calcium	(mmol/l)
Glucose	(mmol/l)
Bicarbonate	(mmol/l)

PRISM III is a third-generation physiology-based method of measuring mortality risk which looks at the child's reason for admission and takes into account events prior to admission to the intensive care unit or PICU (Pollack *et al.*, 1996.)

The PIM (Table 13.4) is based on eight variables measured at the time of first patient contact with intensive care; it includes physiological variables, reason for admission and chronic health (Shann *et al.*, 1997).

Table 13.4   Information to calculate the Pediatric
Index of Mortality (Shann *et al.*, 1997)

Booked or elective admission	
Presence of specified underlying conditions	
Pupillary responses	
Base excess in arterial or capillary blood	(mmHg)
Arterial oxygen tension	(PaO_2)
Fractional inspired oxygen concentration	(FiO_2)
Systolic blood pressure	(mmHg)
Mechanical ventilation during the first hour	
Outcome of intensive care unit admission	

The Therapeutic Intervention Score System (TISS) (Cullen *et al.*, 1974; Malstam and Lind, 1992) is a method for quantifying therapies and may be used to compare interventions for a given illness severity in different units.

The evaluation of the delivery of paediatric intensive care may also include an assessment of adverse events related to intensive care, such as accidental extubations, the blocking of endotracheal tubes, the loss of intravenous arterial lines, line sepsis rates and inappropriate drug doses (Kanter and Tompkins, 1989; Barry and Ralston, 1994).

Using all these validated scoring systems will enable different institutions to be compared on illness severity of the population of children cared for, the process of care delivery and the occurrence of defined adverse events.

Currently, however, there are few validated tools to measure outcomes other than mortality. Because mortality is a relatively uncommon event, large-scale studies are required to enable a valid comparison between units. It can be argued that morbidity in terms of disability, future physical and psychological health, and ultimately economic productivity is a more important measure of the benefits of intensive care, which remains a high-cost area of health care.

Outcome measures used

The main outcome measure used will be death adjusted for predicted mortality calculated from the PRISM score. Secondary outcomes will be length of stay, therapeutic interventions (TISS), POPC (Pediatric Overall Performance Category) and PCPC (Pediatric Cerebral Performance Category) (Fiser, 1992), all adjusted for illness severity, and adverse intensive care events. If there is a difference in outcome between different centres, the data will be analysed for criteria that may identify patients early in their illness who may benefit from transfer to a tertiary centre. This may enable children to be transferred before they become too sick. Centres will be categorised according to 6-monthly audit of trained staff, both medical and nursing, the throughput of children and the availability of paediatric support services.

Several studies carried out in the South West Region over the past 5 years have used similar methods of data collection, relying upon hospitals across the region to notify a central co-ordinator of cases, who then collects the relevant data. The following studies have been successful in receiving regional co-operation and case ascertainment: 'Confidential enquiry into stillbirths and deaths in infancy' (Professor P. Fleming, Bristol) and 'Hearing loss in bacterial meningitis' (Dr M. Richardson, Bath).

Aims of the study

Research questions

- Is there a difference in mortality between critically ill children cared for in a tertiary PICU and in a non-tertiary unit ?
- Can illness severity scoring prospectively identify children who will most benefit from transfer to a tertiary PICU?

Study aims

- To determine the availability of intensive care and high-dependency care facilities for critically ill children in the original South West Regional Health Authority
- To develop methods to prospectively identify children who will most benefit from transfer to a tertiary PICU.

Objectives

- To identify all children in the region who meet the minimum defined criteria of the need for intensive care
- To collect information over the course of their illness to assess objectively their illness severity and the level of intervention
- To record the outcome of all children identified as critically ill over the course of the study
- To collect information on any children transferred between hospitals within and out of the region to determine illness severity pre- and post-transfer, and to identify any adverse events occurring during transfer.

Questions to be considered

At the time that this study was being conducted, conflicting evidence and financial constraints led to little progress being made locally; the BPA working party recommendations had little impact until recently in changing the provision of paediatric intensive care services. In response to the NHS Executive South and West's (1994) discussion paper on the care of critically ill children, several purchasers were unable to identify children receiving critical care; none had separate contracts. Only one supported the development of paediatric intensive care, the remainder developing strategies but expressing concern about the drain on local resources and the development of transport systems. The publication of *Paediatric Intensive Care: A Framework for the Future* and the companion document *A Bridge to the Future* by the NHS Executive (1997) has changed this.

An evaluation of the effects of these documents is not currently available. They provide a clear policy framework, including standards to be met by all hospitals providing paediatric intensive care, principles underpinning the future organisation of these services and means by which to make the best use of available resources, expertise and specialist facilities.

In order to plan to provide critically ill children with efficient and good-quality intensive care, large studies to evaluate the current provisions, outcomes and efficiencies are needed.

Pilot study

A pilot study was carried out in Exeter, a DGH of the South West serving a population of 300,000, in order to assess the use of scoring systems and to ascertain the range of severity of illness in children receiving intensive care in the DGH. This enabled us to make a prediction of the power of the proposed regional study to demonstrate a significant difference in mortality between tertiary and non-tertiary units based on initial illness severity. The power of a study is a calculation of the ability of the study to demonstrate a difference between the outcomes in two populations at a predetermined probability based on the population size, the observed differences between the populations and the variability of measuring the observations.

Children were retrospectively studied by case note review over a 2-year period (1 January 1992 to 31 December 1993). Case mix and outcome, as predicted by the PRISM score, were recorded. One hundred and three children were admitted, records being found for 101 – 40 females and 63 males – with a median age of 37.5 months, ranging from 1 day to 15 years 11 months.

Table 13.5   Number of cases for each diagnosis

Primary diagnosis	Number of cases
Respiratory causes	53
Neurological causes	25
Post-operative	16
Trauma cases	5

Dependency levels were assessed according to the BPA (1993) definitions and Paediatric Intensive Care Society standards (1992). Sixty-two children required level 1 care, 30 children level 2 care and 9 children level 3 care (Table 13.6). No deaths occurred in children needing level 1 or level 2 care, but 7 out of 9 children classified as level 3 died.

Thirty children were ventilated for a mean of 3.45 days (range 0.06–12.33 days). The primary diagnosis of each case is shown in

Table 13.5. From admission-day PRISM score calculations, the probability of death ranged from 0.33 per cent to 95.9 per cent. Seven deaths occurred, compared with a predicted 6.5. The highest risk survivor had a predicted mortality of 33 per cent.

Table 13.6   Number of children, number of deaths and PRISM score for BPA levels 1, 2 and 3

British Paediatric Association	Number of children within criteria	Number of deaths	Mortality risk from PRISM* score (%)
Level 1	62	0	0.33% – 34%
Level 2	30	0	0.45% – 22%
Level 3	9	7	2.75% – 95.5%

*Pediatric Risk of Mortality

There was a wide range of mortality risk within the dependency levels (level 1: 0.33–34.0 per cent; level 2: 0.45–22.0 per cent; level 3: 2.75–95.5 per cent) and the median PRISM score being no different between levels 1 and 2.

To examine which children may have benefited from transfer to a PICU, the following assumptions were made:

1.   The only patients to benefit from transfer to a tertiary PICU were those who subsequently died
2.   Patients who displayed signs of brain stem compromise on arrival (for example, fixed, dilated pupils) would have died in any case.

Based on these assumptions, and using BPA levels 2 and 3 to identify children to be transferred, the sensitivity (the proportion *not* transferred using these criteria of all children who would *not* have benefited from transfer) would have been 75 per cent, and the specificity (the children who would have benefited from and were transferred as a proportion of all those who would potentially have benefited) 64.2 per cent. By using BPA levels 2 and 3 combined with a predicted mortality of greater than 5 per cent (from the day one PRISM score), the number of children for potential transfer is reduced to 12. The sensitivity remains at 75 per cent, but the specificity increases to 90.4 per cent.

The case mix in this study differs from that reported in studies from other countries, supporting the opinion that conclusions on the organisation of care based on these data may not be directly applicable to some areas of the UK population. The results suggest that the care of children with dependency level 1 or 2 and with a predicted mortality of less than 5 per cent can be carried out successfully in a general intensive care unit. None of the four children with a predicted mortality score of greater than 35 per cent survived, but centralised services may improve outcome for this group.

Bristol Children's Hospital has the only tertiary PICU in the South West and at that time cared for an average of 200 patients per annum (1985 figures). Approximately half of these patients are referred for the management of critical illness, the remainder being planned admissions following, for example, cardiac surgery. Statistical calculations have been based on the assumption that 200 patients with acute, critical illness will be managed in the tertiary PICU. This figure has since risen to 600 patients per annum.

Data from the pilot study (Susan Edees and John Tripp, personal communication 1994) suggest that the number of eligible children treated in district hospitals over the 2-year period would be about 800. The distribution of mortality risk in the Children's Hospital was based on unpublished records of patient dependencies in the PICU (1985). The study was predicated upon an 80 per cent power to detect a difference in mortality of 15 per cent between hospitals in subjects with a predicted mortality of 31–100 per cent. A combination of dependency level and PRISM score may provide a method of identifying patients at an appropriate time for transfer to a tertiary centre.

This raises issues for nursing practice. There is a need for nurses on AICUs to maintain staff education and training focusing on paediatric issues, providing an appropriate area for paediatric care and ensuring a safe level of equipment (Bennett, 1997).

Sample

The aim is to collect information prospectively on all children receiving high-dependency and intensive care in the geographically defined South West region over a 2-year period. Information has been collected on disease severity (PRISM, PRISM III and PIM), dependency level (defined by the BPA, 1993, based on previous

Paediatric Intensive Care Society, 1992, definitions), TISS and outcomes (POPC and PCPC). Death is easily defined, but there are few validated tools to measure outcome.

It is likely that long-term follow-up and a detailed knowledge of the pre-morbid state will be needed; no validated tools currently exist for this. It is difficult to assess morbidity associated with paediatric intensive care without a prior knowledge of the pre-morbid state. The PIM, however, does include some limited pre-morbidity data. Although it is acknowledged that morbidity on discharge may not accurately reflect longer-term morbidity, a previously validated tool, the POPC and PCPC, is being used, which will allow some comparison between units based on the initial severity of illness (Fiser, 1992). The absence of validated morbidity tools is a recognised limitation of the study and will provide a direction for future research.

The principal outcome measures used will be mortality using the PRISM, PRISM III and PIM scores, and two validated, six-point performance categories: assessment of neurological and physical status on discharge from hospital using the PCPC and POPC.

Sample size

The South West region has 490,591 children under 17 years of age (OPCS 1991), a figure predicted to rise to 757,938 by 2000. During the pilot study, there were 103 admissions from a population of 81,600 children. Applying this proportion to the regional population, it can be predicted that approximately 1000 children will require intensive care in the 2-year study period. The aim of the study is to collect information on consecutive admissions in the South West region for 2 years; data collection started on 2 December 1996.

Study population

The age distribution chosen for this study is 0–16 years. No lower age limit was applied, but children must have been discharged from hospital since birth in order to exclude neonatal intensive care activity; the upper age limit was less than 16 years on the day of admission.

The inclusion criteria are as follows:

- any child admitted to hospital who reaches the criteria set out in Appendix 13.2

- any child admitted to a designated intensive care or high-dependency care bed
- any child identified by nursing or medical staff as needing 'specialling'
- also, any children admitted through the accident and emergency department who are subsequently transferred out of the region for intensive care facilities or for specialist surgery, and all those who do not survive.

From the data collected in the pilot study, an admission rate of 1 per 800 children over 2 years (1:1600 per annum) is anticipated. This may be a conservative estimate compared with the reported admission rate from another UK region of 1–2 per 1000 per annum (BPA, 1993).

Applying the former frequency to projected figures for the childhood population of the region (OPCS, 1991), it is expected that approximately 1000 children will require high-dependency or intensive care during the prospective 2-year study proposed.

Criteria for inclusion

The criteria for identifying a critically ill child are based on BPA level 1 criteria, a dependency level of one nurse per two patients and recognised clinical descriptions of potentially critically ill children. Although these defined dependency levels are a non-standard assessment and may not be applied consistently across units, there is currently no standard method for identifying such patients at the lower end of the dependency scale. This definition has been selected because it allows the identification of critically ill children who would be missed using more standardised indices of nursing dependency (for example, 'special' nursing). The outcome measure of greatest interest in this study, mortality, is likely to be an extremely rare event in the population of children with the lowest dependency levels.

The inadvertent inclusion or exclusion of occasional subjects in this population is unlikely significantly to affect the primary conclusions of the study. These criteria were evaluated by Dr Susan Edees in the Royal Berkshire Hospital, Reading over a 1-month period to verify that appropriate patients were identified. The aim was to ensure that children requiring high-dependency care on the ward with a BPA dependency level of at least 1 were entered into the study. Some adjustments were made to the original criteria to ensure that most of those entered achieved a PRISM score greater than or equal to 1 per cent.

Design of the study

A team of research nurses co-ordinated the data collection. All hospitals in the original South West region admitting paediatric intensive care patients have been recruited into the study, and data have been collected from these ward areas.

All the hospitals involved in the study were asked to notify the research nurse of all children (under 16 years of age) admitted to:

- PICUs
- AICUs
- HDUs

as well as:

- children on paediatric wards receiving at least high-dependency nursing care
- readmissions to neonatal intensive care units
- any child transferred out of the region for intensive care.

Each ward area was supplied with the criteria for admission, identifying how to enter the child in the study, and guidance for the paperwork.

A link nurse was identified in each ward area to assist in the co-ordination of the study. The study relied on the link nurses to collect and co-ordinate data within each ward area. Where possible, the link nurses have been involved in developing and establishing the study across the region. They are able to provide a vital link between the research team in Bristol and staff in their own area, ensuring that nursing issues have been addressed. The link nurses have been able to identify and highlight problems, assisting in problem solving where possible. They were kept up to date with the study's progress through personal communication and through a quarterly newsletter.

It is anticipated that the identified link nurses will be involved with the research team in utilising and disseminating the findings of the study at a local level. All information collated has been audited by the research team from Bristol.

Nursing staff from the admitting ward completed admission details, day one PRISM score and a daily TISS score. Any adverse events occurring during the child's critical period were identified on the TISS form. Discharge details including length of stay were also provided. The principal consultant involved in the child's care completed a discharge assessment scoring POPC and PCPC. To ensure that data are accurate and complete, all data received from the participating hospitals have been audited by the research nurses, using case notes and intensive care unit charts. This ensures the quality and reliability of all the data used in the study.

It is inevitable that, in some cases, the child's notes or intensive care unit charts were unavailable (as was demonstrated in the pilot study, 2 per cent being unavailable). If particular data have not been audited by the research nurse, that child has been excluded from the study. The use of key initial data will enable comparison of the excluded subjects with the study population to ensure no systematic bias is introduced.

If the child's PRISM score is less than 1 per cent, the child has been excluded, as defined by the previous inclusion criteria. It is inevitable that some children eligible for inclusion in the study may be overlooked. The admission records on the intensive care units involved have been audited to ensure that all children admitted to designated unit beds have been included in the study. Children who have repeated admissions to intensive care during the same illness have been admitted to the study only for the period of their first admission.

Intensive data collection on children in the study was carried out for the first 21 days only; length of stay and outcomes have been recorded. This was done to avoid the amassing of excessive data on very few long-stay patients as the research question is based on resources for acute critical illness.

For each ward area, within each hospital involved in the study, information was collected on the qualifications of staff, their specialty and availability, to identify who was available to look after critically ill children and what hospital facilities were available on a 24-hour basis. Limited information has also been collected on hospital-based estimates of daily costs of care for each patient. This data collection was repeated every 6 months and has provided a profile of each area admitting critically ill children.

Time schedule

The study has run over a 3-year period, the 2 years' data collection being from December 1996 to November 1998. Data analysis, presentation and the publication of results is anticipated from April 2000 onwards.

Conclusion

This study will be one of the largest systematic studies of paediatric intensive and high-dependency care provision and outcome for children to be conducted in the UK. It is anticipated that the results obtained will be representative of other UK populations of children. The scoring systems used – PRISM, PRISM III and PIM – will be validated in a large UK population, which should enable a validated scoring system to be used in other regional studies, thus allowing reliable comparison in the UK.

This study will provide some of the most accurate and up-to-date information available for the development of paediatric intensive care services in the South West, assessing who is currently looking after the children in the region and what services are available to them. The results should allow the allocation of resources to be based on scientific evidence to provide the most appropriate form of intensive care for critically ill children. It may provide a template for a national study to evaluate mortality and morbidity associated with the management of critically ill children.

The results are expected to provide information on the types of child currently being transferred to the regional PICU, and measure the adverse effects that occur during transfer. Developing a method of assessing and identifying those children who would most benefit from transfer to a PICU may be possible following data analysis.

In addition to this, the period of the study spans the introduction of a regional PICU retrieval team (following the NHS Executive's 1997 report). An assessment of the impact of this service on the patterns and outcomes of care before and after its introduction will be made. The study will provide a model, as recommended in the NHS Executive *Framework for the Future* report (1997), for a large-scale study to plan and provide for critically ill children based on the current provision and outcome measures. It is believed that the information generated will form a rational basis to provide the most effective service for critically ill children.

Appendix 13.1

BPA dependency levels definitions

Dependency level 1/ High-dependency care:
The child needing close monitoring and observation, but not requiring assistance from life support machines. Nurse to patient ratio of at least 0.5:1

Dependency level 2/Intensive care:
The child requiring continuous nursing supervision, who is intubated and undergoing IPPV or CPAP. Some unintubated children, whose condition is unstable, may also fall into this category. Nurse to patient ratio of at least 1:1

Dependency level 3/Intensive care:
The child who needs intensive supervision at all times, requiring additional complex and regular nursing and therapeutic procedures. Nurse to patient ratio of 1–2:1

Appendix 13.2

Criteria for inclusion into the critically ill children study

Meningitis
Meningococcal septicaemia
GCS <12 (Glasgow coma score)
Urine output <1ml/kg/per hour
Fitting for over 1 hour

OR

who require one or more of the following:

- Airway intervention/support
- Ventilatory support
- 60 per cent oxygen at one time
- Cardiopulmonary resuscitation
- Nebulised adrenaline
- more than 10ml/kg intravenous fluid bolus

- Continuous monitoring
- Over 40 per cent continuous oxygen for over 12 hours
- Nebulised bronchodilator (more than 1 per hour for more than 6 hours)
- Continuous intravenous drug infusion for over 12 hrs

242   *Siobhan Warne* et al.

References

Balakrishnan G., Aitchison T., Hallworth D. and Morton N. S. (1992) 'Prospective evaluation of the Paediatric Risk of Mortality (PRISM) score', *Archives of Disease in Childhood* 67:196–200.

Barry P. W. and Hocking M. D. (1994) 'Paediatric use of intensive care', *Archives of Disease in Childhood* 70: 391–4.

Barry P. W. and Ralston C. (1994) 'Adverse events occurring during interhospital transfer of the critically ill', *Archives of Disease in Childhood* 71: 8–11.

Bennett J. (1997) 'Critically ill children: the case for short-term care in general intensive care units', *Intensive and Critical Care Nursing* 13(1): 53–7.

British Paediatric Association (1993) *The Care of Critically Ill Children. Report of the Multidisciplinary Working Party on Paediatric Intensive Care*, London, BPA.

Britto J., Nadel S., Maconochie I., Levin M. and Habibi P. (1995) 'Morbidity and severity of illness during interhospital transfer: impact of a specialised paediatric retrieval team', *British Medical Journal* 311: 836–9.

Cullen D. J., Civetta J. M., Briggs B. A. *et al.* (1974) 'Therapeutic intervention scoring system: a method for qualitative comparison of patient care', *Critical Care Medicine* 2: 57–60.

Farley D. E. and Ozminkowski R. J. (1992) 'Volume–outcome relationships and inhospital mortality: the effect of changes in volume over time', *Medical Care* 30: 77–94.

Field D., Hodges S., Mason E. and Burton P. (1991) 'Survival and place of treatment of premature delivery', *Archives of Disease in Childhood*, 66: 408–11.

Fiser D. H. (1992) 'Assessing the outcome of paediatric intensive care', *Journal of Paediatrics* 121: 68–74.

Goddard J. M. (1992) 'Pediatric risk of mortality scoring overestimates severity of illness in infants', *Critical Care Medicine* 20(12): 1662–5.

Kanter R. K, and Tompkins J. M. (1989) 'Adverse events during interhospital transport: physiological deterioration associated with pretransport severity of illness', *Pediatrics* 84: 43–8.

Malstam J. and Lind L. (1992) 'Therapeutic intervention scoring system (TISS) – a method for measuring workload and calculating costs in the ICU', *Acta Anaesthesiologica Scandinavica* 36: 758–63.

NHS Executive (1997) *Paediatric Intensive Care: A Bridge to the Future, Report of the Chief Nursing Officer's Taskforce to the Chief Executive of the NHS Executive*. London, NHSE.

NHS Executive (1997) *Paediatric Intensive Care: A Framework for the Future, Report from the National Co-odinating Group on Intensive Care to The Chief Executive of the NHS Executive*, London, NHSE.

NHS Executive South and West (1994) *Discussion Paper on the Care of Critically Ill Children*. Section 5: 13–20. Bristol.

Office of Population Census and Surveys (1991) *Census Outline Statistics for England and Wales*, London, Government Statistical Service.

Paediatric Intensive Care Society (1993) *Standards for Paediatric Intensive Care*, Mosby Year Book Europe.

Pearson G., Shann F. and Barry P. (1997) 'Should paediatric intensive care be centralised? Trent versus Victoria', *Lancet* **344**: 1213–17.

Pollack M. M., Ruttimann U. E. and Getson P. R. (1988) 'Pediatric risk of mortality (PRISM) score', *Critical Care Medicine* **16**: 1110–16.

Pollack M. M., Alexander S. R., Clarke N., Ruttiman V. E., Tesselaar H. M. and Bachulis A. (1991) 'Improved outcomes from tertiary centre paediatric intensive care: a statewide comparison', *Critical Care Medicine* **19**: 150–9.

Pollack M. M., Kantial M. P. and Ruttiman U. E. (1996) PRISM III: an updated pediatric risk of mortality score', *Critical Care Medicine* **24**(5): 743–52.

Rowan K. (1994) Personal communication in *A Critical Appraisal of the Care of Critically Ill Children*, NHS Centre for Reviews and Dissemination, University of York.

Shann F. (1993a) 'Paediatric intensive care', *Lancet* **342**: 1240.

Shann F. (1993b) 'Australian view of paediatric intensive care in Britain', *Lancet* **342**: 68.

Shann F., Pearson G., Slater A. and Wilkinson K. (1997) 'Paediatric index of mortality (PIM): a mortality prediction model for children in intensive care', *Intensive Care Medicine* **23**: 201–7.

Yeh T. S. (1992) 'Regionalisation of paediatric critical care', *Critical Care Clinics* **8**: 23–35.

14 *The lived experiences of paediatric nurses' enjoyment of caring for sick children*

Marie Bodycombe-James

Introduction

This chapter gives a descriptive account of whether some children are more popular patients than others. Work previously carried out on the topic has concentrated mainly on adult care (Stockwell, 1972). Therefore very little is known about the effect of popularity on nursing relationships and care within paediatric nursing.

The results of the study show that there are, in fact, children who were more popular than others, including children who are brave, can communicate and are uncomplaining. In contrast, unpopular children were uncommunicative, unco-operative, selfish or spoilt. Other factors also influenced the nurses' enjoyment of caring: the relationship of the nurse and the parents, the nurse's own personal experiences and whether the nurse felt that he or she had the expert skills to care for the child. A further important factor was the length of time the nurse had known the child; it appears that the longer the relationship, the more enjoyment the nurse experiences.

The concept of the unpopular adult patient has been well researched (Stockwell, 1972; Baer and Lowery, 1987; English and Morse, 1988; Meadow, 1992; Mathers, 1995). There is, however, a dearth of information and research on the popularity of child patients. Thus, this study focused on the popularity or unpopularity of child patients and its effect on care. Within existing literature, patients who are seen as unpopular are referred to as good, bad, problematic and heartsink (Kelly and May, 1982; English and Morse, 1988; Meadow, 1992).

The research study uses a qualitative method in order to generate nursing knowledge (Field and Morse, 1996). The data are analysed using a thematic approach, and some tentative conclusions are discussed. It is, however, recognised that from such a small-scale study no generalisations can be made from the results. Parahoo

(1997) states that qualitative researchers believe the phenomena under study are specific to time and culture. Therefore, the study cannot be replicated and the findings cannot be generalised to different cultures and settings.

Literature review

From a review of the literature, there was a scarcity of research on the popularity of child patients. The available literature could be analysed within three categories: patient situational factors, physical attractiveness and temperament theory.

Patient situational factors

Research by Stockwell (1972) highlighted factors that could account for patients' popularity. Popular patients were found to be those who were friendly and whom the nurses felt were easy to get on with, as well as those whom they had got to know best. The study identified that the most popular patients were those with whom the nurses had most social contact. Good patients and bad patients can be divided into six categories depending on: illness, disease and symptoms; patient behaviour and staff responses; social and non-clinical factors; perceived patient attitudes; judgements by staff; prescriptions; and remedies (Kelly and May, 1982). Other research studies by Meadow (1992), Baer and Lowery (1987), English and Morse (1988), Mathers *et al.* (1995) suggest there is a definite pattern to patients who are deemed unpopular, these patients often being aggressive, less educated, long-stay patients. Popular patients are cheerful, pleasant and compliant. It would appear that the most important factors in popularity to emerge from these studies are the personality of the individual and compliance to treatment regimes, rather than the illness or level of dependence.

Physical attraction

One of the most obvious and personal characteristics of an individual is his or her personal appearance. Interpersonal attraction has a powerful effect on all human relationships, the precise effect of attraction on quality of care being unknown. However, findings suggest that unattractive patients are neglected by staff, are more isolated and suffer increased psychological and physiological problems (Dion *et al.*, 1972; Corter *et al.*, 1978; Mitsunaga and Hall, 1979; Damrosch, 1982, Bordieri *et al.*, 1984). This, however, is an area that remains inconclusive within paediatric care.

Temperament theory

McLeod and McClowry (1990) and Ruddy-Wallace (1987) suggest that temperament theory could have either a positive or negative effect on the relationship between the nurse and the child. There is, however, no evidence to suggest that a child's temperament affects his or her popularity. From a review of the literature, it is evident that there is a lack of evidence on the popularity of paediatric patients.

The purpose and focus of the study

The literature review revealed that individuals are classed as either popular or unpopular, factors influencing popularity being the personality of the patients, physical attractiveness and the child's temperament (Dion *et al.*, 1972; Stockwell, 1972; Thomas and Chess, 1977; Corter *et al.*, 1978; Damrosch, 1982; Bordieri *et al.*, 1984; McLeod and McClowry, 1990). There was also evidence to suggest that patients who did not conform to the expected norms and values of the nursing and medical profession were viewed as unpopular. There appeared, however, to be a lack of information on paediatric patients' popularity or unpopularity.

It seemed important therefore to discover whether some children are in fact more popular than others with nursing staff. If this appears to be the case, what factors influence nurses' enjoyment of caring for sick children in hospital, and does this affect the quality of care given to children and their families?

A qualitative approach was adopted for this study as the aim was to create a descriptive account of the 'lived experience' of paediatric nurses' enjoyment of caring for sick children in hospital. Qualitative research produces descriptive data that allow the researcher to see people in their immediate environment and witness how they define their world.

Within qualitative analysis there are three established disciplines: anthropology, sociology and existential phenomenology. The phenomenological method is directed towards uncovering the meaning of a phenomenon as it is humanly experienced (Parse *et al.*,

1985). Phenomenology is the kind of thinking that guides one back from the theoretical abstraction to the reality of lived experience (Field and Morse, 1996). Many nurse researchers, for example Benner and Wrubel (1989), Paterson and Zderad (1988), Morrison (1992) and Darbyshire (1994), have used approaches grounded in phenomenology.

Phenomenology was chosen as the theoretical underpinning for the study because the purpose was to make sense of the data so that the world of the informant could be clearly understood (Morrison, 1992). Because the focus of phenomenological research is describing the lived experience, it provided the most appropriate research method to describe the experience of paediatric nurses' enjoyment of caring for sick children in hospital. Phenomenology, according to Munhall and Olier Boyd (1986), is the most appropriate approach to study concepts and issues within nursing whose meanings have remained unclear or unexplained. In order to analyse the data, Giorgi's (1975) framework (Figure 14.1) was used as it was felt that this would ensure that the world of the informant was described in a rigorous manner and offered the opportunity for independent validation. The framework also gave validity and reliability to the study. There is, however, always the possibility of error even when all precautions are taken as the researcher can still describe inaccurately.

---

1. The researcher reads the entire description of the experience in order to get a sense of the whole.
2. The researcher reads the descriptions again, more slowly, identifying transitions or units in the experience, called constituents.
3. The researcher clarifies the units by relating them to each other and to the whole.
4. The researcher reflects on the given constituents, still identified in the concrete language of the subject, and transforms that language into the language or concepts of science.
5. The researcher then integrates and synthesises the insights into a descriptive structure of the meaning of that experience.

(Giorgi 1975, as cited in Omery 1983)

Figure 14.1   Framework of analysis

Setting and research participants

Six participants were chosen at random from a list of Registered Sick Children's Nurses working in three local district general hospitals. This number was felt to be sufficient for the purpose of the study as qualitative methods produce vast quantities of data (Field and Morse, 1996).

Method

The method chosen for this research was the unstructured interview as the intention was to ascertain the feelings and attitudes of the paediatric nurses towards sick children they had enjoyed, or not enjoyed, caring for.

The interview began by asking the participant to describe a child or children whom she had enjoyed nursing. Later in the interview, the participant was asked to describe a child or children whom she had not enjoyed nursing. As the interviews progressed, other questions were asked depending on how the story unfolded. A cassette recorder was used for data gathering during the interviews. Following the interviews, the data were transcribed onto a word processor. The end result was a description of the phenomenon from the accounts given by those who experienced it.

Data analysis and discussion

Seven themes were identified from the new data:

1. age groups
2. conditions
3. getting to know you
4. expert at doing things
5. own experience
6. negative feelings
7. families.

There was some overlap between the themes as it was often a combination of factors that appeared to affect the nurses' enjoyment of caring for sick children.

Age groups

The nurses within the study expressed their enjoyment of caring for children during difference stages of the child's life. To begin with, these preferences were made with no rationale:

> I like adolescents and the school child… but a ward full of toddlers would drive me nuts.

However, there appeared to be commonalities between the nurses' enjoyment of caring for certain children. Babies were very popular because it was felt that they needed a great deal of nursing care. This was reinforced by their belief that the babies were too young to understand who was caring for them:

> I feel they are my favourites because I think I can do all the care for them, where the older children will rely on their parents far more.

This suggests that the nurses enjoy caring for babies because they can do more hands-on nursing care rather than support the parents in caring for their child.

Toddlers were described as difficult and demanding, having temper tantrums and being a handful. The nurses also recognised that these children needed their mothers to be with them constantly during a period of hospitalisation, demonstrating an understanding of the effects of hospitalisation on the young child as described by Robertson (1970). It is indeed of vital importance that paediatric nurses have an in-depth knowledge of child developmental theory and the effects of hospitalisation so that they can be aware of the effects of separation on the young child (Bowlby, 1951; Robertson, 1970).

A popular group with all the nurses were school-aged children because they could communicate by the use of language and were seen as being interested in their environment and 'into everything'. They were viewed as more co-operative because they 'understand more about what is going on'. One nurse expressed this by saying:

> I think mainly because they can listen you can explain things to them and they understand; they are very co-operative, well most of them [laugh] um… or if there is anything they don't understand they are quite willing to listen.

Adolescents, on the other hand, were seen as an unpopular age group, mainly because the nurses felt that they could not communicate with them. This was often because the adolescents were seen to have a poor relationship with their parents and were resentful of being in a ward with younger children. One particular group of adolescents who were described as unpopular were those who had attempted to commit suicide:

> they are difficult to nurse you can't get through to them, especially the overdoses... there is very poor communication.

This was often exaggerated when the parents and the child were in conflict, or the parent appeared to be indifferent to the plight of the adolescent:

> some parents don't give a damn; I have seen some laugh because their child has overdosed on alcohol... it makes me angry.

This nurse stressed that she would not show her anger to the parents or child but would communicate her feelings to other members of staff.

Within the study area, there were no formal avenues of support, stress being dealt with in a very informal way. One nurse's experience was that 'you just talk it through and it comes out that way'. Nurses often give peer support as an example of supervision. However, a few have constructed the opportunity to formalise this support, and the more formal process of clinical supervision gives nurses the opportunity for personal and professional growth (Butterworth and Faugier, 1992).

A further problem with adolescents was that the nurses felt that they were being cared for in the wrong environment:

> they have got to be nursed on this ward but I think it is the wrong place for them.

> these kids have got so many problems... they need their own unit.

It is recognised within this study that this may be a localised problem as adolescents are in many areas cared for within an adolescent unit. The NAWCH report *Setting Standards for Adolescents in Hospital* (1990) states that adolescents require specialist facilities, with staff who are fully conversant with their particular needs. The nurses in the study did not feel that they had these skills, and indeed one nurse said that she would avoid contact with an adolescent patient if she could because of her feelings of inadequacy.

Conditions

A popular child proved to be one with a chronic illness; these children were described as brave, interesting, able to cope and always having a smile on their face. One nurse felt that her experience of caring for these children was very positive, explaining that her enjoyment came from her admiration of them:

> I have so much admiration for them, where you could have a child who is whimpering over something little, when you have these children who might only live for another year or two, anything you do to them they say OK, well do it, I just think they are very special... they take it in their stride.

There would appear to be some commonality in the lived experience of the nurse as both Stockwell (1972) and Baer and Lowery (1987) found a similar description of popular patients within their research studies. However, their participants were nurses caring for adult nurses and baccalaureate nursing students respectively.

The nurses also enjoyed caring for children whom they felt confident to care for:

> children I enjoy caring for have got to be in my speciality.

The nurses expressed an enjoyment of seeing very ill children recover:

> I don't mind when the acute conditions come in like meningitis, most of them make a good recovery and they pick up so quickly, they are so ill when they come in, I know it sounds awful, but it's nice to see.

Another nurse felt satisfaction when a child and family came 'through the trauma'. These nurses seemed to be expressing the enjoyment of witnessing very sick children recover, and their involvement gave them a feeling of job satisfaction.

There were conditions that were not popular with the nurses, including congenital handicap, mainly because of the complexity of the problems:

> some of the cerebral palsy children can be difficult to nurse... I remember this boy he had a hydrocephalus and it was a huge head... I thought I am never going to be able to see to him but with time you do.

Children with special needs were unpopular because the nurses felt that on an acute paediatric ward there was often insufficient time to care for these children.

I don't like them because I don't give them enough care.

When discussing children who were unpopular, the nurses looked for reasons other than the child, such as not having time or expertise to care for them, to try to explain their feelings.

Getting to know you

Some of the feelings of enjoyment of caring for a child came from the nurses getting to know the child and family. They used phrases such as 'building up a rapport', 'closeness of relationship', 'building up a bond' and 'depth of relationship'. A relationship is an elusive concept but is well recognised as being of central importance within nursing (Darbyshire, 1994). Most of the nurses felt that the longer the child was in hospital, the easier it was to form a relationship with him or her. One nurse explained that:

the longer they are here, they get to know us... if you have just got a few hours you don't get to know them or the parents.

Two nurses stressed that, because of the shorter length of stay on the ward and the nurses' shift patterns, it was possible to see children for a brief period during admission and then 'never see them again'. This was felt to be very unsettling for the child and difficult for the nurse to accept. However, another nurse felt that, as a short hospital stay is better for the child, she just had to accept it and 'make the most of the child when he is here'.

Many of the nurses talked about building up a rapport with the child and family. Within paediatric care, it is important to recognise that the relationship is triangular, involving the nurse, the parents and the child. Parents are encouraged to become partners in caring for their sick child, a philosophy described by Casey (1988) as a partnership with child and family.

All of the nurses in the study worked in areas of high patient turnover and felt that they were able to adapt to the situation of needing to form a relationship quickly with the child and family. One nurse stressed that she enjoyed the families needing 'input' from her, which included advice and preparation before theatre, post-operative care and discharge advice. She felt that although the children were discharged relatively quickly, there was still the opportunity to get to know the family through education and by giving them support. This nurse described these patients as her 'bread and butter work'.

Two of the nurses said that they used the named nurse concept to help to build up a rapport with the child and family. The DoH (1993) document *The Named Nurse, Midwife and Health Visitor* discusses the implementation of the named nurse concept across the spectrum of occupations. Its philosophy involves providing continuity of care, patient empowerment, professional accountability and autonomy. Another nurse, however, felt that this was impossible to achieve as her experience was that:

> we try to do a named nurse system but the kids are not in long enough for you to do a profile on them really.

It would seem that the named nurse concept was not really helpful in getting to know patients if their admission period was going to be very short.

Care was often felt to be fragmented, and communication between professionals could affect whether the nurses enjoyed caring for a child. Also important to the nurses' feelings of enjoyment was having continuity of care. Many expressed a wish to follow up a child's care at home. Deeper and longlasting relationships seemed to develop with children and families for whom they cared over a long period of time. Darbyshire (1994) describes this as a special relationship, more of a friendship that develops between the family and the nurse. None of the nurses in the present study said that having children in for short periods made them unpopular. It would, however, seem that enjoyment came from caring for a child and family whom they were able to get to know.

Expert at doing things

An enjoyment of caring for a child came from having the expertise and opportunity to 'do things' with or for the child and family. One nurse said that she enjoyed caring for children who were:

> within my speciality, and maybe it's because of my knowledge base I feel more confident with them, and the care I will give them is of my best knowledge.

It was very important to all the nurses that they felt confident to give nursing care. One nurse felt that this was recognised by other members of staff, who used it at times to their advantage:

> recently there was a child on the ward with lots of problems... I very quickly got put in there because [name] relates to these parents.

This nurse felt that her expertise was used by other nurses to avoid a 'difficult' family. All of the nurses stressed that they enjoyed caring for a child who needed a great deal of nursing care. One nurse, however, felt that when the family became involved in care, this changed her role and affected her enjoyment of caring for the child. She explained:

> if it's me seeing to the child I enjoy that, but when the parents are there they take over the role and I feel my role is halved if not quartered, I am really there for the parents... I don't feel I am there for the child as much as when mum isn't coming in.

This nurse felt that her role had changed with the advent of family-centred care. She said that she now saw her role as the link for the family rather than as the carer of the child. She also admitted to being poor at delegation, stressing that 'I like to do it myself.' This can be very difficult in the clinical area when the philosophy of care is one of partnership. This 'wanting to do it myself' may be one of the barriers to providing true partnerships in care with families so it is important for nurses to examine their own needs before dealing with the needs of families (Darbyshire, 1994).

However, other nurses in the study had a positive attitude to parents becoming involved in care. One nurse said that she enjoyed educating and teaching parents how to care for their child in hospital. She explained that she:

> Usually pounced on the parents when they come in, finding out what they know and what they feel, and would they like any input from me...

Casey (1988) refers to the role of the nurse within the partnership model as one who supports and teaches the parents, and that the paediatric nurse complements the care given by the parents to meet the needs of the child. One nurse in the study felt that the problem was that 'what everyone thinks of family-centred care varies'; her understanding was expressed as:

It's the sort of deciding between you... so deciding what they are going to do and what we are going to do; they can all be taught skills eventually.

Here is a demonstration of the need to negotiate with the parents in order to facilitate partnerships in care. Darbyshire (1994), however, suggests that the demarcation of care is not always explained to parents.

If the nurses felt that they lacked the expertise to care for the child, this made caring for the child less rewarding and a more stressful experience. Families were at times avoided because the nurse felt inadequate; one nurse gave her account of feeling intimidated by a family because a relative was a 'neuro sister' and the nurse felt that this aunt had more knowledge than she did. The nurse did, however, recognise this fact and tried to meet the needs of the family.

Inadequacy in caring for certain patients was expressed. Again, adolescents were seen as being problematic. The nurses felt ill prepared to care for them, especially if they had psychological problems. One difficulty seemed to be that the nurses felt that they lacked theoretical knowledge and needed a course to help them care for the adolescent. One nurse, however, felt that after so many years of experience, one got 'used to doing it'. Benner (1984) makes the distinction between theoretical knowledge and practical knowledge. This 'knowing that' and 'knowing how', develops through clinical practice.

All the nurses felt that they enjoyed caring for the child and family when they were able to 'do things'. By this, they meant providing nursing care, information and support. It was also of great importance to these nurses to feel that they had the expertise to provide the care to the child and family.

Own experience

A significant factor regarding the popularity of a child appeared to be the experiences of the individual nurse. This was expressed as empathy or feeling drawn to children who were the same age as their own children. One nurse felt that, as her children grew up, she would develop a better understanding of the needs of adolescents.

The nurses also stressed that personal experiences could influence their level of involvement with a child and family. One nurse enjoyed caring for children with a certain condition because a friend's child had the same problem. There does not seem to be a logical explanation for this except that the nurse is possibly transferring her feelings from her private life to her professional role. In this situation, the outcome was positive, but the scenario could have a very different outcome if the nurse's experience were of a negative nature. Personal feelings of commonality were also identified by Smith (1992) in her research into the emotional labour of nursing.

The nurses expressed empathy towards the parents, one nurse saying that she often tried to put herself in the parents' position and think of how she would feel:

> I try and put myself in their position, what would it be like if it was my child or my mother... how would I want her cared for?

One nurse stated that she felt 'resentful' and 'used' when parents used the ward for respite care. However, following the births of her own children, she stated that her views had changed, as she realised how much parents of children with special needs required such a service.

One nurse felt that her own inner feelings could affect whether or not she liked a child. She expressed this by saying:

> sometimes you can tolerate them, sometimes you can't, whether that's got anything to do with PMT...

The nurses appeared to be aware that their own personal feelings and experience could influence their enjoyment of caring for children and families.

Negative feelings

Children were described in negative terms if they were unco-operative; this was also found by Stockwell (1972). These children were the 'hysterical toddler, silly boy, spoilt child, the child who lacks behavioural skills and the adolescent'. Deviant behaviour was seen as very negative and made the child very unpopular. One nurse describes her experience of some adolescents thus:

> a lot of them smoke; if you won't let them they go off the ward. I am afraid if I say no they will smoke on the ward; they are difficult to nurse.

Adolescents with psychological problems were highlighted as difficult because they 'resented being in hospital' and 'just want to get out'. These patients were viewed as threatening and abusive, although one nurse recognised that adolescents were often attention seeking and needed someone to take notice of them.

Children who were 'giggly' or 'spoilt' were also unpopular:

> I disliked him because all he ate was sweets, and his parents only ever brought him sweets.

This nurse felt there was no partnership with the parents even when she explained the need for a good diet: as she saw it, all that the family wanted to do was spoil the child.

It was also felt by the nurses that they could over-compensate if they felt a dislike for a child and that it was very important not to ostracise the unco-operative child but to find ways of coping with them.

Within this theme, some nurses appeared to be expressing value judgements of children and families that were based on their own values and beliefs. One nurse described an unpopular child as:

> the sort of child I don't enjoy nursing is the younger child from the lower social classes. They don't want anything done, and they are hysterical when you go to do things to them... they are just hard work.

It is important for nurses to recognise that their own value and belief systems can affect the way in which they perceive patients in a positive or negative way.

Families

Partnership

All of the nurses in the study felt that developing a partnership with the family improved their enjoyment of caring for the child. The Platt Report (MoH, 1959) states that the care of the sick child requires the involvement of the family if it is to be effective. One nurse stated that she 'got more satisfaction when the parents wanted to be involved'. It was also important for the nurses to teach the parents skills so that they could care for their sick child.

These feelings of partnership and negotiation between parent and nurse seemed, however, to work in favour of those families who were willing to conform to the 'ward routine and way of life'. Families were unpopular if they had different values and beliefs regarding child-rearing practices:

> they were trying to bring him up with a different view point to the way most people would bring their children up... and it caused quite a few problems.

Unpopular parents

These were often seen as difficult, rude, aggressive, fussy and unco-operative with medical advice. For two nurses, professional parents, especially doctors, nurses and teachers, were unpopular. However, another nurse felt that she disliked 'thick' parents because they did not listen, and many, in her experience, did not want to be involved in their child's care, being there just to 'do nothing'. Casey (1988) suggested that parents can be labelled as being unable to manage complex skills because of their socio-economic background. This could, however, be a reflection of the nurses' attitude to the parents rather than the ability or motivation of the parents. Nurses are making value judgements on parents' ability and therefore often preventing them becoming active partners in care.

The attitude of the parents was a very important factor for the nurses in the study. One nurse stated that a child could become unpopular because of the parents:

> where there are problems with the parents; I mean often on the ward it's oh god that baby is coming in, but it's not the baby it's the parents who we know will kick up a fuss, will cause trouble on the ward for us.

Demanding parents were viewed as a 'big strain', and the relationship with the parents often became one of love and hate.

It appeared to be very important to the nurses to be able to give advice and support to parents, but one nurse felt that some parents would not act on any advice but 'want to do it their way'.

Developing a partnership model of care was for some nurses viewed as a threatening experience. One felt that her role was less important when the parents were involved in care. She most enjoyed caring for young babies when their mothers were not resident with them. Family-centred care constitutes a major change in nursing practice. In order to be rewarded with enjoyment and satisfaction, nurses will need to accept a partnership model. Within family-centred care, the nurse is seen as a support for the family, providing care only when it cannot be given by the parents, being able to teach parents the skills necessary to meet their needs and acting as a referral agent when necessary (Casey, 1988).

Discussion and conclusion

The results of the study showed that there were similarities to previous research identified in the literature review (Stockwell, 1972; Kelly and May, 1982; Baer and Lowery, 1987; English and Morse, 1988; Meadow, 1992; Mathers *et al.*, 1995). Popular children were those who were brave, could communicate, were uncomplaining and with whom the nurses felt they had a good relationship. Unpopular children were unco-operative, uncommunicative, selfish or spoilt.

New evidence to emerge from the study indicated the importance of the age of the child, babies and schoolchildren being most popular, and toddlers and adolescents least popular. This evidence suggests a need for paediatric nurses to be specifically educated to deal with the complex needs of the adolescent patient.

Throughout the study, the nurses' commitment to a philosophy of 'family-centred care' was evident (Casey, 1988). All of the nurses identified parental participation in care as a vital factor in their enjoyment of caring for sick children. There were, however, problems identified by the nurses in that some families were seen as 'difficult' to work with. The findings of the study suggest that the nurses would avoid contact with parents if they were viewed as unpopular. However, the unpopularity of the parents did not necessarily lead to the unpopularity of the child. From the results of the study, it would appear that some nurses still make critical decisions and assumptions based on nothing more than their own personal feelings.

This research suggests that the nurses felt that they worked within a philosophy of family-centred care and provided non-judgemental care. The evidence suggests, however, that some child patients were more popular and that the nurses therefore gained more enjoyment from caring for them. The nurses also felt that they valued parents as partners in care. However, the most popular parents were those who 'conformed' to the nurses' expectations. This was also evident in the work of Stockwell (1972), in which patients who conformed were deemed to be more popular.

Therefore there is a need for nurses to look critically at their practice and question whether the care they provide is influenced by their like or dislike of the child and family. Nurses have to put the needs of the child and family before their own need to be the 'expert doer', in order to fulfil the role as described by Casey (1988) as one of supporter, teacher and referral agent.

References

Baer E. D. and Lowery B. J. (1987) 'Patient and situational factors that affect nursing students' like or dislike of caring for patients', *Nursing Research* 36(5): 298–302.

Benner P. (1984) *From Novice to Expert*, Reading, MA, Addison-Wesley.

Benner P. and Wrubel J. (1989) *The Primacy of Caring*, California, Addison-Wesley.

Bordieri J., Solodky M. and Mikos A. (1984) 'Physical attractiveness and nurses' perceptions of paediatric patients', *Nursing Research* 34(1): 24–6.

Bowlby J. (1951) *Maternal Care and Mental Health*, Geneva, WHO.

Butterworth T. and Faugier J. (eds) (1992) *Clinical Supervision and Mentorship in Nursing*, London, Chapman & Hall.

Casey A. (1988) 'A partnership with child and family', *Senior Nurse* 8(4): 8–9.

Corter C., Trehub S., Boukydis C., Ford L., Celhoffer L. and Minde K. (1978) 'Nurses' judgements of the attractiveness of premature infants', *Infant Behaviour and Development* 1: 373–80.

Damrosch S. P. (1982) 'More than skin deep: relationship between perceived physical attractiveness and nursing students' assessments', *Western Journal of Nursing Research* 4(4): 423–33.

Darbyshire P. (1994) *Living with a Sick Child in Hospital*, London, Chapman & Hall.

Department of Health (1993) *The Named Nurse, Midwife and Health Visitor*. London, HMSO.

Dion K., Berscheid E. and Walster E. (1972) 'What is beautiful is good', *Journal of Personality and Social Psychology* 24(3): 285–9.

English J. and Morse J. (1988) 'The "difficult" elderly patient: adjustment or maladjustment', *International Journal of Nursing Studies* 25(1): 23–39.

Field P. and Morse J. (1996) *Nursing Research. The Application of Qualitative Approaches* (2nd edn), London, Chapman & Hall.

Giorgi A. (1975) 'An application of phenomenological method in psychology'. In Giorgi A., Fisher C. and Murray E. (eds) *Duquesne Studies in Phenomenological Psychology*, vol. 12, Pittsburgh, Duquesne University Press.

Kelly M. and May D. (1982) 'Good and bad patients: a theoretical critique', *Journal of Advanced Nursing* 7: 147–56.

McLeod S. and McClowry S. (1990) 'Using temperament theory to individualise the psychological care of hospitalised children', *Children's Health Care* 19(2): 79–84.

Mathers N., Jones N. and Hannay D. (1995) 'Heartsink patients: a study of their general practitioners', *British Journal of General Practice* 45: 293–6.

Meadow R. (1992) 'Difficult and unlikeable patients', *Archives of Diseases in Childhood* 67: 697–702.

Ministry of Health (1959) *The Welfare of Children in Hospital*, (Platt Report), London, HMSO.

Mitsunaga B. and Hall B. (1979) 'Interpersonal attraction and perceived quality of medical-surgical care', *Western Journal of Nursing Research* 1(1): 5–26.

Munhall P. and Olier Boyd C. (1993) *Nursing Research: A Qualitative Perspective*, 2nd edn, New York, National League for Nursing Press.

Morrison P. (1992) *Professional Caring in Practice*, Aylesbury, Ashgate.

National Association for the Welfare of Children in Hospital (1990) *Setting Standards for Adolescents in Hospital*.

Omery A. (1983) 'Phenomenology: a method for nursing research', *Advances in Nursing Science*, Jan.: 49–62.

Parahoo A. K. (1997) *Nursing Research: Principles, Process and Issues*, Basingstoke, Macmillan.

Parse R., Coyne A. and Smith M. (1985) *Nursing Research Qualitative Methods*, Maryland, Brady Communications.

Paterson J. and Zderad L. (1988) *Humanistic Nursing*, New York, National League for Nursing Press.

Robertson J. (1970) *Young Children in Hospital* (2nd edn), London, Tavistock Press.

Ruddy-Wallace M. (1987) 'Temperament assessing individual differences in hospitalised children', *Journal of Paediatric Nursing* 2(1).

Smith P. (1992) *The Emotional Labour of Nursing*, Basingstoke, Macmillan.

Stockwell F. (1972) *The Unpopular Patient*, London, RCN.

Thomas A. and Chess S. (1977) *Temperament and Development*, New York, Brunner Mazell.

15 Nurses' management of fever in children: rituals or evidence-based practice?

Maureen R. Harrison

Introduction

In most instances when children have had febrile convulsions, they are admitted to hospital (Morgan, 1991), and once admitted the patterns of their body temperature and other symptoms will be monitored and managed by medical and nursing staff in order to establish a cause for the convulsion. Febrile seizures are extremely distressing for parents (Addy, 1991; Balslev, 1991; Monsen *et al.*, 1991), and management is often concerned with the prevention of a recurrence, which, if it should happen, is not necessarily harmful to the child (Hunter, 1973; Ellenberg and Nelson, 1980; Neville, 1991; Ross, 1991; Bethune *et al.*, 1993). Management strategies often include pharmacological treatment of the fever using antipyretics such as paracetamol (acetaminophen) or ibuprofen. Among physicians and nurses, the rationale for this procedure appears to be that fever is deemed harmful and should be treated, because antipyretics are thought to provide comfort to a child and prevent febrile convulsions, and finally, because parents often expect to see some treatment administered, usually in the form of medication, for their child (El-Radhi and Carroll, 1994). Despite research findings that support the positive immunological and diagnostic role of fever (Hull, 1991; Kluger, 1995), and that argue against the use of antipyretics, El-Radhi and Carroll (1994) state that the reality in practice appears to be their continued liberal use.

An investigative study in the form of an audit was undertaken to determine how children's nurses manage fever, with particular reference to the use and administration of the antipyretic paracetamol (acetaminophen). The main purpose of the study was to review *when* and for *what reason* nurses administer paracetamol for the treatment of fever. This would confirm whether or not antipyretic medication was administered liberally, and why. The study was able

262

to acknowledge areas of good practice and also those situations in which practice was rote rather than evidence based.

Literature review

Is fever harmful? How do nurses define fever and decide when or when not to treat a child? What are nurses' rationales for administrating antipyretics? How efficacious are the actions of antipyretics: do they provide comfort and prevent febrile seizures? Is the pharmacological management of fever based on rituals or evidence-based practice? All of these questions are highly pertinent to a nurse managing a child with fever, and they formed the basis for the investigative study.

Understanding the nature of fever

Fever is one of the oldest, best-known and best-observed manifestations of disease (Atkins, 1984), manuscripts from as early as the fifth century BC having been found that debate the topic. Fever is defined as a rise in the body temperature resulting from an elevation in the temperature set point, which is controlled by the body's thermoregulatory centre in the hypothalamus (Kluger, 1995). The normal body temperature set point is maintained by the thermoregulatory centre at between 36.1 °C and 37.5 °C (McCance and Huether, 1994).

During fever, there are a number of factors that influence the regulation of body temperature, factors raising the thermoregulatory set point (endogenous pyrogens, which are internal heat-producing substances), and those lowering the set point or preventing its rising too high (endogenous cryogens, or internal heat-cooling substances). When activated by infection or trauma, cells within the body respond by producing endogenous pyrogens, such as interleukin-1α, interleukin-1β, interleukin-6 and tumour necrosis factor (Kluger, 1991, 1995). These substances initiate two main responses: the mobilisation of the immune response and the local inflammatory response. The presence of endogenous pyrogens in the blood circulation causes the thermoregulatory centre in the anterior hypothalamus to secrete prostaglandins of the 'E' series, which cause a rise in the thermoregulatory set point (Hull, 1991; McCance and Huether, 1994; Kluger, 1995). Prostaglandins are produced from a protein called arachidonic acid and are one of the end-products of the cyclo-oxygenase metabolic pathway.

Once the higher temperature (determined by the new set point) has been reached and the individual has a fever, arginine vasopressin (AVP), alpha-melanocyte-stimulating hormone, and corticotrophin-releasing factor are released and act at the level of the anterior hypothalamus, working as endogenous cryogens (antipyretics), preventing the body temperature rising further and also reducing the febrile response. As these substances ensure that the body temperature will not rise relentlessly but will remain at a level at which tissue damage through heat is minimised, they may account for the common fluctuations of temperature manifested during fever (McCance and Huether, 1994). When pyrogens are no longer released from the immune cells, the hypothalamic thermoregulatory centre will be reset back to normal.

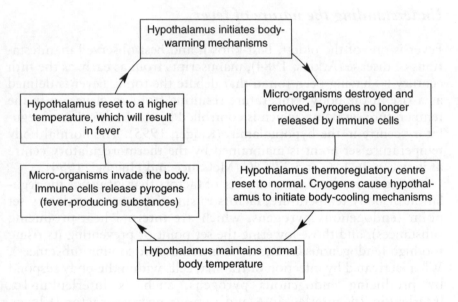

Figure 15.1   The fever cycle

The efficacious nature of fever has been shown through research studies demonstrating that when various species of the animal kingdom were subjected to infectious agents, the chances of recovery and survival were increased if fever was allowed to develop (Carmichael *et al.*, 1969; Bernheim and Kluger, 1976; Haahr and Mogenson, 1977) (Table 15.1).

Table 15.1   Positive immunological role of fever

- Increased antibody and cytokine production (Hanson *et al.*, 1983)

- Increased neutrophil mobility (Nahas *et al.*, 1981, cited in Kluger, 1991)

- Proliferation of certain populations of T lymphocytes (Nahas *et al.*, 1991, cited in Kluger, 1991)

- Enhanced production and pyrogenic effects of interferons (Dinarello *et al.*,1984)

- Reduction in plasma iron concentration, which reduces the proliferation rate of bacteria (Weinberg, 1978)

- Reduction in bacterial growth rate and increased bactericidal effect of serum during fever (Small *et al.*, 1986; Sande *et al.*, 1987, both cited in Kluger, 1991)

- Production of acute-phase proteins from the liver, which stimulate the hypothalamus to raise its set point and also induce anorexia, drowsiness and lethargy. It is believed that this 'enforced' rest is an important aspect of the healing process (Kluger, 1995)

Fever is very important to the overall defence strategy of the body. Because modest fevers are thought to be beneficial and a normal adaptive response to infection, it is thought that caution should be exercised when using antipyretic drugs, many of which are cyclo-oxygenase inhibitors and thus prevent the release of prostaglandins within the anterior hypothalamus that cause the rise in the thermoregulatory set point.

The interpretation of fever

Important considerations in the management of fever are at what body temperature the definition of fever can be imposed, and what promotes the treatment of fever. El-Rahdi and Carroll (1994) have recommended that there should be no pharmacological intervention to treat fever unless the temperature is greater than 38.5 °C or 39.0 °C. This policy, however, is by no means universal. Some studies have recommended managing fever when the temperature is higher than 37.0–37.9 °C (Ipp and Jaffe, 1993), or above 37.9–38.0 °C (Eskerud and Brodwall, 1993; Schnaiderman *et al.*, 1993). Wilson *et al.* (1982) have proposed the commencement of treatment when the body temperature exceeds 38.5 °C, and Walson *et al.* (1992) and Addy (1983) suggest a temperature above 39.0 °C. These studies highlight the inconsistencies in the definition of fever and in the advice given for the administration of antipyretics for fever. Consequently, the response of treatment or non-treatment varies.

Morley *et al.* (1992) have indicated that any temperature higher than 2 standard deviations above the mean in normal circumstances could be considered to be fever (interpreted as 37.9–38.5 °C). This definition is probably one of the more accurate ones, given the observation that body temperature does have a 24-hour (circadian) fluctuation pattern. Anderson *et al.* (1990), for example, have described the normal circadian range of infants' temperatures during the day, which varied between 36.0 °C at night and 37.8 °C during active periods of the day. Therefore, if a pyrexia is interpreted as being above 37.5 °C, it might include those temperature variations that are 'normal' daytime occurrences.

The physiological action of the antipyretic paracetamol

The antipyretics most commonly used on paediatric units in the UK are paracetamol and ibuprofen, paracetamol having been the choice of antipyretic under investigation. As well as understanding fever physiology when managing fever in children, evidence-based practice should have its foundation in a sound knowledge of the physiological action of antipyretics.

Paracetamol is a metabolite of both acetanilid and phenacetin, both of which have analgesic (pain-relieving) and antipyretic (temperature-reducing) effects but very weak anti-inflammatory ones (Goodman and Gilman, 1980). The weak effects arise because paracetamol is only a weak inhibitor of prostaglandin synthetase (one of the enzymes in the cyclo-oxygenase pathway), unlike aspirin or ibuprofen, which are very potent prostaglandin synthetase inhibitors. It has been thought that paracetamol has more action against enzymes of archidonic acid metabolism in the central nervous system (CNS) rather than those in the periphery, although little as yet is known about its properties (Smith and Reynard, 1995).

In endotoxin-induced fever, (that type of fever caused by bacterial infection), there has been found to be a considerable rise in the prostaglandin (PGE1) concentration of the cerebrospinal fluid, this rise being prevented by the administration of paracetamol; however, in experiments in which PGE1 was injected directly into the cerebral ventricles, there was a marked and longlasting increase in body temperature that was not affected by the administration of paracetamol (Bowman and Rand, 1980; Uhari *et al.*, 1995). To explain this simply, these studies demonstrate that, following the stimulation of endogenous pyrogens, which are produced when bacteria or viruses invade the body, paracetamol can stop the early production of prostaglandins in the CNS. However, once a large amount of prostaglandin is already present in the brain, the administration of paracetamol cannot reduce the level, so the temperature will remain high.

Following Wilson *et al.*'s (1982) study, which revealed an absolute antipyretic efficacy of paracetamol in the quick onset of temperature reduction and the duration of the temperature decrement over a period of 4 hours, the recommendation to administer 10 mg/kg paracetamol every 4–6 hours as a maintenance dose was adopted. Antipyretic efficacy also relates to the route of administration, oral liquid producing an effect in 30 minutes regardless of dose, with a duration of effect of between 4–6 hours. Rectal suppositories have a slower effect – between 2 and 3 hours, with a maximal effect at 2.5–4.0 hours (Rylance, 1991) – demonstrating that oral medication has a faster rate of action than that administered rectally. However, the presence of food in the stomach and changes in gut perfusion can affect the oral absorption rate.

Bonadio *et al.* (1993) found that temperature patterns following the administration of therapeutic doses of paracetamol are age rather than disease dependent. Their results demonstrated that highly febrile young children with or without an invasive bacterial infection experienced a significant temperature drop following the administration of paracetamol, but these authors showed that the temperature did not return to that of an afebrile state, the children in some instances still having a fever of greater than 38.0 °C. This correlated with Bowman and Rand's (1980) findings that once there is an increased prostaglandin level in the CNS, the temperature will remain high. Thoughts worthy of consideration are whether the body has other mechanisms to maintain a state of fever in the presence of bacteria, regardless of whether antipyretics are administered, or whether paracetamol is not effective on all the control mechanisms of fever.

Wilson *et al.* (1991), following a study comparing the efficacy of ibuprofen and paracetamol, concluded that although age was an important variable, the most significant variable was the height of the initial temperature, which influenced the magnitude of the reduction in temperature: the lower the initial fever, the greater the efficacy. Those children with a initial temperature of less than 38 °C demonstrated a twofold increase in efficacy. The reason for this apparent efficacy needs explaining further. If the rationale is that the paracetamol blocks the production of prostaglandins, which cause the hypothalamus to reset its temperature, the results perhaps demonstrate a reduced production of heat owing to a lower thermoregulatory set point, rather than that the administration of paracetamol indirectly stimulates the body's heat loss mechanisms.

The administration of paracetamol to provide comfort to a child

Most children admitted to hospital with fever will demonstrate at some point the acute-phase response to infection. The effect of antigens, either bacteria or viruses, on macrophages and T lymphocytes (immune cells) results in these cells releasing a range of cell messengers, or cytokines. Many of these cytokines enhance the inflammatory response and induce the symptoms of malaise associated with infections. Adding to the malaise and 'misery' seen in a child, prostaglandins are produced from tissue cell walls, lowering the threshold of pain receptors to substances that cause pain, such as bradykinin, and also sensitising peripheral nociceptors, triggering their activity and thus producing hyperalgesia (Bowman and Rand, 1980; Needleman and Isakson, 1998). As paracetamol (unlike aspirin) is only a very weak anti-inflammatory agent and is only a weak inhibitor of the biosynthesis of prostaglandin from arachidonic acid, researchers are still not totally sure how it produces its reported beneficial effects. It has been thought that phenacetin, like acetaminophen a para-aminophenol derivative, causes relaxation, drowsiness and euphoria, although these have again not been explained (Goodman and Gilman, 1980).

In a very interesting study, Kramer *et al.* (1991) set out to examine what benefits, for example improved comfort and behavioural responses, paracetamol therapy was associated with. Their study was a randomised, double-blind, placebo-controlled trial of paracetamol. The cohort comprised 225 children aged between 6 months and 6 years, all of whom presented with an acute fever of 38 °C or greater. Parents were asked to give the paracetamol suspension (in a recommended dose of 10–15 mg/kg) or the placebo for fever greater than 38 °C every 4 hours, as required ('prn') and to administer no other cooling treatment. Parents kept temperature and symptom diaries, and recorded changes in child comfort and behaviour according to a Likert-type questionnaire. Only a third of the paracetamol-treated children were rated by their parents as having an improvement in alertness and activity, and no significant differences between the two groups were noted in mood, comfort, appetite or fluid intake. A very interesting point made was that the overall improvement in comfort with paracetamol was not impressive because when parents were asked which drug their child was taking, a correct guess was obtained in only 45 per cent of the paracetamol group and 52 per cent of the placebo group. Other parents either gave the incorrect response or felt unable to attempt a guess. The authors concluded that the clinically relevant benefits and hazards of paracetamol antipyresis have been grossly exaggerated.

Hull (1991), reviewing the rationale for the administration of antipyretics, maintained that fever itself does not make metabolic demands but that it is the environmental adjustment of the body to raised temperature set points that make the demands and cause feelings of discomfort. He advocated 'wrapping up' a fever by keeping a child in a comfortable thermoneutral range, thus minimising metabolic demands and ensuring that the child's behaviour and temperature remain vital signs for observation.

This point requires a careful explanation because it is a significant factor in knowing how to manage fever correctly. When the hypothalamus has reset the body's thermostat to a higher temperature point, the sympathetic nervous system and various hormones are activated to start increasing the body temperature. For example, the child will start feeling 'cold' even though, if the body temperature were taken, the nurse might well find it raised to a point higher than normal. Peripheral vasoconstriction helps to minimise heat loss from the body surface and the shivering of skeletal muscle helps to increase body heat production, as does increased metabolic activity. At this point, the nurse should do nothing to disrupt the body's 'warming' mechanism; hence the child should be kept lightly 'wrapped up'. This procedure will minimise some of the uncomfortable symptoms, such as 'feeling cold', during this phase. As the peripheral skin temperature receptors help to inform the hypothalamus of whether the new temperature set point has been reached, a higher temperature will be registered by the temperature receptors if the skin is covered, than if it is uncovered. This means that efforts made by the body to raise the body temperature would be reduced and some of those uncomfortable symptoms moderated. Hull (1991) expressed the view that if a child has fever but is nursed in a comfortable environment, the administration of antipyretics is unnecessary.

The administration of antipyretics to comply with parents' wishes

Paracetamol is not only in widespread use in hospitals, but can also easily be bought at a variety of chemists and superstores, as well as being found in most homes (Sanz *et al.*, 1996). Prior to admission to hospital, many parents have already administered one (or more) doses to their child. If a child is admitted to hospital following a febrile seizure, many parents might be unhappy if no treatment is given, especially if they have been treating their child at home. Despite paracetamol's easy availability in many stores, there is evidence to suggest that the general population also have a poor knowledge of this drug (Gubermann, 1990; Eskerud and Brodwall, 1993), and it is one of the responsibilities of a paediatric nurse when giving discharge advice for the management of fever that the advice is relevant and providing sufficient information for parents to cope with a possible febrile seizure.

Other studies have suggested that it is not only the general population and nurses who have a poor knowledge of fever management and the benefits and risks of paracetamol: pharmacists and GPs have also been seen to give out conflicting and inconsistent advice (Eskerud and Brodwall, 1993; Eskerud *et al.*, 1993; Ipp and Jaffe, 1993).

Guberman (1990) reviewed the use of paracetamol in the Israeli community. He asked 101 parents of children 5-years old or younger to describe the dose of paracetamol, mode of administration and maximal frequency given for fever. The main recommendation from his findings were that parents need more education regarding the use of this drug. He found that the average single dose administered was 13.8 mg/kg (+/– 5.5 mg/kg). Only 61 per cent of the children had received a reasonable quantity; 12 per cent had had an overdose and 27 per cent an underdose.

The role of antipyretics in preventing febrile convulsions

The effect of antipyretics alone in reducing the recurrence of febrile seizures is currently unknown (Rylance, 1991). It has been suggested that vigorous early treatment is unlikely to be effective because parents are in many cases unaware of the fever when the convulsion first occurs, and the convulsion frequently occurs with a lower temperature (El-Radhi and Banajeh, 1989). There is now a question of whether there is a correlation at all between temperature and febrile convulsions. For example, Lewis *et al.* (1979) surmise that a febrile convulsion could be a response to the invasion of the bloodstream or CNS by a viral agent. Not all children are at risk of febrile convulsions, factors that might predispose children including a genetic predisposition, those children who are slow in their development or neurologically impaired and day nursery attendees (Bethune *et al.*, 1993).

In recent years, studies have been undertaken to determine whether or not paracetamol does influence the recurrence of febrile seizures. Schnaiderman *et al.* (1993), in a controlled clinical study (undertaken in Israel) on a cohort of 104 children presenting with simple febrile seizures, compared the antipyretic effectiveness of paracetamol syrup administered at regular 4-hourly intervals at a dose of 15–20 mg/kg (Group 1) with that of sporadic usage with a similar dose and subject to a body temperature above 37.9 °C (Group 2). The results found the body temperature to be statistically similar in both groups in spite of significantly larger amounts of paracetamol being given to Group 1. The clinical diagnosis was similar in both groups, with viral infections predominating. The authors concluded that the prophylactic administration of paracetamol was not effective in the prevention of temperature elevation, the reduction of the degree of fever or preventing the early recurrence of febrile convulsions. No other measures were undertaken to reduce fever in either project, although nothing is mentioned regarding the intake of fluids. As a result of their findings, Schnaiderman *et al.* advocated that the excessive use of antipyretics in children with febrile convulsions could be reduced and, whenever clinically indicated, tepid water baths might be as effective as acetaminophen.

Tepid bathing is a means of sponging children down with water that is just warm. A thin layer of water is left on the body, and as this water evaporates from the surface of the body, heat is also lost from the body, therefore cooling the child down. Fevers greater than 41 °C must be treated (Rowsey, 1997), and these often require more active measures such as tepid sponging combined with antipyretic administration. Even though Schnaiderman was dubious of the efficacious nature of paracetamol, Agbolosu *et al.* (1997) suggest that the administration of paracetamol is more effective than just tepid sponging in reducing the body temperature of highly febrile children in tropical countries. The current recommendation for the UK is warm rather than tepid bathing (Kinmonth *et al.*, 1992), but fevers greater than 41 °C are rarely seen in this country.

Wilson *et al.* (1982) reviewed the efficacy in temperature reduction following only a single oral dose, whereas Schnaiderman's cohort received more than one dose and the analysis of temperature patterns followed a number of hours. Schnaiderman *et al.* (1993), like Lewes (1979), make the comment that febrile seizures may be purely coincidental and independent of temperature elevation; these are unique views and have currently not been widely expressed, although there is evidence that they are being considered (El-Radhi and Banajeh, 1989).

Uhari *et al.* (1995) evaluated the effect of paracetamol and of low intermittent doses of diazepam on the prevention of recurrence of febrile seizures. In a 2-year trial, 180 patients were divided into four groups: those receiving two kinds of a placebo, those receiving diazepam and a placebo, those receiving paracetamol and a placebo, and those receiving both diazepam and paracetamol. During this time, there were 641 fever events, and 21 per cent of the children suffered a recurrence of their febrile seizures. The results showed that paracetamol had no effect on the recurrence rate. The combination of antipyretic agents with anticonvulsant medication did not reduce the recurrence of febrile seizures. In this study, paracetamol was not given prophylactically but at a dose of 10 mg/kg 4-hourly when the temperature exceeded 40 °C. The authors found that although parcetamol reduced the mean temperature, it had no effect on the highest temperatures or on the temperatures of those patients who had febrile seizures.

To conclude, it has been demonstrated that fever is not harmful but very beneficial to the body's healing process. The definition of fever varies from author to author, and it seems important that when managing fever, a high body temperature alone should not be the only sign to initiate treatment – the nurse should treat according to metabolic clues. Antipyretics are administered for a number of symptoms, yet it has been found that if they are administered for comfort purposes and if administered to prevent temperature rise and prevent febrile seizures, the rationale for this is highly questionable.

The study identified what nurses' management of fever practices were during the period of the audit. The question of whether the pharmacological management of fever is based on rituals or evidence-based practice will be considered.

Methodological approaches

The manner by which nurses make decisions to treat and care for patients is complex and multidimensional. Antipyretics are often prescribed on an 'as required' basis. It is thus the nurse who decides when and if to administer them. This process was audited in the investigation of how nurses manage fever. Making sense of the reality of the way in which nurses managed fever required two main methodological approaches. Research methods included an analysis of a temperature chart designed specifically for the study (Figure 15.2),

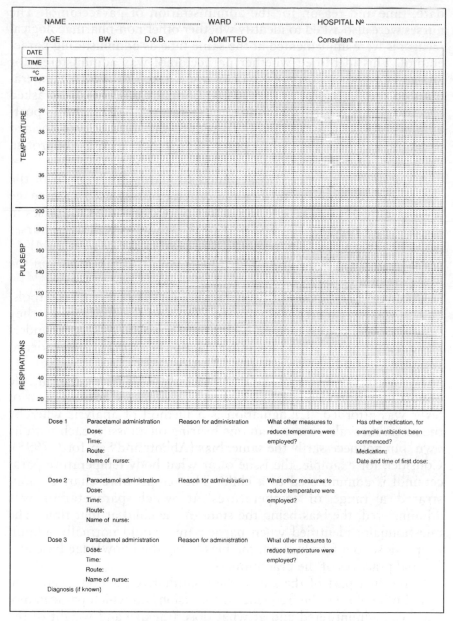

Figure 15.2   Temperature chart

which was distributed and used on three units in two different hospitals. The chart was similar in style to the charts used by the different hospital Trusts, but in addition to the normal data on the chart, there was on the base of the chart a series of questions concerning dose, date, time and reason for the administration of paracetamol. The nurses were also asked to identify whether other non-pharmacological measures were implemented at the same time as administering parac-etamol. This identified whether paracetamol was administered for analgesic or other purposes. Nurses were asked to record tempera-tures on the charts just as they would normally do. They were asked specifically to record the child's temperatures half an hour post-administration of paracetamol. To reduce variables, it was decided to ignore any occasions when other antipyretics, such as ibuprofen, were administered.

A questionnaire was also designed to clarify findings from the charts and to establish further the criteria nurses used to manage fever (Figure 15.3). The questionnaires were distributed to nurses in the hospitals used for the first part of the study, as well as to nurses from 12 other units. The response rate was 35 per cent (n = 44) 15 per cent of these being from individuals who had taken part in the first part of the study.

Qualitative and quantitative data were established from the tools, and it was considered valuable to combine the findings as they supported and complemented each other: it was necessary to under-stand the rationale behind the nurses' actions (qualitative) in order to support the findings on the temperature charts (quantitative). By analysing the two sets of data together through triangulation, the opportunity to review a realistic view of the nurses' management of fever was afforded. Triangulation is a method of analysis whereby the researcher takes more than one bearing on an issue, each with its own, but not necessarily the same, bias (Abbott and Sapsford, 1998). Consider, for example, the issue of at what body temperature para-cetamol is administered to a child. The temperature chart demon-strated a range of temperatures at which paracetamol was administered, the bias being the state of the child at that time. The questionnaire identified when participants would normally admin-ister a dose to a febrile child, the bias being the knowledge base and normal practices of the practitioners.

In the first part of the study, the quantitative methods were well suited to exploring the frequency of occasions on which paracetamol had been administered and at what dose (the age and weight of the child being recorded on the charts), the effect of paracetamol on body temperature, and at what temperature paracetamol was administered. The second part of the project was needed to verify issues identified from the charts, such as the rationale behind the decision to treat a fever pharmacologically, and what the nurses' understanding of the pharmacodynamics of paracetamol was. A flaw in the research

1. Does your hospital have a policy for the administration of paracetamol?
2. What is this policy?
3. What are some of the symptoms with which a child might present that would make you consider administering paracetamol?
4. How important do you consider the administration of paracetamol in the treatment of pyrexia in children? Please give your reasons.
5. In what circumstances would you administer paracetamol regularly on a 4–6-hourly basis? Give examples.
6. In what circumstances would you administer paracetamol on an 'as required' basis? Give examples.
7. If paracetamol is prescribed on an 'as required' basis, list the factors that might influence you to administer the medication.
8. Above what temperature do you consider a patient pyretic?
9. If a child is admitted with a history of febrile seizures, and up to two initial doses of paracetamol have reduced the temperature to normal, would you continue the use of paracetamol to maintain stability?
10. What other medications are prescribed for pyrexia on your unit?
11. Are these medications administered in conjunction with paracetamol, for example alternately or on their own? Please give examples of their use.
12. Apart from medication, what other methods do you employ to reduce fever in children?
13. What determines your choice in implementing the above methods?
14. Do you monitor and record the temperature on a regular basis?
15. If 'yes', what is the frequency of recording the temperature?
16. If your answer was 'no', what determines your decision to monitor temperature?
17. What advice do you give to parents regarding the administration of paracetamol and the treatment of fever?
18. Can you describe the physiological action of paracetamol?

Figure 15.3 Paracetamol administration questionnaire

method was that it was impossible to determine the rationale for individual incidents demonstrated on the charts, but the nurses who filled in the charts were encouraged to answer the questionnaire; thus, their answers reflected only general principles and modes of practice. If a hypothesis such as 'Paracetamol is administered liberally to reduce fever' was being tested, it is argued that quantitative methods alone would possibly have answered the question, but the administration of paracetamol for other reasons would have been ignored and the process of how and why a nurse makes the decision to administer a drug which is prescribed 'as required' would not be tested, hence the inclusion of qualitative methods of research,

Three health authorities were approached for permission to conduct the study, which was granted, hence avoiding any in-house 'cultural' bias from one authority. Permission was sought from senior nurses, and meetings were held with representatives from all grades of staff, to discuss the project. The nurses were all enthusiastic about being involved, but the project was unfortunately not established in one unit owing to opposition from medical colleagues.

Many of the facets investigated cannot be discussed comprehensively in this chapter; thus, only the nurses' definition of fever, the understanding of the pharmacodynamics and the uses of paracetamol, for example to provide comfort and to prevent febrile seizures, will be discussed. While non-pharmacological measures to reduce fever were investigated in the study, the discussion will concentrate solely on the use of the antipyretic paracetamol to treat fever.

Discussion of selected findings

Definition of fever

In the literature reviewed, the definition of fever appeared to be problematic, and the same was demonstrated in the study. Responses from the questionnaires demonstrated that many of the nurses (54 per cent) considered a child to be pyrexic with a temperature of 37.5 °C and above. This information was verified when analysing data from temperature charts, with indications that antipyretic therapy was commenced when the temperature was even as low as 36.6 °C, a temperature that can hardly be defined as a fever. This was an incident for which it would have been useful to verify why the paracetamol was given for fever. It is important to mention that all those occasions on which the nurse stated that paracetamol was given for analgesia were not included for analysis. Symptoms such as pallor caused by vasoconstriction, tachycardia, tachypnoea, lying in a curled up position and miserable behaviour, nausea and sleepiness are all indicative of sympathetic nervous system activity, body warming mechanisms and impending fever, but there was no place to identify all these symptoms on the charts. Kluger (1991) stated that when the thermoregulatory set point is raised, deep body temperature may or may not be raised at the same time, depending on whether the body is invoking its heat gain or heat loss mechanisms.

The range of temperatures in which nurses were most frequently seen to administer medication lay between 38.0 °C and 39.4 °C. When asked to clarify what was considered an appropriate temperature at which to administer antipyretics, the temperatures cited were those over 37.7 °C, over 38.0 °C or over 38.5 °C. Again, a lack of consistency was demonstrated. Given that the recommendations from the literature on what constitutes fever, and at what temperature to administer medication, are vague, it is not surprising that the temperatures at which nurses suggested giving and actually gave paracetamol were inconsistent. Most literature recommendations indicate that antipyretics should only be administered if the body temperature exceeds 38.5 °C; 54 per cent of the doses reviewed during the study were, however, given to children whose temperatures were less than 38.5 °C.

Table 15.2 Signs and symptoms that indicate fever

Symptoms observed during heat gain mechanisms	Symptoms observed during heat loss mechanisms
Pallor and possible cyanosis of the peripheries	Flushed, hot skin
Shivering	Sweating
Skin over the peripheries cool, but skin at the back of the neck warm	
Child lying in curled up or fetal position. Child says he or she feels cold	Child in a splayed out position. Covers kicked off
Raised heart and respiratory rates	Vital signs within normal ranges
Anorexia and/or nausea	Thirsty, willing to drink
Generally miserable, irritable and/or sleeping	More relaxed, happier in behaviour

A problem with the method of study was that it was impossible to determine why nurses administered the antipyretic for fever when the child's body temperature was less than 38.5 °C. It might have been because there was evidence of sympathetic nervous system activity with the body temperature rising, or it might have indicated rote practice, that is, paracetamol being administered simply because the child appeared to have a fever. In the questionnaire, some nurses were able to provide a rationale for the pros and cons of administering antipyretic medication whereas others were not.

While Morley *et al.*'s (1992) definition does acknowledge the daily fluctuations of fever, very few nurses would be able to interpret what might be 2 'standard deviations' higher than a normal temperature, and no nurses in the study acknowledged that, in diagnosing fever, the time of day and the child's level of activity should be considered.

Understanding the pharmacodynamic action of paracetamol

Having established that all nurses regularly administered paracetamol for the treatment of fever, it was important to establish the nurses' understanding of the action of paracetamol. However, 77 per cent of the respondents, who were all nurses working with children, could not describe or did not know the action of paracetamol, and only 9 per cent of the responses were correct. This does not comply with the UKCC's (1992) standards for the administration of medications.

The advice given to parents for the management of fever using paracetamol was vague, despite evidence to suggest that the general population has a poor knowledge of this drug. Most respondents stated that parents were advised 'to give paracetamol regularly and not to exceed the dose stated on the bottle'. Regularity was not defined, nor were parents given any indication of when to commence treatment. The advice that was seen to be given would do little to dispel 'fever phobia of parents' described by Kramer *et al.* (1985) and Schmitt (1980).

Nurses should be seen to give parents an understanding of the nature of fever, acknowledging and emphasising its benefits. Paracetamol can be recommended for its analgesic effects (the aches and pains often associated with fever), and it should only be recommended for its antipyretic properties if the fluctuating thermoregulatory responses are distressing or harmful to the child (Hull, 1991). It might help to be more specific about the drug's action. For example, Wilson *et al.* (1991) found ibuprofen and acetaminophen to be most efficacious when administered at a temperature of less than 38 °C; thus, should the fever be undesirable, the antipyretic should be given before the child feels hot and while he or she is demonstrating evidence of the body going into a 'warming mode'. However, it is more important for the child to have the fever, and establish a cause for the fever prior to the administration of antipyretics. Once children have a raised temperature, parents can be reassured that paracetamol can produce a decrease in higher temperatures, although the amount of defervescence varies (Wilson *et al.*, 1982) and they must be warned that paracetamol will not prevent further rises of temperature (Uhari *et al.*, 1995).

Rationales given for administration of paracetamol

One of the problems encountered in this study was that pyrexia was not the only reason identified for administering paracetamol, and the administration of the drug for pain and comfort had to be acknowledged. Ipp and Jaffe (1993), reviewing the use of antipyretics among GPs, found that 70 per cent of the participants would administer antipyretics for the relief of discomfort, and only 30 per cent used temperature alone as the indicator for giving these drugs. Following the results of the research on temperature charts, it was necessary to ask the question, 'What are (were) the symptoms a child might present with that would make you consider administering paracetamol?', the results to this question being shown in Figure 15.4.

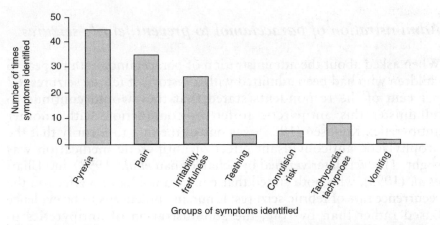

Figure 15.4   Reasons identified for the administration of paracetamol

As can be seen, the main single reason cited for the administration of paracetamol was pyrexia, and the second, pain. Sixty-five per cent of the respondents stated that they would administer paracetamol for comfort reasons. These categories included irritability, fretfulness, lethargy and teething, although Kramer *et al.* (1991) found that the clinically relevant benefits have been greatly exaggerated. Even though most nurses could not fully explain the action of paracetamol, it was apparent that some nurses believed in paracetamol as a drug to cure all manner of ills.

When asked how important the nurses considered the administration of paracetamol for the treatment of pyrexia to be, a group of 52 per cent stated 'very important'. The reasons given for its importance were for its fever-reducing properties, because it was thought to prevent seizures, and because of its action as a mild analgesic agent that relieves the associated aches and pains. It was interesting to note that a group of 29 per cent of respondents thought that paracetamol had only moderate importance because they would only administer it if the temperature was above 38 °C and persistent. These nurses stated that paracetamol would only be given in conjunction with other cooling methods, some responding that they did not always find it effective; not all individuals answered this question. The latter group's observations were more consistent with views from literature, whereas the former group's views are largely based on tradition. A fault with the questionnaire method was that the grade of the nurse or length of experience was not identified so it was impossible to state why there might have been a difference in opinion regarding the importance of administering paracetamol for fever.

Administration of paracetamol to prevent febrile seizures

When asked about the administration of paracetamol with respect to children who had been admitted with a history of febrile seizures, 67 per cent of the respondents stated that they would continue to administer this antipyretic (often in conjunction with another antipyretic). Knudsen (1988) was one of the first to identify that the prophylactic anticonvulsant effect of antipyretic medication was slight. This was later verified by Schaiderman *et al.* (1993) and Uhari *et al.* (1995), who both stated that paracetamol had no effect on the recurrence rate of febrile seizures. If nursing practice is to be evidence based rather than by rote, the administration of antipyretics to reduce or prevent febrile seizures must now cease.

Implications for clinical practice

1. Nurses need to have an understanding of the nature of fever and be aware that, in most instances, fever is highly beneficial to the human body. In understanding the physiological mechanisms of fever, the nurse should understand the physiological rationale behind the increases and decreases of temperature seen during fever. This can then be interpreted by the symptoms observed in patients.

2. When managing fever, a decision to treat or not to treat should not be made on temperature alone but on the basis of the variety of symptoms displayed by children.

3. Nurses should have a very good understanding of the risks, benefits and mode of action of the drugs they commonly admin-

ister. A nurse should have a very good understanding of any medications that are prescribed 'as required', as these are the drugs whereby nurses are using their judgement on when and if to administer. Despite its regular use, the understanding of the drug paracetamol was seen in this study to be very limited.

4. Antipyretics should not be given unless the child is distressed by the fever. If antipyretics are needed to prevent fever, they should be given at a temperature lower than 38.0 °C. However, owing to the beneficial nature of fever, and the need for a diagnosis of the cause of fever, antipyretics should not otherwise be given unless the temperature exceeds 38.5 °C.

5. Febrile convulsions in children are extremely distressing for parents, and nurses need to discuss at length with carers what fever is and what febrile convulsions are. Parents should not be given false assurances that the administration of paracetamol will prevent the recurrence of a seizure; instead, time should be taken to ensure that parents could cope should such a situation reccur.

Conclusion

In conclusion, studies are currently being undertaken that demonstrate the immunological benefits of fever. Despite this, antipyretics are widely used in paediatric practice and at home. Practitioners vary in their definitions of what body temperature constitutes a fever as well as in their ideas of the temperature at which antipyretics should be administered. Many authors (for example, Kramer *et al.*, 1991; Schnaiderman *et al.*, 1993; El-Radhi and Carroll, 1994) indicate that antipyretic use is unnecessary unless the temperature exceeds 38.5–39 °C and unless there are clinical indications of discomfort in the child, in which case their administration is for their analgesic properties. It is apparent that nurses need a greater understanding of the physiology and benefits of fever. If administering an antipyretic, a clear rationale should be given that shows an understanding of the drug's action and corresponds to research recommendations.

Most drug trials have found that both paracetamol and ibuprofen are efficacious in reducing temperature, but some studies are reporting that that efficacy is demonstrated more in fevers of below 38 °C. The evidence that the administration of antipyretics enhances the comfort of the child is very limited. In some clinical trials, paracetamol has not been found to influence either the prevention of temperature elevations or the reduction of the degree of fever, or to prevent the recurrence of febrile convulsions. Many authors (for example, Hull, 1991; Schnaiderman *et al.*, 1993) are now recommending a return to 'traditional methods' such as warm bathing to reduce high fevers and increasing the intake of fluids orally, in addition to the administration of antipyretics.

Nurses need to receive more education regarding the advantages and disadvantages of using antipyretics. Advice given to parents regarding fever management should include a simple explanation of the nature of fever, including its benefits, as well as give parents an understanding of the action of paracetamol.

An interesting follow-up study would be to analyse in greater depth the specific symptoms a nurse would use to make a diagnosis of fever, and which symptoms viewed together warrant pharmacological intervention. Also helpful would be a study to explore a parent's understanding of fever and pharmacological management, as well as of the pre and post advice being given.

References

Abbott P. and Sapsford R. (1998) *Research Methods for Nurses and the Caring Professsions* (2nd edn), Buckingham, Open University Press.

Addy D. P. (1991) What information and advice should be given to parents? Background paper, Research Unit of the Royal College of Physicians in association with British Paediatric Association.

Agbolosu N. B., Cuevas L. E., Millingan P., Broadhead R. L., Brewster D. and Graham S. M. (1997) 'Efficacy of tepid sponging versus paracetamol in reducing temperature in febrile children', *Annual Trop. Paediatrics* (6AH) 17(3): 283–8.

Anderson E. S., Peterson S. A. and Wailoo M. P. (1990) 'Factors influencing the body temperature of 3–4 month-old infants at home during the day', *Archives of Disease in Childhood* 65: 1308–10.

Atkins E. (1984) 'Fever: the old and the new', *Journal of Infectious Diseases* 149(3): 339–48.

Balslev T. (1991) 'Parental reactions to a child's first febrile convulsion', *Acta Paed. Scand.* 80: 466–9.

Bernheim H. A. and Kluger M. J. (1976) 'Fever: effect of drug-induced antipyresis on survival', *Science* 16 July (193): 237–9.

Bethune P., Gordon K., Dooley J., Camfield C. and Camfield P. (1993) 'Which child will have a febrile seizure?' *American Journal of Diseases in Children* 147: 35–9.

Bonadio W. A., Bellomo T., Brady W. and Smith D. (1993) 'Correlating changes in body temperature with infectious outcome in febrile children who receive acetaminophen', *Clinical Pediatrics* 32(6): 343–6.

Bowman W. C. and Rand M. J. (1980) *Textbook of Pharmacology*, Oxford, Blackwell.

Carmichael L. E., Barnes F. D. and Percy D. H. (1969) 'Temperature as a factor in resistance in young puppies', *Journal of Infectious Disease* 120: 669–78.

Dinarello C. A., Bernheim H. A., Duff G. S. *et al.* (1984) 'Mechanisms of fever induced by recombinant human interferon', *Journal of Clinical Investigation* 94: 906–31.

Ellenburg J. H. and Nelson K. B. (1980) 'Sample selection and the natural history of disease', *Journal of American Medical Association* 243(13): 1337–40.

El-Radhi A. S. and Banajeh S. (1989) 'Effect of fever on reoccurence rate of febrile convulsions', *Archives of Disease in Childhood* 64: 89–90.

El-Radhi A. S. and Carroll J. E. (1994) *Fever in Paediatric Practice*, Oxford, Blackwell.

Eskerud J. R., Andrew M., Stromnes B. *et al.* (1993) 'Pharmacy personnel and fever: a study on perception, selfcare and information to customers. General practitioners and fever: a study on perception, self care and advice to patients', *Pharmacy World and Science* 15(4): 156–64.

Goodman A., Gilman A. and Goodman L. S. (1980) *The Pharmacological Basis of Therapeutics* (6th edn), New York, Macmillan.

Guberman D. (1990) 'Use of acetaminophen in the community', *Harefuah*, 118(1): 17–19.

Haahr S. and Mogensen S. (1977) 'Function of fever', *Lancet* 2: 613.

Hanson D. F., Murphy P. A., Silicano R. and Shin H. S. (1983) 'The effect of temperature on the activation of thymocytes by interleukins I and II', *Journal of Immunology* 130: 216–21.

Heron I., and Berg K. (1978) 'The actions of interferons are potentiated at elevated temperature', *Nature* 274: 508–510.

Hull D. (1991) How important is it to control fever? How is it best controlled? Does control of fever affect febrile convulsions? Background paper, Research Unit of the Royal College of Physicians in association with the British Paediatric Association.

Hunter J. (1973) 'Study of antipyretic therapy in current use', *Archives of Disease in Childhood* 48: 313–15.

Ipp M. and Jaffe D. (1993) 'Physician's attitudes toward the diagnosis and management of fever in children 3 months to 2 years of age', *Clinical Pediatrics* 32(2): 66–70.

Kinmonth A. L., Fulton H. and Campbell M. J. (1992) 'Management of feverish children at home', *British Medical Journal* 305(6682): 1134–6.

Kluger M. J. (1991) 'Fever: role of endogenous pyrogens and cryogens', *Physiology Reviews* 71: 93–127.

Kluger M. J. (1995) 'The mechanism of fever'. In David T. J. (ed.) *Recent Advances in Paediatrics* London, Longman Group.

Knudsen F. U. (1988) 'Optimum management of febrile seizures in childhood', *Drugs* 36: 111–120.

Kramer M. S., Naimark L. Leduc D. J. *et al.* (1985) Parental fever phobia and its correlates', *Paediatrics* 75: 1110–13.

Kramer M. S., Naimark L. E., Roberts-Brauer R., McDougall A. and Leduc D. G. (1991) 'Risks and benefits of paracetamol antipyresis in young children with fever of presumed viral origin', *Lancet* 337(8741): 591–4.

Lewis H. M., Parry J. V., Parry R. *et al.* (1979) 'Role of viruses in febrile convulsions', *Archives of Disease in Childhood* 54: 869–76.

McCance K. L. and Huether S. E. (1994) *Pathophysiology: The Biologic Basis for Disease in Adults and Children*, St Louis, Mosby Year Book.

Monsen R. F., Graham W. M. and Snell G. F. (1991) 'Febrile seizures: caring for the patients and their parents', *Post Graduate Medicine* 90(2): 217–23.

Morgan D. R. (1991) How are febrile convulsions best managed in general practice? Background paper, Research Unit of Royal College of Physicians in asso-
   ciation with British Paediatric Association.
Morley C. J., Hewson P. H., Thornton A. J. and Cole T. J. (1992) 'Axillary and
   rectal temperature measurements in infants', *Archives of Disease in Childhood*
   67: 122–5.
Needleman P. and Isakson P. C. (1998) 'Selective inhibition of cyclo-oxygenase 2',
   Science and Medicine Jan./Feb.: 26–35.
Neville B. (1991) What do we mean by febrile convulsions? Background paper,
   Research Unit of Royal College of Physicians in association with British Paedi-
   atric Association.
Ross E. M. (1991) What is the prognosis following a febrile convulsion? Background paper, Research Unit of Royal College of Physicians in association with
   British Paediatric Association.
Rowsey P. J. (1997) 'Pathophysiology of fever. 2: Relooking at cooling interventions', *Dimensions of Critical Care Nursing* 16(5): 251–6.
Rylance G. W. (1991) What do we know about the drugs which may be used in
   children with febrile convulsions? What are the potential toxic effects of the
   drugs? Background paper, Research Unit of the Royal College of Physicians in
   association with the British Paediatric Association.
Sanz E. J., Bush P. J. and Garcia M. (1996) 'Medicines at home: the contents of
   medicine cabinets in eight countries'. In Bush P., Trakas D., Sanz E. *et al.* (eds)
   Children, Medicines and Culture, New York, Haworth Press.
Schmit B. D. (1985) 'Fever phobia: misconception of parents about fevers', *American Journal of Disease in Children*.
Schnaiderman D., Lahat E., Sheefer T. and Aladjem M. (1993) 'Antipyretic effec-
   tiveness of acetaminophen in febrile seizures: ongoing prophylaxis versus
   sporadic usage', *European Journal of Pediatrics* 152: 747–9.
Smith C. M. and Reynard A. M. (1995) *Essentials of Pharmacology*. Philadelphia,
   W.B. Saunders, pp. 147–63.
Uhari M., Rantala H., Vainionpaa L. and Kurttila R. (1995) 'Effect of aceta-
   minophen and of low intermittent doses of diazepam on prevention of recur-
   rences of febrile seizures', *Journal of Pediatrics* 126(6): 991–5.
UKCC (1992) *Standards for the Administration of Medicines*, London, UKCC.
Walson P. D., Galletta G., Chomilo F., Braden N. J., Sawyer L. A. and Scheinbaum
   M. L. (1992) 'Comparison of multidose ibuprofen and acetaminophen therapy
   in febrile children', *American Journal of Diseases of Children*, 146(5): 626–32.
Weinberg E. D. (1978) 'Iron and infection', *Microbiology Reviews*, 42: 45–66.
Wilson J. T., Brown D., Bocchini J. A. and Kearns G. L. (1982) 'Efficacy, disposi-
   tion and pharmacodynamics of asprin, acetaminophen, and choline salicylate
   in young febrile children', *Therapeutic Drug Monitoring* 4: 147–180.
Wilson J. T., Brown, R. D., Kearns G. L. *et al.* (1991) 'Single-dose, placebo-
   controlled comparative study of ibuprofen and acetaminophen antipyresis in
   children', *Journal of Pediatrics* 119(5): 803–11.

16 *Measuring effectiveness: the paediatric diabetes specialist nurse role*

Lesley Lowes

Introduction

In Cardiff, a multidisciplinary team approach underpins paediatric diabetes care. In 1995, a new paediatric diabetes specialist nurse (PDSN) post was implemented, and was continuously evaluated to measure the impact of interventions introduced to meet expected outcomes. Data collected retrospectively for the 2 years preceding the PDSN appointment were measured against data collected contemporaneously over the first 4 years of the post. The findings demonstrated that collaborative teamwork with a substantial input from the PDSN resulted in:

- the avoidance of hospitalisation for newly diagnosed children
- a significantly reduced length of stay for hospitalised children
- subsequent increased bed availability
- improved clinic attendance
- the introduction of innovative methods of education and support.

The evaluation also identified areas in which further interventions were needed to achieve specific objectives. The demonstration of positive outcomes resulted in the new post being made substantive and the paediatric diabetes team receiving a Quality Award for improvement to service provision.

The paediatric diabetes service at the University Hospital of Wales (UHW), Cardiff, cares for 174 children with diabetes, with approximately 24 newly diagnosed children each year. The aim of our service is to incorporate diabetes into the daily routine of children and their families, minimising disruption to their lifestyle while maintaining the glycaemic control necessary to ensure normal growth and development and reduce the risk of complications in later life.

A team approach underpins the care that we provide. Our paediatric diabetes team comprises a consultant paediatric endocrinologist, a specialist registrar, a part-time clinical assistant, a lecturer in child health, a paediatric dietitian, a paediatric diabetes specialist nurse (PDSN), two diabetes specialist nurses (DSNs) with adult and paediatric caseloads, a growth nurse specialist, a clinical child psychologist and a social worker. To provide an efficient, consistent and co-ordinated service, there is a continual liaison between team members, children and their families and related professional groups. Innovative work undertaken by our team to improve and evaluate service provision resulted in our paediatric diabetes service receiving the UHW Chairman's Quality Award 1998. Thus, while this chapter focuses on the specialist nurse role, the work described is primarily attributable to effective interdisciplinary teamwork.

The PDSN post was implemented at UHW in April 1995 on a 2-year fixed term contract, funded jointly by a pharmaceutical company and the health authority. To justify the continuation of the post beyond this period, there were specific outcomes previously agreed with the health authority that needed to be achieved by the PDSN. The main objectives were:

- home management for newly diagnosed children
- a minimal length of stay for hospitalised children
- fewer readmissions for children with established diabetes
- a reduction in the number of clinic non-attenders
- the introduction of age-banded education sessions.

Initially, role justification was the main reason for evaluating this new post. It was essential to demonstrate value and effectiveness over the first 2 years of the post by measuring the impact of interventions introduced to achieve the objectives. However, as evaluation is also necessary to examine current practice and service provision in order to identify areas for improvement and role development (Smart, 1994), this PDSN role has been continually evaluated since its implementation.

Each of the specific objectives merits individual discussion; these include relevant background information, the interventions introduced, the measurement of the outcomes and the subsequent findings. In order to permit a valid measurement of any outcomes, where appropriate, data were collected retrospectively for the 2 years preceding the commencement of the post (group 1: 1.4.93–31.3.95); these were subsequently compared with similar data collected contemporaneously during the first 4 years of the post (group 2: 1.4.95–31.3.99). Significant differences were tested for by the

Mann–Whitney U test using the Statistical Package for the Social Sciences (SPSS, 1993). Differences were considered to be significant if $p < 0.05$.

Home management for newly diagnosed children

In Leicestershire, where the outpatient management of children with newly diagnosed diabetes was pioneered in the early 1950s (Walker, 1953), home care is firmly established, and from 1979–1988 only 98 (42 per cent) of 236 newly diagnosed children were admitted at diagnosis (Swift *et al.*, 1993). Similarly, in Birmingham, the introduction of a home care unit in 1981 resulted in 60 per cent of newly diagnosed children being managed entirely at home by 1994 (McEvilly, 1996). This approach to initial management was, however, not generally adopted in the British Isles, to the extent that 96 per cent of children under 15 years of age diagnosed in 1988 were admitted to hospital at diagnosis (Lessing *et al.*, 1992). Historically, a lack of local community resources has inhibited the introduction of home management in the UK, and out of 87 per cent of British paediatricians who admitted more than 80 per cent of all newly diagnosed children, 47 per cent would have changed this policy if better community services had been available (British Paediatric Association Working Party, 1990).

Home management has been shown to be cost-effective (Banion *et al.*, 1987; Lee, 1992), to be as safe and effective as inpatient treatment (Chase *et al.*, 1992; Dougherty *et al.*, 1998), to reduce significantly bed occupancy (Hamman *et al.*, 1985; McEvilly, 1991; Lowes and Davis, 1997) and to be associated with a reduction in the number of subsequent readmissions (Swift *et al.*, 1993, Cowan *et al.*, 1997). The avoidance of hospitalisation is believed to be in children's best interests (DoH, 1991; RCN, 1994). Research has shown that children are particularly vulnerable to the emotional impact of illness and hospitalisation (Visintainer and Wolfer, 1975; Tiedeman and Clatworthy, 1990; Rossen and McKeever, 1996), although there are multiple influences on any particular child's short- or long-term reaction to hospitalisation (Muller *et al.*, 1994).

Furthermore, if children with newly diagnosed diabetes are clinically well at presentation, it is perhaps more appropriate for stabilisation to take place at home rather than in hospital. Glycaemic control is affected not only by insulin dosage, but also by carbohydrate intake and exercise. Hospital food is not always what children are used to, which may affect the amount they eat, and children may be less active in hospital. Any difference in diet and activity between hospital and home can result in the insulin dosage prescribed in hospital needing to be substantially readjusted after the child goes home. Home-managed children have also been found to have fewer readmissions, perhaps because active involvement in their child's diabetes management from diagnosis gives parents the confidence to cope more effectively with subsequent problems (Swift *et al.*, 1993).

Home management in Cardiff

In Cardiff, before the PDSN appointment, paediatric diabetes nursing care was undertaken by four part time DSNs, who worked predominantly within the adult service. They were community based and unable to offer a service to paediatric inpatients or outside normal working hours (Cowan *et al.*, 1997). All children were admitted at diagnosis and were not discharged at weekends. The diabetes education programme was commenced in hospital, where ward-based nurses taught the child and parents the practical skills of diabetes management. A DSN visited the child at home on the day of discharge from hospital.

Home management for newly diagnosed children was introduced in August 1995 (Lowes and Davis, 1997). Protocols were drawn up that identified specific criteria for assessing the appropriateness of home management for any particular child and family. Assessment included the clinical condition of the child at presentation, the child's age and the willingness and ability of the family to care for the child at home with intensive support from the PDSN. Home management was also dependent on the availability of the necessary members of the paediatric diabetes team. Children who needed to be admitted were hospitalised for as short a time as possible, and if ketoacidotic at presentation, were discharged on normalisation of their plasma biochemistry.

When home management was instigated, the PDSN monitored the blood glucose level and started insulin therapy and the education programme in the child's home. During the first few days, the PDSN always visited at the time of insulin administration, either to give the insulin or to supervise the child or parents. Many families were keen to take control of the practical skills quite soon after diagnosis, but some families needed a longer period of support. Therefore, the intensity of nurse intervention was tailored to meet the specific needs of individual families. As the number of home visits decreased, regular contact was maintained by telephone and during clinic visits.

In addition to the practical skills of diabetes management, initial education focused on the aetiology and physiology of diabetes, and of necessity, following the administration of exogenous insulin, on the avoidance and treatment of hypoglycaemia. Subsequent education included information about hyperglycaemia, ketoacidosis, illness and exercise, insulin (its action, dosage and storage), personal identification and available benefits. Dietary education was provided by the hospital-based paediatric dietitian, who devised a leaflet giving simple dietary advice to families at diagnosis to help to alleviate parents' concerns about what their children were able to eat. Advice included the restriction of sugary foods while emphasising the importance of regular meals and snacks, and examples were given of everyday carbohydrate-containing foods.

To avoid overwhelming children and their families with information at diagnosis, two booklets were issued for future reference. One booklet gave information about diabetes and its management (Paediatric Diabetes Teams, Newcastle and Gateshead 1993), the other provided an outline of the Cardiff paediatric diabetes service, which included:

- an explanation of the initial management methods
- identification of the team members
- what families can expect from the service
- what happens at clinics
- an outline of organised activities
- useful telephone contact numbers.

To coincide with the introduction of home management, a 24-hour emergency on-call service was introduced. Using a mobile telephone as the point of contact, partly funded by charitable donations, this voluntary out-of-hours service was provided by the consultant paediatrician, the lecturer in child health and the PDSN. Families of children with newly diagnosed and established diabetes were able to contact the paediatric diabetes team for advice and support at evenings and weekends, which empowered families to manage crises at home. Anecdotal evidence suggests that this service gave the families of newly diagnosed children a sense of security at a time when they felt confused and unsure of their ability to cope.

The PDSN had flexible working hours as many home-managed children were diagnosed in the evenings or at weekends. Furthermore, some families required up to four visits a day initially until they felt confident in their ability to carry out the practical skills of diabetes management. Medical colleagues could be contacted at any time for advice on management issues and changes to insulin dosage. This team approach allowed the PDSN to feel comfortable about her role, an important consideration as the relative autonomy of this specialist role can result in feelings of isolation and ultimate responsibility for the welfare of the newly diagnosed child (Lowes, 1997)

Approach to the evaluation

To evaluate one specific aspect of home management, that is, length of stay, a quantitative approach was chosen, measuring the length of hospitalisation for newly diagnosed children in groups 1 (1.4.93–31.3.95) and 2 (1.4.95–31.3.99). Data collected included:

- the date of diagnosis
- the age at diagnosis (in years)
- the gender
- the clinical condition at diagnosis (blood pH/intravenous therapy)
- the length of admission (in days).

It should be noted that the blood pH indicates the clinical condition by establishing the presence and/or extent of acidosis. For the purpose of this study, children with a blood pH of less than 7.35 were deemed to be clinically unwell.

Results

There was no significant difference between the two groups in the number of newly diagnosed children each year (Figure 16.1).

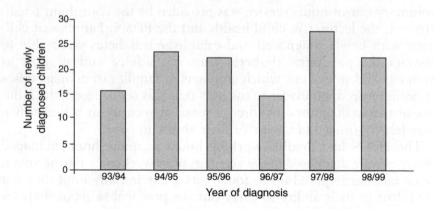

Figure 16.1   Number of newly diagnosed children by year

The findings showed that, from 1.4.95 to 31.3.99, 51 (57 per cent) of 89 newly diagnosed children were managed at home from diagnosis (Figure 16.2).

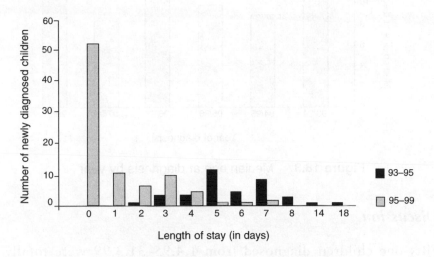

Figure 16.2 Length of stay pre and post the establishment of the paediatric diabetes specialist nurse post

For the 38 hospitalised children, 2 were referred initially to the adult service, 1 had co-existing cystic fibrosis, 7 were diagnosed before home management was introduced, 27 required intravenous therapy for dehydration or ketoacidosis, and 1 was diagnosed while the PDSN was on annual leave.

For all newly diagnosed children, the median length of stay was significantly reduced ($p < 0.001$) from 5 days (range 2–18 days) to 1 day (range 0–7 days) after implementation of the PDSN post. Similarly, for hospitalised children, the median length of stay was significantly reduced ($p < 0.001$) from 5 days (range 2–18 days) to 2.5 days (range 1–7 days).

There was no significant difference between the groups for age at diagnosis ($p < 0.5$) (Figure 16.3), gender ($p > 0.5$) and clinical condition at diagnosis ($p < 0.5$). Blood pH values were missing for nine children diagnosed before 1.4.95, but because intravenous therapy was not required, it was assumed that these children were clinically well at presentation.

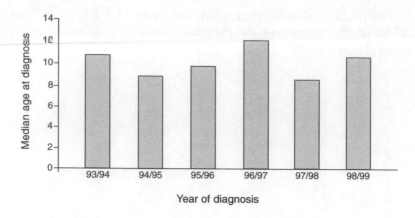

Figure 16.3   Median age at diagnosis by year

Discussion

Fifty-one children diagnosed from 1.4.95–31.3.99 were totally home managed, thereby avoiding a hospital stay of up to a week, and the percentage of home-managed children was found to increase over consecutive years (95/96 = 43 per cent; 96/97 = 53 per cent; 97/98 = 64 per cent; 98/99 = 65 per cent). The findings also demonstrated a reduced length of stay for children admitted at diagnosis. Therefore, findings from this evaluation suggest that the implementation of the PDSN post, and the introduction of home management, had a considerable impact on the avoidance or minimisation of hospitalisation for children with newly diagnosed diabetes. The achievement of these objectives was possible because the PDSN was able to cross the boundary between hospital and community, providing a seamless and integrated service for children with diabetes and their families.

In contemporary health care, there is a need to consider the cost implications of any new post or initiative. An analysis of cost benefit in relation to home management is complex and difficult to determine with any certainty. Evidence of cost savings from home management is found in studies undertaken predominantly in countries such as America or Canada (Strock *et al.*, 1987; Lee, 1992; Dougherty *et al.*, 1998), where the complication of various hospital, government, insurance and social costs make it difficult to relate findings to health care costs in the UK. At a basic level, it could be suggested that all costs resulting from home management need to be measured against all costs resulting from a period of hospitalisation.

It is necessary to consider, however, whether avoiding a child's admission makes a difference to hospital costs in real terms; that is, are heating, lighting or staffing costs reduced? However, although cost-effectiveness is difficult to prove, one obvious advantage of home management is increased bed availability, which alleviates the pressure on paediatric wards by freeing beds for other acutely ill children. The significant reduction in length of stay for newly diagnosed children after the implementation of the PDSN post represented a considerable reduction in bed occupancy (Figure 16.4).

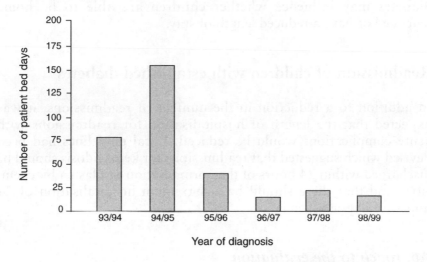

Figure 16.4   Bed occupancy by year of diagnosis

The clinical condition at presentation was the main determinant when assessing for initial management. Children under 3 years of age were thought to be more likely to be admitted at diagnosis, as a result of their limited metabolic reserves and a possible preference for an initial hospital stay by parents of such young children. From 1.4.93 to 31.3.95, 6 (15 per cent) newly diagnosed children were under 3 years of age, 5 of whom presented in ketoacidosis. From 1.4.95 to 31.3.99, there were 9 (10 per cent) children less than 3 years old, 6 of whom were ketoacidotic at diagnosis and 2 of whom were home managed. A high incidence of ketoacidosis at diagnosis is not uncommon in this age group (Swift *et al.*, 1993), perhaps because of a delayed clinical recognition of the disease (Gregory and Taylor, 1995). It was interesting to note that, over this 6-year evaluation, 38 (29 per cent) of 129 newly diagnosed children were under 5 years of age, which supports other reports of an increasing incidence in this age group (Metcalfe and Baum 1991; Gardner *et al.*, 1997). From 1.4.95 to 31.3.99, only 11 (8 per cent) of 139 readmissions were attributable to home-managed children. No conclusions can be drawn from this, however, because of many possible unexamined biases, such as duration of disease.

Although no significant difference was found between the two groups for age or clinical condition at diagnosis, it is acknowledged that other factors, such as the educational status of parents, family structure (a single- or two-parent family) and a prior knowledge of diabetes may influence whether children are able to be home managed or have a reduced length of stay.

Readmission of children with established diabetes

In addition to a reduction in the number of readmissions, it was expected that the length of hospitalisation for readmissions with acute complications would be reduced. Local guidelines had been devised which suggested that readmissions for ketoacidosis should be discharged within 24 hours of the normalisation of plasma biochemistry, and that there should be a maximum hospitalisation of 24 hours for hypoglycaemia.

Approach to the evaluation

To measure the readmission rate, data were collected retrospectively for group 1 (1.4.93–31.3.95) and contemporaneously for group 2 (1.4.95–31.3.99). Data collected included:

- the number of children readmitted
- the age of children readmitted
- the reasons for readmission
- the length of hospitalisation
- the clinical condition on admission (blood pH).

Results

For clarity of presentation, the findings are tabulated below (Tables 16.1 and 16.2).

Table 16.1 Readmissions 1.4.93–31.3.99

Year readmitted	93/94	94/95	95/96	96/97	97/98	98/99
Number of readmissions	26	35	50	36	23	30
Number of patients readmitted	19	23	23	18	21	21
Age range of readmissions (years)						
0–2	1	0	9	6	2	4
3–5	5	6	3	8	3	5
6–8	2	8	6	3	5	7
9–11	3	6	17	15	5	3
12–18	15	15	15	4	8	11
Reasons for readmission						
Diabetic ketoacidosis	8	11	27	19	5	12
Hypoglycaemia	8	13	12	4	6	6
Hyperglycaemia	8	8	5	4	2	1
Vomiting	2	3	3	8	10	11
Investigations	0	0	3	1	0	0
Number requiring intravenous therapy	11	24	40	23	16	21

Table 16.2 Length of hospital stay for readmission

	Median number of days in hospital (range)		
Year admitted	All readmissions	Hypoglycaemia	Ketoacidosis
93/94	1 (0.5–5)	1 (0.5–2)	2 (2–5)
94/95	2 (0.5–6)	1 (0.5–6)	2 (1–6)
95/96	2 (0.5–13)	1 (0.5–3)	2 (1–13)
96/97	1 (0.5–5)	1 (0.5–2)	1 (1–5)
97/98	1 (1–2)	1 (1–3)	1 (1–2)
98/99	1 (1–7)	1 (1–2)	1 (1–3)

There was no significant difference between the two groups in the length of hospitalisation ($p < 1.0$), pH on admission ($p < 0.5$), number of readmissions requiring intravenous therapy ($p < 0.1$), gender ($p < 0.5$) or reason for admission ($p < 0.5$). There was a significant difference in the age of readmissions ($p < 0.01$), reflecting an increased number of readmissions in the 0–2-year and 9–11-year age groups in 95/96 and 96/97 (Table 16.1). There were extremes in the length of stay for both groups (Table 16.2).

Discussion

A reduction in the number of readmissions was not achieved, perhaps because, as Cowan *et al.* (1997) suggest, established views and behaviour are less amenable to change. However, the findings demonstrated an overall adherence to the guidelines for the length of stay of readmissions for ketoacidosis and hypoglycaemia.

The increased readmission rate from 1.4.95 to 31.3.97 could be attributable, in part, to the introduction of the 24-hour emergency on-call service. An improved accessibility to the paediatric diabetes team may have resulted in children being referred to hospital during the late evening and admitted overnight as a precautionary measure, whereas previously parents may have coped at home rather than contacting the hospital directly (Lowes, 1997). Data relating to the timing and subsequent treatment of readmissions were not collected, but the reduced number of readmissions from 1.4.97 to 31.3.99 might suggest that the initial impact of the on-call service has diminished over time.

To address further the number of readmissions, dedicated educational home visits will be undertaken in 2000 by the PDSN to all children over 8 years of age and their families. The programme will reinforce education on the management of illness and the avoidance and treatment of hypoglycaemia and ketoacidosis. For children, the education will be age appropriate. This initiative is particularly pertinent for children who were too young at diagnosis to receive diabetes education. There is, perhaps, an expectation from health professionals that, as children grow up, they will learn about diabetes management from their parents, but this cannot be assumed. The role of the PDSN includes the provision of ongoing diabetes education (RCN Paediatric Diabetes Special Interest Group, 1993). The effectiveness of this initiative will be audited by examining readmission rates for the acute complications of diabetes after the programme has been completed.

Many readmissions cannot, however, be addressed proactively. In addition to periods of acute illness, psychosocial issues frequently

underlie recurrent readmission. The increased readmission rate in the
0–2-year and 9–11-year age groups from 1.4.95 to 31.3.97 reflected
repeated readmission for three particular children. One child, readmitted on nine occasions, was found to have been subjected to sexual
abuse, and another, with six readmissions, was using the omission of
insulin to lose weight. This diabetes-specific 'eating disorder' can
result in significant weight loss when body fat is broken down as an
alternative energy source (Barber and Lowes, 1998). Another family,
with a newly diagnosed toddler, found it difficult to fit the diabetes
management into their lifestyle. From personal experience, families
with a chaotic lifestyle often find it difficult to achieve good diabetes
control. Successful diabetes management requires a fairly organised
approach to, for example, the timing of meals and insulin injections,
regular blood glucose monitoring, and thinking ahead about the
avoidance of hypoglycaemia. A resistance to change may result in
poor diabetes control, which has implications for diabetes-related
health problems in later life.

In group 2, a child admitted for 6 days with hypoglycaemia in
1994 was secretly self-administering extra insulin, and another
admitted for 13 days with ketoacidosis in 1996 was awaiting a foster
placement. These examples demonstrate how any child's individual
circumstances may influence the frequency and length of readmission, as well as highlighting some of the difficulties often associated
with recurrent readmission, in which psychosocial issues can affect
diabetes control. Repeated readmission or consistently poor control
may necessitate a referral to other agencies, such as the psychological, psychiatric or social services.

Psychological support

The clinical child psychologist is an important member of the paediatric diabetes team. Many children and their families with problems
are referred to, and have benefited from, this service. The introduction of psychological support also resulted from a need to disseminate
basic psychological techniques to team members, so that patients who
would most benefit from this interaction could be identified.

Clinic attendance

The Cardiff paediatric diabetes service holds three paediatric clinics
and one adolescent clinic each month. Children and teenagers are

invited to attend clinic every 3 months, although the frequency of attendance varies according to individual needs. The adolescent clinic is held after school hours because many teenagers are studying for examinations or have started full-time employment. Teenagers attend without their parents, which encourages a shift towards independence in the management of their diabetes, and they have the opportunity to consult an adult physician in preparation for the transition to the adult diabetes service.

The paediatric diabetes team holds a 10-minute pre-clinic meeting and receives feedback after the clinic in order to share information about patients. Clinic attendance and patient information from clinics is transferred onto a diabetes database.

The non-attendance (DNA) rate in the paediatric and adolescent clinics needed to be reduced. The clinic is an important part of diabetes management because it allows a regular monitoring of glycaemic control, growth and development, as well as screening for the early signs of complications. Poor glycaemic control can adversely affect growth and development, and has been shown to increase the risk of long-term diabetes-related complications such as retinopathy, nephropathy and neuropathy (Diabetes Control and Complications Trial Research Group, 1993). Clinic non-attendance also has implications of cost- and time-effectiveness for staff.

Approach to the evaluation

After becoming familiar with clinic routine, the PDSN hypothesised that appointments given to patients 3 months in advance were being forgotten. Consequently, clinic reminder cards were introduced and sent to all patients a week before their appointment. To measure the effectiveness of this intervention, data were collected on the number of DNAs, retrospectively from 1.4.93 to 31.3.95 and contemporaneously from 1.4.95 to 31.3.99.

Results

The results showed a significant reduction in the percentage of DNAs for the paediatric ($p < 0.01$) (Figure 16.5) and adolescent clinics ($p < 0.01$) (Figure 16.6) following the introduction of the clinic reminder cards.

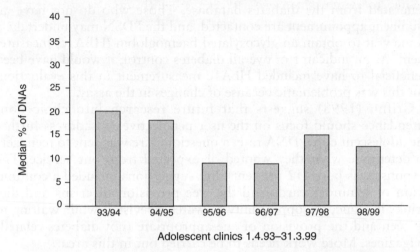

Adolescent clinics 1.4.93–31.3.99

Figure 16.5   Paediatric clinic non-attendance (DNA) rate by year

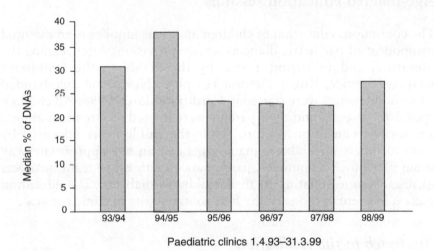

Paediatric clinics 1.4.93–31.3.99

Figure 16.6   Adolescent clinic non-attendance (DNA) rate by year

Discussion

An evaluation of the introduction of clinic reminder cards has demonstrated a significantly improved outcome over the past 4 years. However, the initial positive effect on the DNA rate resulting from this intervention has waned slightly over time, as found by others (Griffin, 1998). There are a number of persistent non-attenders in both clinics. Every month, a list of patients who have not been seen for 6 months is generated from the diabetes database. Those who do not have an imminent appointment are contacted, and the PDSN may undertake a home visit to obtain an glycosylated haemoglobin (HBA1c) measurement. As an indicator of overall diabetes control, it would have been beneficial to have included HbA1c measurement in this evaluation, but this was problematic because of changes in the assay.

Griffin (1998) suggests that future research into clinic non-attendance should focus on the user perspective. To address further the adolescent clinic DNA rate, a questionnaire was sent to teenagers to determine what they wanted or expected from our service. The response was poor (12 per cent), but suggestions included a continuation of reminder cards and the free provision of crisps and diet drinks in clinic, the opportunity to watch television while waiting to be seen and the provision of age-appropriate (not diabetes-related) magazines. More work needs to be carried out in this area.

Age-banded education sessions

The continuous education of children and their families is an essential component of paediatric diabetes service provision. After reading the literature, and following a visit by the PDSN to the Children's Diabetes Service, Royal Victoria Hospital, Newcastle, age-banded education sessions were started in Cardiff in March 1996. All children aged 5 to 14 years and their parents were invited to attend an annual age-specific education session. While the children are educated by team members on diabetes management in an age-appropriate way using play-based techniques, parents meet with other team members to discuss issues relating to their children's diabetes. The education session has replaced one of the four routine visits to clinic per year.

Approach to the evaluation

Attendance was recorded contemporaneously. After the first seven education sessions, separate evaluation sheets were sent to participating children and their parents. The questions were semi-structured, and the replies were anonymous.

Results and discussion

Attendance at most of the education sessions was excellent, with a median attendance rate of 91 per cent (range 50–100 per cent). Twenty-three out of 56 (41 per cent) evaluation sheets were returned.

Most children and parents appreciated being given the opportunity to share their experiences with others in the same situation. Many parents found it reassuring that others were coping with similar problems and found it beneficial to hear how other parents dealt with specific age-related issues. Almost all parents found the sessions 'comforting', 'well focused' and 'interesting', requesting more frequent and longer sessions. All parents felt that it helped their children to meet others of the same age with diabetes, some commenting that, before the session, their children had believed that 'they were the only ones of their age with diabetes'. Children benefited from learning about specific diabetes issues, such as blood glucose monitoring and diet, as well as sharing tips from others about the change to secondary education, and said that 'it helped to share moans about parents nagging about diabetes management'. Some parents and children suggested that the groups were too large, inhibiting open expression. Smaller, more-frequent groups would be difficult to organise within the available resources, but as the groups become established, with the same children and parents attending, those who feel inhibited about speaking may become more comfortable within their group.

In addition to evaluating these sessions from the perspective of participating families, it would in retrospect have been helpful also to have determined reasons for non-attendance. However, the evaluation suggested that age-banded education sessions were successfully introduced, and many parents gave very encouraging feedback on the work undertaken by the paediatric diabetes service, saying that they greatly valued the help and support provided.

Conclusion

This PDSN role was initially evaluated to help to ensure continued funding of the post, and the outcomes from 1.4.95 to 31.3.97 resulted in the post being made substantive. However, other equally important benefits resulted from the role evaluation. As Smart (1994) suggests:

> so often, a new role is started with a clear perception of what is required and two years down the road the specialist has become so absorbed with the mechanics of the job that sight of the overall plan has been lost. (p. 71)

The continuous evaluation of this specialist post over 4 years included the submission of 6-monthly progress reports until 31.3.97. This allowed the PDSN to keep sight of the overall plan, formulated in a 2-year projection of workload devised at the commencement of the post. Every 6 months, outcomes from the evaluation were compared with the initial expectations of achievement, allowing an assessment of the rate and level of progress and guidance for the next 6 months' work.

Children with diabetes and their families contributed to the evaluation of certain interventions. Ultimately, the quality of service provision and the appropriateness of any service development can only be measured by ascertaining the views of patients and their families or carers. For example, it is widely recognised that, because of the adverse effects of hospitalisation, children should only be admitted to hospital when absolutely necessary (DoH, 1991; RCN, 1994). However, it is currently not known how parents experience or cope with the home management of children with newly diagnosed diabetes. To address this, the author is currently undertaking a longitudinal qualitative study exploring this phenomenon.

Recommendations for practice

- A team approach to paediatric diabetes care
- A seamless, integrated service between hospital and community
- Care tailored to the needs of individual families
- Easy accessibility to team members for help and advice
- An awareness of underlying psychosocial issues
- The development of communication and counselling skills
- A consideration of the needs of different age groups
- Innovative methods of providing education
- A continual qualitative and quantitative evaluation of service provision
- Undertaking, or an involvement in, research about paediatric diabetes
- The implementation of more paediatric diabetes specialist nurse posts
- Ongoing professional development.

Acknowledgements

The author would like to acknowledge Dr J. W. Gregory, Consultant Paediatric Endocrinologist, for his constant support, Lilli Pharmaceuticals and South Glamorgan (Bro Taf) Health Authority for their financial support, and the *British Journal of Nursing* for their permission to reproduce some of the text included in this chapter.

References

Banion C., Klingersmith G., Giordano B. and Radcliffe J. (1987) 'Efficacy of outpatient management of new onset diabetes in children (abstract)', *Diabetes* (supplement 1): 118A.

Barber C. J. and Lowes L. (1998) 'Eating disorders and adolescent diabetes: is there a link?', *British Journal of Nursing* 7(7): 307–10.

British Paediatric Association Working Party (1990) 'The organisation of services for children with diabetes in the United Kingdom', *Diabetic Medicine* 7: 457–64.

Chase H. P., Crews K. R., Garg S. *et al.* (1992) 'Outpatient management versus in-hospital management of children with new-onset diabetes', *Clinical Pediatrics,* Aug.: 450–6.

Cowan F. J., Warner J. T., Lowes L., Ribeiro J. P. and Gregory J. W. (1997) 'Auditing paediatric diabetes care and the impact of a specialist nurse trained in paediatric diabetes', *Archives of Disease in Childhood* 77: 109–14.

Department of Health (1991) *Welfare of Children and Young People in Hospital,* London, HMSO.

Diabetes Control and Complications Trial Research Group (1993) 'The effect of intensive treatment of diabetes on the development and progression of long-term complications in insulin dependent diabetes mellitus', *New England Journal of Medicine* 329(14): 977–86.

Dougherty G. E., Soderstrom L. and Schiffrin A. (1998) 'An economic evaluation of home care for children with newly diagnosed diabetes. Results from a randomised control trial', *Medical Care* 36(4): 586–98.

Gardner S. G., Bingley P. J., Sawtell P. A., Weeks S., Gale A. M. and the Barts-Oxford Study Group (1997) 'Rising incidence of insulin dependent diabetes in children aged under 5 years in the Oxford region: time trend analysis', *British Medical Journal* 315: 713–17.

Gregory J. W. and Taylor R. (1995) 'Biochemistry and intermediate metabolism'. In Kelnar J. H. (ed.) *Childhood and Adolescent Diabetes,* London, Chapman & Hall.

Griffin S. J. (1998) 'Lost to follow-up: the problem of defaulters from diabetes clinics', *Diabetic Medicine* 15 (supplement 3): S15–S24.

Hamman R. F., Cook M., Keefer S. *et al.* (1985) 'Medical care patterns at the onset of insulin dependent diabetes mellitus: association with severity and subsequent complications', *Diabetes Care* 8 (supplement 1): 94–100.

Lee P. D. K. (1992) 'An outpatient-focused program for childhood diabetes: design, implementation and effectiveness', *Texas Medicine/The Journal* 88(7): 64–8.

Lessing D. N., Swift P. G. F., Metcalfe M. A. and Baum J. D. (1992) 'Newly diagnosed diabetes: a study of parental satisfaction', *Archives of Disease in Childhood* 67: 1011–13.

Lowes L. (1997) 'Evaluation of a paediatric diabetes specialist nurse post', *British Journal of Nursing* 6(11): 625–33.

Lowes L. and Davis R. (1997) 'Minimizing hospitalisation: children with newly diagnosed diabetes', *British Journal of Nursing* 6(1): 28–33.

McEvilly A. (1991) 'Home management on diagnosis', *Paediatric Nursing* 3(5): 16–18.

McEvilly A. (1996) 'Setting standards for the home care of children with diabetes', *Cascade* Dec.: 4–5.

Metcalfe M. A. and Baum J. D. (1991) 'Incidence of insulin dependent diabetes in children aged under 15 years in the British Isles during 1988', *British Medical Journal* 302: 443–7.

Muller D. J., Harris P. J., Wattley L. and Taylor J. D. (1994) *Nursing Children. Psychology, Research and Practice* (2nd edn), London, Chapman & Hall.

Paediatric Diabetes Teams, Newcastle and Gateshead (1993) *Diabetes. A Book for Children and their Families*, Sussex, Boehringer Mannheim.

Rossen B. E. and McKeever P. D. (1996) 'The behaviour of preschoolers during and after brief surgical hospitalizations', *Issues in Comprehensive Pediatric Nursing* 19: 121–33.

Royal College of Nursing (1994) *The Care of Sick Children. A Review of the Guidelines in the Wake of the Allitt Inquiry*, London, RCN.

Royal College of Nursing Paediatric Diabetes Special Interest Group (1993) *The Role and Qualifications of the Nurse Specialising in Paediatric Diabetes – A Working Party Report*, London, RCN.

Smart S. (1994) 'Evaluating the impact: using a business planning approach'. In Humphris D. (ed.) *The Clinical Nurse Specialist. Issues in Practice*, London, Macmillan.

SPSS (1993) *Statistical Package for the Social Sciences for Windows. Release 6.0*, Surrey, SPSS.

Strock E., Spencer M., Sandell J. and Hollander P. (1987) 'Reimbursement of an ambulatory insulin programme (abstract)', *Diabetes* (supplement 1): 33A.

Swift P. F., Hearnshaw J. R., Botha J. L., Wright G., Raymond N. T. and Jamieson K. F. (1993) 'A decade of diabetes: keeping children out of hospital', *British Medical Journal* 307: 96–8.

Tiedeman M. E. and Clatworthy S. (1990) 'Anxiety responses of 5- to 11-year-old children during and after hospitalization', *Journal of Pediatric Nursing* 5(5): 334–42.

Visintainer M. A. and Wolfer J. A. (1975) 'Psychological preparation for surgical patients: the effect on children's and parent's stress responses and adjustment', *Pediatrics* 56: 187–202.

Walker J. B. (1953) 'Field work of a diabetic clinic', *Lancet* ii: 445–7. Cited in Swift P. F., Hearnshaw J. R., Botha J. L. *et al.* (1993) 'A decade of diabetes: keeping children out of hospital', *British Medical Journal* 307: 96–8.

Further reading

Charron-Prochownik D., Siminerio L., Maihle T. and Songer T. (1997) 'Outpatient versus inpatient care of children newly diagnosed with IDDM', *Diabetes Care* **20**(4): 657–60.

Dunning M., Abi-Aad G. and Gilbert D. (1998) 'Turning evidence into everyday practice', *Nursing Times* **94**(47): 60.

Kelnar J. H. (ed.) (1995) *Childhood and Adolescent Diabetes*, London, Chapman & Hall.

Lowes L. and Davis R. (1998) 'Ambulatory care for children with newly diagnosed diabetes'. In Glasper A. and Lowson S. (eds) *Innovations in Paediatric Ambulatory Care – A Nursing Perspective*, Basingstoke, Macmillan.

17 Decision analysis in evidence-based children's nursing: a community nursing perspective

Dorothèe J. H. O'Sullivan-Burchard

Introduction

In this chapter, decision analysis is explored as a model in support of the clinical judgement and decision making necessary for the transfer of care from the hospital to the home environment. The need to be able to demonstrate accountability in a health care arena such as community children's nursing is argued. Decision analysis is suggested as a process that may enable children's nurses to provide the evidence of their judgement and decision making when working in increasingly complex care settings and within multiprofessional health care teams.

Consideration is given to the complex relationships and variables involved that influence the cognitive processes in clinical judgement and decision making. By using a case study, the process of decision analysis will be applied in the context of home care for a child with a chronic illness. The evidence in support of how and why a decision for discharge has been reached is made explicit in working through the analysis. The judgement and decision-making processes are uncovered and the uncertainties of outcomes acknowledged. Both process and outcomes are linked to the decision making. The implication of decision analysis for practice is discussed in relation to its appropriateness and ethical significance.

Framing the problem

Professional bodies and the public now demand that health care professionals demonstrate competence and accountability in service provision. The ability to base judgements on evidence and to justify decisions requires not just knowledge and skill, but also exposure to and practice in clinical reasoning and problem solving. Throughout their pre-registration education, prospective children's nurses are required to give a rationale for the nursing care that they propose. In clinical practice, however, decisions are not always made on the basis of such an explicit rationale. In reality, a care situation tends to be complex and dynamic. Information may be limited. As a result, constraints influence the nurse's clinical judgement and decision-making processes. Despite these limitations, rapid responses are often required. The transfer of care from hospital to home, however, requires careful consideration by those who initiate and accept such a change. In this context, decision analysis may offer some scope, for example, to aid the referral of a family to a community children's nursing service.

To be able to demonstrate how and why a decision has been reached is particularly important in community children's nursing. The context of care is, indeed, complex and uncertain, calling for a reciprocal working relationship. Given the long-term implications of undertaking new tasks and commitments on the part of the family, facilitating parental choice in the decision-making process for early discharge is essential. The emotional investment of the parent is likely to be high, and the community children's nurse has to accept considerable uncertainty in the outcome of the nursing input. In addition, issues related to safety and compliance have to be borne in mind, as the control and the primary position of authority shift in favour of the family (Hogue, 1992; Lantos and Kohrman, 1992; Klug, 1993).

The discharge of a child with complex nursing needs depends on the provision of a community children's nursing service. Fundamentally, however, it rests on the willingness and commitment of the parents to participate in the ongoing nursing care of their child. Participation enables the parent and child to be in control of their health care, but it also means taking on the extra burden in responsibility and the demands of a significant role change (Hill, 1993; Bond *et al.*, 1994; Whyte, 1994). To initiate the early discharge of a child with special needs in such circumstances presents a challenge in judgement and decision making for all concerned, that is, the multiprofessional health care team and the family involved. How can the community children's nurse demonstrate accountability for clinical judgements and decision making in such an unstable context of care? What variables have to be considered in situations where challenging clinical and management judgements are called for and decisions need to be reached?

Variables affecting the decision-making process

Any problem solving requires the skill of processing information, defining the problem, asking productive questions, using logical reasoning and making judgements in order to arrive at decisions (Blagg *et al.*, 1988; Soden, 1994; Watson, 1994). These are all processes of higher-order thinking skills.

A framework for classifying cognitive processes as a continuum is offered by Hammond *et al.* (1980) in which modes of enquiry range from an ill-structured task to a well-structured task. The former corresponds to an intuitive cognitive mode, and the latter lends itself to a more analytical mode of cognition. Along this continuum, a system-aided judgement is placed at a pivotal position, in which verbal quantifiers of magnitude or severity are replaced by numerical quantifiers. Figure 17.1 provides an adapted and simplified concept map showing the relationships of judgements leading to decision analysis.

A variety of judgements need to be made for the referral of a family to a community children's nursing service, for example:

- a diagnostic judgement – the classificatory assessment of whether the parent is ready to take on extra responsibility and what nursing interventions are required
- a therapeutic judgement – how to support the parent in this new task
- an ethical judgement – why the referral should be initiated, what is in the best interest of child/parent and how they perceive the potential outcomes
- an evaluative judgement – when the referral has taken place and of what value it has been.

These clinical judgements appear to match the assumptions made by Gordon *et al.* (1994) in their integrated model based on information-processing theory. Diagnostic, therapeutic and ethical reasoning is assumed and suggested for every act in nursing judgements. Hence, these diagnostic, therapeutic, ethical as well as evaluative dimensions are all brought to bear on the clinical judgement and decision-making processes.

The question arises of how children's nurses arrive at these judgements. From observation and experience, the children's nurse may be able to assess whether a parent is ready to take on the extra burden of responsibility. The nurse may notice subtle changes in parental behaviour and infer from these a parent's readiness for a greater participation in complex care. Such judgements are made intuitively based on cues. From these cues, it is possible to deduce and hypothesise further. Such a process takes place very rapidly and relates to the hypothetico-deductive model of cognition as described by Elstein and Bordage (1988). The expert nurse is likely to be accustomed to this intuitive mode of cognition, which can be promoted through reflection in and on practice (Benner, 1984; Emden, 1991; Schön, 1991). However, one needs to remember that intuitive judgements are subjective.

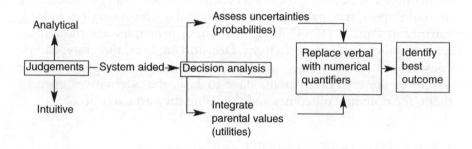

Figure 17.1   Concept map (adapted from Hammond *et al.*, 1980)

In addition, parents may demonstrate in much more overt ways their willingness to undertake home care, for example by asking questions, by demonstrating greater confidence, by their eagerness to learn technical nursing procedures – in short, by generally wanting to overcome any knowledge deficit. These events can also be taken as cues indicating the timeliness of exploring issues of home care and can be considered to be less subjective for influencing the nurse's clinical judgement. The most obvious process is, of course, to explore and negotiate verbally the level of participation in care that is desired by the parent.

Home care is associated with extra pressure for parents. These demands may well be filtered out from their perception as the desire to have their child at home may outweigh any potential limitations. By using decision analysis, the community children's nurse may be able to facilitate a more transparent decision-making process while incorporating parental input. Nonetheless, ownership of the decision will firmly remain with the parent.

In order to make an early discharge possible, a range of factors will need to be considered, all of which influence such a management decision. The community children's nurse needs to bring into the encounter with the family a sound knowledge base, sufficient experience, the ability to reflect on this experience, analytical skills, clinical judgement and decision-making skills. These are all processes necessary for effective problem solving (Roberts *et al.*, 1993, 1995). By introducing a decision analysis, the potential options, the evidence for the likelihood of possible outcomes, the parental preference and the chosen action can be identified.

The relationship between the community children's nurse and the family needs to be a reciprocal one. Such reciprocity can be fostered by mutual respect, true participation and shared decision making. Indeed, Zarin and Pauker (1984) imply that these principles are the ethical underpinnings in decision analysis. Decision analysis, therefore, can be considered to be a suitable analytical framework for appraising the nature of the task that parents have to face, the alternatives open to them, the potential outcomes and the value they attach to it.

Decision analysis – a model and a process

Decision analysis is a model that may be used for the benefit of both the family and the nurse practitioner. It is also a process that involves problem analysis, logical action and explicit judgement. Decision analysis is an applied approach of statistical decision theory and relates to probability and utility theories (Harbison, 1991). Applied decision analysis is more commonly associated with business and industry, where it is used to identify risk management; with economics, to aid planning decisions in resource allocation processes; and with medicine, to support clinical judgements. The medical application of decision analysis comprises mainly hypothetical situations (Eraker and Politser, 1988).

Decision analysis involves (Zarin and Pauker, 1984):

- the three inputs of structure, probabilities and values
- a process by which they are combined
- a decision leading to action as the output.

Applied decision analysis allows the construction of a problem, in which potential options are considered, each being assessed in terms of its respective consequences. These possible outcomes are assigned a probability. The probability of each of the outcomes is based on either the evidence obtained from research or expert opinion. The likelihood that the outcome will occur is expressed in numerical terms and a value is assigned to each possible outcome. It should be noted that this value should be elicited from the decision maker in order to secure the integration of his or her perspective. It should also be expressed in numerical terms reflecting the desirability of the outcome. The probability of each outcome is combined with each assigned value, revealing the 'expected value' of each option. The best option to choose would be the one with the highest 'expected value' (Harbison, 1991) (Figure 17.2).

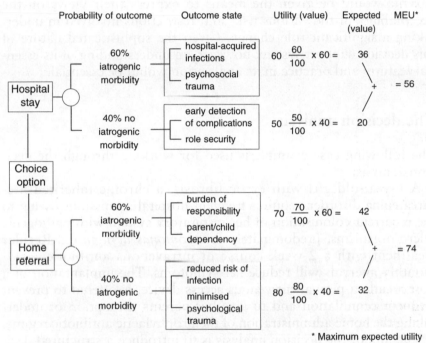

1. Identify the available options
2. Identify the consequences of following each (qualitative quantifiers)
3. Estimate the probability of possible outcomes (numerical quantifiers of chance events)
4. Elicit the assigned value of chance events from the client/parent (quantified and ranked)
5. Calculate the probability along with assigned value revealing the expected value of each outcome
6. The option with the highest expected value, that is, maximum expected utility, is the best outcome

Figure 17.2   Decision flow diagram

The quantification and calculation in decision analysis are an attempt to make a more detached analysis of clinical decisions possible. It simultaneously identifies the course of action that is in the best interest of the client. This process facilitates the normative analysis of how judgements and decisions should be made. A comparison of outcomes can be achieved that will aid their evaluation. Emphasis is given to the cognitive processing of information in order to reach a decision for action. Decision analysis aids the formal reasoning necessary for making judgements and decisions. Using it, the logical analysis of uncertainties (probabilities) and the integration of values (utilities) can both be accommodated (Dowie, 1993).

In the context of negotiating home care for the child and family, parents would be given the means to express their views on the acceptability of the various risks and restrictions involved in undertaking a significant role change. Given the sophisticated nature of this decision support system, however, an understanding of its essential features and practice in its application would be essential.

The decision analysis

The following case example is used for working through the decision analysis:

A 6-year-old girl with cystic fibrosis, a chronic inherited life-threatening disorder, requires frequent hospital admissions owing to the recurrent colonisation of her respiratory system with pathogenic micro-organisms, predominately *Pseudomonas aeruginosa*. Regular treatment with a 2-week course of intravenous antibiotics at 3-monthly intervals will reduce her symptoms. The implantation of a Port-a-cath, a permanent venous access device, is offered to prevent frequent cannulation and to give her parents the option of undertaking the home administration of the prophylactic antibiotic regime.

The aim of the decision analysis is to introduce a structured decision support system for the referral of a family to a community children's nursing service. The objectives are:

- to assess the consequences of this transfer of care
- to integrate the parental perspective
- to identify the best client valued outcome from the given alternatives.

Step 1

The decision flow diagram (see Figure 17.2 above) shows a binary decision tree for structuring the problem. The choice option is either for the child to stay in hospital, where the treatment will be given by hospital staff, or for her parents to learn to give the intravenous therapy at home with support from the community children's nurse. Each considered option – 'hospital stay' or 'home referral' – is identified and assessed with two incompatible opposing branches. The possible chance events for both options have been called 'iatrogenic morbidity' and 'no iatrogenic morbidity'. An iatrogenic disorder can be defined as any condition that is caused by medical personnel or procedures, or indeed by an exposure to the environment of a health care facility (Anderson *et al.*, 1994). The term classifies appropriately the potential outcome states, which are associated with each branch of the respective options. These outcome states should ideally be based on frequency data, statistical evidence and/or other research findings in order to raise the level of objectivity in the analysis. However, insufficient research evidence would have to be complemented by expert knowledge and experience.

Branch: option hospital stay

The outcome states relating to iatrogenic morbidity for the option 'hospital stay' can be identified as hospital-acquired infection based on research by Signorelli *et al.* (1991) and Mehtar (1992), and psychosocial trauma caused by frequent hospital admission. Evidence for psychosocial trauma can be found in While (1991), Müller *et al.* (1993) and Whyte (1994).

Potential outcome states relating to 'no iatrogenic morbidity' can be identified as the early detection of complications and a sense of role security for the parent and child as clear boundaries in nursing tasks will be maintained. In this case, the judgement that these outcomes may occur is based on expert knowledge and experience gained through the decision facilitator's clinical practice.

Branch: option home referral

For the option 'home referral', the probabilities of outcome states relating to *iatrogenic morbidity* can be identified from the literature as burden of responsibility (Sterling, 1990; Bond *et al.*, 1994; Hill,

1993; Whyte, 1994) and parent/child dependency. For the latter, the judgement is again based on expert knowledge and experience gained through clinical practice. The outcome state 'no iatrogenic morbidity' associated with 'home referral' can be identified as a reduced risk of infection (Atwell and Gow, 1985; Couriel and Davies, 1988) and minimised psychosocial trauma (Fields *et al.*, 1991; DoH, 1993; Müller *et al.*, 1993).

Once the outcome states have been identified, the likelihood that they will occur is estimated by the decision facilitator from a sum of 1–100 per cent and assigned to each branch of each option. One could say that 'qualitative quantifiers' are now transposed into 'numerical quantifiers'. The estimation of the probability of the identified outcomes has to be equal for each branch. However, the degree of probability that they may occur may change with each analysis, depending on the knowledge and experience of the decision facilitator, as well as the nature of bias and error inherent in human cognition. The estimation of probabilities should ideally be based on objective frequency data, as mentioned earlier. Without such data, the estimation would have to be attempted based on expert knowledge.

The following estimation of probabilities is put forward for the analysis.

Branch: option hospital stay

If the child stays in hospital for treatment, there is a 60 per cent chance of the child experiencing iatrogenic morbidity. This may show itself in a hospital-acquired infection and/or psychosocial trauma. A probability of 40 per cent is assigned to 'no iatrogenic morbidity', which is linked to the early detection of complications and role security.

Branch: option home referral

If the child is referred home, with the family accepting giving the treatment, there is a 60 per cent chance of the child experiencing iatrogenic morbidity. This can be associated with an increased burden in terms of responsibility and parent/child dependency. A 40 per cent probability assigned to 'no iatrogenic morbidity' is linked to a reduced risk of infection and minimal psychological trauma.

Step 2

Moving along the decision tree carries the analysis forward. As parents are the assumed owners of the decision, their expressed value of the four sets of outcomes needs to be elicited. Parents will be asked to quantify and rank the outcomes on a scale of 0 to 100 in order of preference. To reiterate, a value based on the parent's perception of each probable outcome state has to be elicited; parents will have to quantify and rank each potential outcome. By assigning a numerical value to each outcome state, the subjective parental perception of each is transposed into a framework, which makes further mechanical calculation possible.

The best outcome in this case is attributed to the option 'home referral' with a probability of 'no iatrogenic morbidity' rated at 80. Minimising the psychological trauma and reducing the risk of infection is valued the highest. The burden of responsibility and the potential parent/child dependency are also given considerable significance and ranked at 70. The probability of contracting a hospital-acquired infection and experiencing psychosocial trauma is ranked as being fairly important and assigned a value of 60, whereas the early detection of complications and role security are seen as the least important outcome and given a value of 50.

Step 3

This step involves the calculation of the analysis. In order to reveal the expected value of each outcome, the assigned value of each outcome state is divided by 100 and multiplied by the estimated probability of each branch, giving an expected value for each branch. For example, the calculation for 'hospital stay' in the top branch would thus read:

$$\frac{\text{assigned value}}{100} \times \text{estimated probability} = \text{expected value}$$

for the *Branch: option hospital stay*, this would read:

$$\frac{60}{100} \times 60 = 36 \text{ and } \frac{50}{100} \times 40 = 20$$

To be able to identify the highest expected value, or maximum expected utility (MEU), the expected values of each branch have to be added up, thus giving the optimal outcome. The option with the maximum expected utility is the one to be chosen as the best outcome. Figure 17.2 outlines a calculation of the analysis.

A comparison of the two expected utilities reveals an MEU of 74 in favour of 'home referral', taking into account all probabilities and values assumed at this point in time for this exercise. It should be noted that the MEU might change over time as values are characterised by instability (Fischhoff *et al.*, 1980). Furthermore, depending on how the decision analysis is presented, how questions are asked or how environmental factors impinge on the situation, the value of outcomes may be weighted differently by the same parent.

To conclude, a system-aided referral would open up the decision-making process to all participants, bringing to light the variables that need to be taken into account for this management problem. By applying a decision analysis, the community children's nurse may be able to facilitate an informed choice for the family, support the quantification of outcomes and demonstrate accountability for the decision taken. In addition, the best client-valued outcome would be explicitly identified, the transparency of the decision-making process encouraged and evidence-based practice advanced.

Assumptions and limitations

When working through a decision analysis, the decision facilitator attempts to synthesise objective and subjective data by assigning probabilities to chance events in order to arrive at the best outcome as perceived by the parent. For example, sources of objective frequency data and information on the home administration of intravenous antibiotics can be found in the literature (David, 1986; Catchpole, 1989; Ellis, 1989; Gill, 1993) and have been used to inform the decision facilitator for structuring the problem.

Luker and Kenrick (1992) suggest that community nurses in general base their decisions less on evidence supported by research than on past experience and situational factors. Grounding variables, which influence decisions predominantly in the realm of subjectivity, leave the nursing profession open to criticism. Hence, decision analysis, as a more systematic process to complement the intuitive mode of reasoning, is suggested for aiding the integration of cognitive faculties essential for problem solving.

Despite the analytical effort of raising the level of objectivity, one needs to acknowledge that the integration of complex information for decision making remains largely a subjective process. This is particularly so when it is difficult to separate judgements from actions in interpreting outcomes, as noted by Einhorn (1980). He proposes that discerning the structure of tasks when the content is rich in detail adds to the problem of judgement and decision making.

This relates well to observations made when working through the above decision analysis. While structuring the decision analysis, the writer, in her dual role of decision facilitator and decision-maker/owner, initially felt overwhelmed by the amount of information that needed to be incorporated. She also experienced conflict in balancing professional role values with personal values associated with her role as a parent. The task demanded that explicit meaning be given to values in order to achieve decomposition (Fischhoff *et al.*, 1980). 'Knowing what to want' for the analysis became a lived experience. The need to attend to dis-confirming evidence or to overcome selective attention to certain aspects is, therefore, a noteworthy recommendation by Einhorn. An awareness of cognitive bias, over-confidence and hindsight may also help to minimise contamination with influences that are too subjective or with one's own values. Although heuristics, used in the form of trial and error and informal reasoning, help to speed up the cognitive processes, they do lead to misperceptions. One needs to bear in mind that value judgements are affected by intellectual and emotional filters such as motivational biases, cognitive limitations and situational factors (Komaroff, 1979; Tversky and Kahneman, 1982; Zarin and Pauker, 1984; Baumann *et al.*, 1991).

It is also possible to revise the probability estimates by conducting a sensitivity analysis. Such a sensitivity analysis would allow the calculation of error in the problem structure, incorrect probabilities or inappropriately ranked values, but it has not been pursued for this simple binary decision. Furthermore, a more sophisticated analysis could be attempted by widening the range and emphasising the positive and negative values attached to each single outcome from −100 to +100.

However, the aims and objectives of the decision analysis for this case example have been achieved. The process of linking judgements to the decision making has been made more transparent, and action on the further management of the case could now be taken. A full assessment of the potential consequences has been achieved, the hypothesised parental perspective has been integrated into the analysis and the best client-valued outcome from the given alternatives has been identified.

This prescriptive and analytical approach acknowledges the uncertainties of outcome that need to be borne in mind in a shared care context. Decision analysis allows linking processes to outcomes in decision making. At the same time, uncertainties are fully acknowledged. Although the assessment of the problem may change depending on the expert knowledge available, outcome states remain. This makes comparison and measurement possible.

Implications for practice

A case study was used to demonstrate decision analysis as a model and process of intervention for the transfer of care from hospital to home. The use of decision analysis may support the professional judgement and decision making of a specialist practitioner within an autonomous role and setting such as community children's nursing. As the decision-making process would be opened up to scrutiny, issues of negligence and compliance might be less threatening in a context of care that was likely to be complex and unstable.

The impact of taking on an extended role for parents in the health care of their child with a chronic illness is likely to be substantial and, more importantly, unpredictable. It can be argued that the parental decision to undertake this commitment may be implicitly driven by a number of factors. These may be the desire to meet the unique needs of the child for emotional security, the professional goal of therapeutic nursing care, the present resource-driven health care system and/or a covert collective utilitarian ethos characterised by technological advances in medicine.

The question arises of whether applied decision analysis is an appropriate method for uncovering these implicit propositions, and furthermore, of whether the use of decision analysis is ethically acceptable or indeed desirable. Transparency in decision making means inevitably accepting exposure, uncertainty and vulnerability. Opening up the decision-making process may be perceived – by the family as well as the nurse – as being very threatening. Spelling out the likelihood of chance events may either prompt a more decisive response from parents or may worry them more. However, as the parental perspective would be explicitly incorporated into the decision-making process, the consequences of their decisions would rest on a foundation of ownership.

Nursing decision making has been identified as a significant area of outcome research (McCormack, 1992). Little is, however, known about how nurses arrive at clinical judgements and decisions, how client preferences are established and how compliance is maintained in the context of home care. Further research that examines whether decision analysis can be used as an appropriate and scientifically defensible nursing intervention option needs to be undertaken.

References

Anderson K. N., Anderson L. E. and Glanze W. D. (1994) *Mosby's Medical, Nursing and Allied Health Dictionary*, 4th edn, St Louis, Mosby.

Atwell J. D. and Gow M. A. (1985) 'Paediatric trained district nurse in the community: expensive luxury or economic necessity?', *British Medical Journal*, **291**: 227–9.

Baumann A. O., Deber R. B. and Thompson G. G. (1991) 'Overconfidence among physicians and nurses: the "micro-certainty, macro-uncertainty" phenomenon', *Social Science of Medicine* **32**(2): 161–74.

Benner P. (1984) *From Novice to Expert: Excellence and Power in Clinical Nursing Practice*, Menlo Park, CA, Addison Wesley.

Blagg N., Ballinger M. and Gardner R. (1988) *Somerset Thinking Skills Course*, Oxford, Basil Blackwell.

Bond N., Philips P. and Rollins J. A. (1994) 'Family centered care at home for families with children who are technology dependent', *Pediatric Nursing* **20**(2): 123–30.

Catchpole A. (1989) 'Cystic fibrosis: intravenous treatment at home', *Nursing Times* **85**(12): 40–2.

Couriel J. M. and Davies P. (1988) 'Costs and benefits of a community special care baby service', *British Medical Journal* **296**: 1043–6.

David J. T. (1986) 'Potential practical and legal problems with home administration of intravenous antibiotics for children with cystic fibrosis'. In Davis J. T. (ed.) *Cystic Fibrosis in Children. Practical and Legal Aspects of Intravenous Antibiotic Administration in the Home*, Amsterdam, Elsevier.

Department of Health (1993) *Children First – a Study of Hospital Services*, London, Audit Commission/HMSO.

Dowie J. (1993) 'Clinical decision analysis: background and introduction'. In Llewelyn H. and Hopkins A. (eds) *Analysing How we Reach Clinical Decisions*, London, Royal College of Physicians.

Einhorn H. J. (1980) 'Overconfidence in judgment. New directions for methodology of social and behavioral science' *New Directions for Methodology of Social and Behavioural Science* **4**: 1–16.

Ellis J. M. (1989) 'Let parents give the care: IV therapy at home in cystic fibrosis', *Professional Nurse* **4**(12): 589–92.

Elstein A. S. and Bordage G. (1988) 'Psychology of clinical reasoning'. In Dowie J. and Elstein A. (eds) *Professional Judgment: A Reader in Clinical Decision Making*, Cambridge, Cambridge University Press, pp. 109–29.

Emden C. (1991) 'Becoming a reflective practitioner'. In Gray G. and Pratt R. (eds) *Towards a Discipline of Nursing*, Edinburgh, Churchill Livingstone.

Eraker S. A. and Politser P. E. (1988) 'How decisions are reached: physician and patient'. In Dowie J. and Elstein A. (eds) *Professional Judgement: A Reader in Clinical Decision Making*, Cambridge, Cambridge University Press, pp. 379–94.

Fields A. I., Hardy Coble D., Pollock M. M. and Kaufman J. (1991) 'Outcome of home care for the technology-dependent children', *Pediatric Pulmonology* 11, 310 17.

Fischhoff B., Slovic P. and Lichtenstein S. (1980) 'Knowing what you want: measuring labile values'. In Wallsten T. S. (ed.) *Cognitive Processes in Choice and Decision Behaviour*, USA, Lawrence Erlbaum.

Gill S. (1993) 'Home administration of intravenous antibiotics to children with cystic fibrosis', *British Journal of Nursing* 2(15): 767–70.

Gordon M., Murphy C. P., Candee D. and Hiltunen E. (1994) 'Clinical judgement: an integrated model', *Advances in Nursing Science* 16(4): 55–70.

Hammond K. R., McClelland G. H. and Mumpower J. (1980) *Human Judgement and Decision Making*, New York, Hemisphere.

Harbison J. (1991) 'Clinical decision making in nursing', *Journal of Advanced Nursing* 16: 404–7.

Hill D. S. (1993) 'Co-ordinating a multi disciplinary discharge for the technology-dependent child based on parental needs', *Issues in Comprehensive Paediatric Nursing*, 16: 229–37.

Hogue E. (1992) 'Parental noncompliance in home care', *Pediatric Nursing* 18(6): 603–6.

Klug R. M. (1993) 'Clarifying roles and expectations in home care', *Pediatric Nursing* 19(4): 374–6.

Komaroff A. J. (1979) The variability and inaccuracy of medical data, *Proceedings of IEEE* 67: 1196–207.

Lantos J. D. and Kohrman A. F. (1992) 'Ethical aspects in pediatric home care', *Pediatrics* 89(5): 920–4.

Luker K. A. and Kendrick M. (1992) 'An exploratory study of the sources of influence on the clinical decisions of community nurses', *Journal of Advanced Nursing* 17: 457–66.

McCormack K. (1992) 'Areas of outcome research in nursing', *Journal of Professional Nursing* 8(2): 71.

Mehtar S. (1992) *Hospital Infection Control*, Oxford, Oxford Medical Publications.

Müller D. J., Harris P. J., Wattley L. A. and Taylor J. (1993) *Nursing Children: Psychology, Research and Practice* (2nd edn), London, Chapman & Hall.

Roberts J., While A. E. and Fitzpatrick J. M. (1993) 'Problem solving in nursing practice: application, process, skill acquisition and measurement', *Journal of Advanced Nursing* 18: 886–91.

Roberts J., While A. and Fitzpatrick J. (1995) 'Information-seeking strategies and data utilisation: theory and practice', *International Journal of Nursing Studies* 32(6): 601–11.

Schön D. A. (1991) *The Reflective Practitioner* (2nd edn), San Francisco, Jossey Bass.

Signorelli C., D'Alessandro D., Collina D. and Fara G. M. (1991) 'Prevalence survey of nosocomial infections in a paediatric hospital', *Journal of Hospital Infection* 18: 139–43.

Soden R. (1994) *Teaching Problem Solving in Vocational Education*, London, Routledge.

Sterling Y. (1990) 'Resource needs of mothers managing chronically ill infants at home', *Neonatal Work* 9(1): 55–9.
Tversky A. and Kahneman D. (1982) 'Judgment under uncertainties and biases'. In Kahneman D., Slovic P. and Tversky A. (eds) *Under Uncertainty: Heuristics and Biases*, Cambridge, Cambridge University Press.
Watson S. (1994) 'An exploratory study into a methodology for the examination of decision making by nurses in the clinical area', *Journal of Advanced Nursing* 20: 351–60.
While E. A. (1991) 'An evaluation of a paediatric home care scheme', *Journal of Advanced Nursing* 16: 1413–21.
Whyte D. A. (1994) *Family Nursing: The Case of Cystic Fibrosis*, Aldershot, Avebury.
Zarin D. A. and Pauker S. G. (1984) 'Decision analysis as a basis for medical decision making: the tree of Hippocrates', *Journal of Medicine and Philosophy* 9: 181–213.

Further reading

Bakken H. S. (1995) 'Nursing informatics: state of the science', *Journal of Advanced Nursing* 22: 1182–92.
Corcoran S. (1989) 'Decision analysis: a step-by-step guide for making clinical decisions', *Nursing and Health Care* Mar.: pp 149–54.
Edwards B. (1994) 'Telephone triage: how experienced nurses reach decisions', *Journal of Advanced Nursing* 19: 717–24.
Gray J. A. Muir (1997) *Evidence-based Health Care*, Edinburgh, Churchill Livingstone.
O'Neill E. and Dluhy N. M. (1997) 'A longitudinal framework for fostering critical thinking and diagnostic reasoning', *Journal of Advanced Nursing* 26: 825–32.
Thomas S., Wearing A. and Bennett M. (1991) *Clinical Decision Making for Nurses and Health Professionals*, New York, W. B. Saunders/Baillière Tindall.

18 Home sweet home – examining the interface between hospital and home

Margaret Lane and Sarah Baker

Introduction

Most episodes of hospitalisation will incorporate some form of discharge planning in the quest for enhancing clinical practice and facilitating satisfactory transitional care for the child and family. (Smith, 1995). The outcome of discharge planning can have irrevocable effects on both the child and family, so it is essential *to get it right*. There has been much discussion regarding how and when this should happen, but is it rhetoric or reality?

With the publication of the Children's Charter (DoH, 1996a), the child and family now have the opportunity to read for themselves what good practice should involve. The chapter draws on previous theories and current research to examine the art of discharge planning, identifying principles of good practice.

The increasing number of community paediatric teams enhances the opportunity for interfacing between the hospital and community. There has never been a better time to redefine the art of discharge planning, and this chapter utilises results from a recent survey to illustrate some of the issues and complexities for children and families. Discharge planning will be more successful if it is based upon the best evidence available. Muir Gray (1997, p. 9) states that:

> Evidence-based clinical practice is an approach to decision making in which the clinician uses the best evidence available, in consultation with the patient, to decide upon the option which suits the patient best.

Discharge planning, a key target in the Community Care Act 1990 and the *Patient's Charter* (DoH, 1992), can effectively reduce anxiety for the child and family, and may herald an early return to the child's normal home environment. It may be incorporated into the preparation for hospitalisation long before admission takes place, although is most likely to commence at some point following admission. It may be attended to at the point of discharge only, with little evidence of planning. It would appear that there are in the community a number of children who are discharged home with little apparent planning, leading to limitations of resources and frustrations for the child, family and practitioner alike (Thornes, 1993).

Reflective discussion highlights an apparent discrepancy in the implementation of discharge planning in some clinical situations. An exploratory study was undertaken to identify what planning for discharge actually occurs. The rationale for the study was related to the apparent dearth of evidence on what appeared to be an important aspect of clinical practice; the key aim of the work was to identify and develop good models for practice.

As with all sound examples of evidence-based practice, the study included a literature review. While much of the work appears to hail from North America, it was apparent that the issue of discharge planning was not new on the health agenda. However, robust literature on the subject was not available, and a lateral approach was required. Furthermore, an over-emphasis on some prominent pieces of work is evident but should be noted as a consequence of limitation rather than an over-reliance on some authors (Kongelbeck, 1990; McClowry, 1993; Thornes, 1993).

A historical exploration illustrated the relevance of planning for continuing care for children and their families. Other themes revolved around communication, teaching, psychological issues and discharge planning. A further aspect was concerned with co-ordination and continuing care associated with discharge planning.

Literature review

Historical overview and contextual position

From the time of the Report of the Platt Committee (Ministry of Health, 1959), it has been clear that the most essential place for children to be is within their family environment, unless there is just cause for this not to be the appropriate choice. It follows, therefore, that the key components of a hospital admission must of necessity encapsulate the notion of a speedy return to home. Within this notion rests the importance of discharge planning.

Similarly, the Report of the Committee on Child Health Services (DoH, 1976) advocated a child- and family-centred service. By their very nature, services must include a careful planning of the hospital experience from commencement to conclusion. Furthermore, the Court Report (DoH, 1976) recommended the expansion of the children's community service, emphasising the need to collaborate and co-ordinate between hospital and community services.

In spite of these key proposals, the Department of Health (DoH) found it necessary in 1989 to re-assert the requirement for health authorities and children's services to have in place up-to-date discharge procedures. The report made three key recommendations, advising districts to ensure that the units from which children's services were to be purchased had the following procedures in place:

- *a definition of the responsibility of all those involved*, including different hospital staff teams, primary care team members, ambulance and local authority staff and any voluntary organisations involved
- *timely communication* between the staff involved, which was to be clear in the arrangements for discharge
- an allocation of responsibility for discharge planning to a named person who could *ensure that all procedures had been completed* before a patient was discharged (DoH, 1989).

In 1991, the DoH published the report *The Welfare of Children and Young People in Hospital*. This reiterated previous reports associated with planning discharge for children and again highlighted the need for timely arrangements ensuring that discharge was not delayed. These recommendations evolved from the conclusion that little had changed since 1959 (DoH, 1991).

Thornes (1993) described the evidence gathered during the inquiry into caring for children in the health services and included information identifying the core principles of discharge planning for children. The report also highlighted that the implementation of the recommendations contained in the DoH circular of 1989 had been woefully slow. Evidence also illustrates that the complexity of care for children with multiple and technologically dependent needs is a growing element. It is thus even more critical that the discharge planning process is incorporated into the day-to-day care environment (Thornes, 1993). It is apparent from the literature review undertaken that this report is the most substantial piece of UK evidence available. It is for this reason that the work is extensively referred to in this chapter.

The Audit Commission (1993) advocated that hospitals should review the length of hospital admission and have in place guidelines for effective case management promoting early discharge, thereby enhancing the organisation of efficient discharge planning. Improved procedures are likely to result in a shorter hospital stay, and the Audit Commission recommended that a named discharge co-ordinator be allocated to each child. This equates with the DoH (1989) expectation alluded to earlier.

The 'Children's Charter' (DoH, 1996a) and Child Health in the Community (DoH, 1996b) continue the theme, emphasising the quest for timely and effective discharge planning in the desire to promote the delivery of acute secondary care outside the district general hospital.

In response to the issues raised through this historical exploration, the literature review continues utilising health studies related to the care of the child and their impact upon the discharge planning process. An exploration of the reports and evidence on discharge planning identified that much of the discussion is embedded within the hospital verses home debate. Consequently, the researchers were obliged to take a lateral stance when reviewing the literature in order that a holistic picture could be established.

At a time of rationalisation of scarce resources, it is imperative that each health care professional is able to justify the care package: it seems at times that monetary value is given greater emphasis than quality of service delivery. Studies have attempted to justify the cost-effectiveness of home versus hospital care (McClowry, 1993). Although the debate within the field continues, it is imperative that its focus is based upon the needs of the child and family (Kongelbeck, 1990). Indeed, the approach to health care in the USA appears to be so money orientated that there is no doubt, from the families' point of view, that discharge planning must commence as soon as the child is admitted to hospital if not before (Kongelbeck, 1990).

Furthermore, McClowry (1993) reports that earlier discharge may be associated with the high cost of hospitalisation. As a consequence, it could also be argued that time is limited for both assessment and planning of discharge information needed by individual families (Snowden and Kane, 1995).

McClowry (1993) explores the changing nature of admission to hospital for children. She suggests that those who are admitted are often sicker, may have conditions that would previously have proved fatal and may need a more sophisticated range of technological treatment. Repeated admission may be the norm, children with chronic conditions being hospitalised ten times more frequently. One of the key factors included by a number of authors on the provision of continuing care for children is that of information and communication (Bradford and Singer, 1991; Kanneh, 1991; Cox, 1992; Arthur, 1995). This aspect is pertinent to peruse here.

Communication

Communication is the key element for ensuring that discharge planning is facilitated effectively and is more than just the provision of
information. In a number of studies, families report general satisfaction
with the information they have received. However, Kanneh (1991), in a
study looking specifically at communication, found that there were a
number of areas in which communication was poor. She reports that
65 per cent of the parents in the study were dissatisfied with information about shared care. Similarly, 60 per cent were less than satisfied
with the explanations they were given about their child's condition.
Bradford and Singer (1991) also reported a high level of dissatisfaction
in a specialist liver unit, as many as 50 per cent of parents feeling that
they did not know enough about their child's prognosis.

It is evident from these studies that communication can be directly
associated with satisfaction, which can also be linked to compliance
and involvement in the continuing care of children (Morgan *et al.*,
1988). This is particularly important as the hospitalisation experience moves towards discharge home. The shifting locus for child
health care has an immediate impact upon the communication
networks required for successful transfer from secondary to primary
health care (Kelly *et al.*, 1995).

Thornes (1993) illustrates some of the difficulties of information
transfer experienced by families that can result in poor follow-up and
a less than adequate provision of support. For example, families
report conflicting advice, lack of information on general patterns of
care, uncertainty about prognosis and limited or non-existent plans
of care to assist in the decision-making process. Furthermore,
Thorne's study identifies the consequences of a lack of communication between secondary and primary health professionals in
supporting families caring for their child at home. This deficit could
be greatly minimised by the provision of written treatment plans
clearly articulating the care required (Thornes, 1993).

Arthur (1995) reinforces the notion that communication is a two-
way process and that it is pertinent to identify just what the child and
family want to know. It would appear that an unwanted consequence
of not addressing this basic question may be information overload,
further compounding a potentially stressful situation.

Cox (1992) described the development and use of an information
leaflet designed for the parents of children with burns and scalds.
The leaflet provided parents with information related to how the
burn affected their child's activities of living and how to manage
these following a thermal injury. The study (Cox, 1992) identified

that out of a possible 23 children, only five received the leaflet during the evaluation period. Cox suggested that one reason for the poor circulation was a lack of staff awareness of the need for written discharge information.

It would be pertinent to assume that the period approaching discharge is the most critical time for comprehensive information. Snowden and Kane (1995) report a dearth of literature examining the needs of parents following the discharge of their child. Kelly *et al.* (1991) identify increased parental satisfaction in the care-giving arena when their need for information is anticipated and met. Future research should focus on when and how discharge information is managed in order to ensure the best possible health outcome for the child.

It can thus be said that the information and communication process is fraught with complexity. This may mar attempts by health professionals to assist families to continue caring for their child from admission to hospital and beyond.

Teaching and discharge planning

Parental and child teaching is a key component of successful discharge planning and may be a significant factor in the reduction of anxiety. Kongelbeck (1990) identifies that the negotiation of teaching an aspect of health care must commence from the first day of admission. Parents and children alike differ significantly in what they feel comfortable taking on. Some parents have first to come to terms with the emotional aspects of assuming a health care role, alongside their acceptance of the child's diagnosis and prognosis (Kongelbeck, 1990). The impact of the diagnosis prevents some parents assuming a nursing role for their child until some time at or following discharge (Kongelbeck, 1990). The child, too, varies in the acceptance of the health problem, the understanding of the impact and the involvement in the self-care required.

It can fall to the continuing care team to provide the teaching input that facilitates the transition of care giving to the parents/primary carer or child. While (1992) looked at consumer views of health care, comparing hospital and home care. The study included 40 families and identified parental satisfaction with the support and guidance of the home care nurses. This reinforces the need for the health care professional to be competent in taking a significant nursing role as the care is transferred from one care setting to another. This may, however, change in light of the child's condition, with the knowledge that for some families, it is more therapeutic for them to be the parent than the nurse. In other cases, the family become expert practitioners, the health professional acting as the supporter and guide. Caution, however, is needed. While (1992) identified that some parents felt 'pressurised' into the health-giving arena. The health care professional must thus be proficient at recognising the needs of the family to opt in or out of direct nursing intervention as the situation dictates.

Coombes (1995) suggests that the provision of information to parents about their child's condition and treatment may assist them in gaining control and thus empower them. Similarly, parents' thirst for knowledge is evident (Darbyshire, 1994), and the parents of a sick child will be no different in their desire to acquire information. It is essential that the health care professionals working with the family are able to quench this thirst.

Much of the preceding literature explores information, teaching and collaboration between parents and health care professionals. However, as indicated, it is important to consider the child who is experiencing the heath problem. Botting (1995) suggests that children may have limited access to the health care services and information specifically geared towards them. This is another facet of the complexities involved in planning discharge and continuing care for children. Stacey (1991) confirms that the shift of environment from home to hospital can exert an unnecessary burden on the child and diminish coping. The area of teaching and collaboration should form the basis of a more extensive qualitative investigation.

Psychological issues and discharge planning

The major influence on the child and family when confronting a health problem is likely to be that associated with anxiety and the psychological impact of the experience. A wealth of literature exists exploring the psychological impact of a hospital admission for the child and family, and the necessity of preparation for that experience (Visintainer and Wolfer, 1975; Hayes and Knox, 1984; Glasper and Straddling, 1989; Ellerton and Merriam, 1994).

While seminal research by Jessner *et al.* (1952) and Vernon *et al.* (1966) focused on the pre-school child, Glazebrook and Sheard (1994) suggest that the school child is just as likely to experience increased stress when admitted to hospital. It is important to note that the effects of hospitalisation span the childhood years and increasing age does not necessarily diminish vulnerability. Similarly, it is essential to consider the impact upon parents as their level of anxiety affects the emotional security of the child (Snowden and Kane, 1995).

McClowry (1993) intimates that because of the psychological impact upon the child and family, hospitalisation should only be used when no alternative exists. Even if hospitalisation is required, prompt discharge home is advocated to minimise the adverse effects. Thus, a planned discharge co-ordinated from the point of admission, if not before, should be the cornerstone of the successful provision of care. As Snowden and Kane (1995) suggest, a critical element is the provision of information for parents to reduce the stress of the experience. However, these authors also state that there is minimal literature exploring parental need for information at the point when preparation for discharge occurs.

It is pleasing to note that the literature examining the needs of families when a child is discharged from hospital is growing. However, this demands a wider exploration to enhance the understanding of just what parents want. Kelly *et al.* (1991) indicate that parental satisfaction can be associated with anticipatory guidance and information giving. Unfortunately, as suggested earlier, economic constraint affecting the length of hospital stay limits the time for nursing staff to assess, plan and implement discharge procedures and may impact upon the quality of information given and internalised by parents. In addition, literature indicates that the stressful nature of a hospital environment can inhibit the learning of new information, compounding the effect even more (Morgan *et al.*, 1988; McClowry, 1993).

Continuing care for the child at home is not without its stresses too. Leonard *et al.* (1993) explore parental distress when caring for medically vulnerable children at home. This may involve a major change in family lifestyle, including a loss of jobs and a reduction of social activity as parents take on the caring role. The psychological cost is at times awesome.

Kongelbeck (1990) explores the sharing and teaching of information and health care in the discharge of a child with infantile spasms. She identifies the value of community health care professionals networking with the nurse specialist to promote a seamless transfer of care. Similarly, Whyte (1994), from her study of children and families with cystic fibrosis, has developed a systems approach to meet the needs of the family and child. Having identified each family member, she explores how each interacts within a larger social system to meet their individual health, social and psychological needs. It is thus appropriate to consider these approaches and their relevance in the discharge planning process.

Co-ordinating discharge and continuing care

Much of the preceding discussion has identified some of the factors associated with both admission to hospital and planning for continuing care. Another aspect critical to success is the collaboration and co-ordination of the care process. Without a concerted and planned approach between all parties, discharge home is likely to result in significant failure in one or more domains.

The complexity of hospitalisation for children is such that it is important to consider the experience in its entirety. Co-ordination and collaboration between the primary, secondary and tertiary health care services is essential (Jennings, 1994). This is particularly critical for children with chronic conditions, whose families are encouraged to contribute extensively to meeting their child's care needs. Hill (1993) intimates that parents can experience overload with teaching yet are fearful of admitting that they do not understand everything placed in front of them. The key role of the nurse will be to have insight into the individual child and family's ability to cope with the information presented to them at any point during the admission period.

Thornes (1993) suggests that the best person to organise discharge is the named nurse, although official responsibility will lie with the consultant. It is often the nurse who seeks out information relating to the availability of appropriate help. Furthermore, the nurse will also be in a position to consider the competence and confidence of the parent's nursing skills. However, as While (1992) has noted, it can be potentially damaging to the parents' confidence and self-esteem to expect them to 'acknowledge their weaknesses'. The most effective handover will be between the nurse who has been caring for a child, the carer and child, and the nurse who will be continuing that care.

Thornes (1993) explores the interface between admission and discharge. While the interface at admission may be easy to determine, it is less well defined at the time of potential discharge. The process from the primary to the secondary level of health care can follow a readily auditable pathway, but the reverse is not necessarily evident once discharge home is proposed. Shorter and more focused hospitalisation episodes may mean that a child continues to require nursing intervention once discharged. Therefore, a secondary level of care can still be required in the primary care setting.

A review of the literature has identified four key areas that impact on the success of the discharge planning process. First, all those involved need to be fully conversant with the purpose of discharge planning and each individual's role within the process. Second, communication in all its guises is essential between all the participants. Third, the needs of children and their families before, during and after discharge must be identified and addressed. Finally, a greater recognition and acknowledgement of the psychological impact of ill-health, hospitalisation and follow-on care for the child and family is required if the discharge planning process is to be evaluated as being successful.

The review identifies a dearth of literature from the UK, and there are inherent difficulties in applying US nursing practices to our own. Consequently, it has been necessary to rely heavily on the most substantial piece of work available (Thornes, 1993). The scarcity of literature has precluded an examination of existing definitions and models of good practice and has confirmed the need to study the discharge planning process at a time when the UK government is creating a primary care-led National Health Service (NHS) and reducing the number of hospital beds.

Methodology

The role of research in nursing is aimed at confirming or refuting ideas (Morse and Field, 1996), discovering new knowledge and the development of theory for the advancement of nursing practice. Morse and Field (1996, p. 2) suggest that qualitative research is aimed at the exploration of areas in which 'relatively little is known'. One supposes that much is known about the discharge planning process, yet there docs appear to be a theory–practice gap. The use of a questionnaire provided the researchers with the opportunity to quantify the occurrence phenomena and at the same time gain descriptions of nursing behaviour. Through the exploration of previous research on discharge planning, the researchers were able to formulate a questionnaire from which to develop a greater understanding of current practice and generate a theoretical framework to advance nursing practice.

Aims and objectives

The aim of the study of discharge planning was:

- To examine the contribution that discharge planning makes to the enhancement of nursing care for the sick child and family, identifying the roles and responsibilities of health care professionals in the process.

The objectives were to:

- critically examine communication networks for achieving successful discharge planning
- explore current research findings illustrating the significance of discharge planning in meeting the holistic health care needs of the child and family
- identify models of discharge planning, evaluating their effectiveness.

Methodological approaches

The design utilised a postal questionnaire that focused on the key aspects of the discharge planning process as reflected in the literature. McGibbon (1997) has provided some insight into the development of the questionnaire, and it is important to consider some of the potential pitfalls when developing the tool. McGibbon highlights the necessity of having a clear definition of the issue being investigated; this provides essential guidance for questionnaire development. Questions were developed using statistically proven approaches (McGibbon, 1997) in an attempt to enhance reliability and validity.

The aim in formulating questions is to ensure that they are clear and unambiguous. Clarity of the question, minimising ambiguity, is essential in order to avoid various interpretations and hence inaccurate data collection (Polit and Hungler, 1983). The questionnaire design utilised this approach. Simple phrasing, succinctly expressed, which does not lead the respondent, engenders successful completion. However, an invitation to develop responses through additional comments will enhance the potential richness of the data collected. The purpose of this exploratory study was to test this out with a pertinent population. The questions formulated evolved from both the literature and the desire to explore the issues in a more scientific way. It also included elements from reflection on practice.

The questionnaire responses will be referred to in the discussion (see Appendix 18.1).

Sample

While it may have been pertinent to target all children's units, the study was seen as a pilot study to test the reliability and validity of the questionnaire. The geographical location selected was within the Thames region of the UK. With the above point in mind, 74 children's wards and units were targeted. Community children's nursing teams were also included and contributed to the study sample. The questionnaire was sent to a named senior practitioner in each location used.

Ethical consideration

Ethical consideration was given to the work. Following discussion with one of the ethical committees, it was agreed that as the views of children or carers were not being sought, ethical approval was not required at this point. However, any subsequent work would follow the recommended ethical guidelines.

Data analysis

An analysis of the data was undertaken by the researchers individually and subsequently independently by an administrator.

The response rate was 53 per cent, with 39 questionnaires returned. This is not inconsistent with response rates of questionnaire approaches and exceeds expectations of the response rate for postal surveys (Waltz *et al.*, 1991).

A closer examination of the results indicated that the responses came from paediatric wards in district general hospitals (DGHs; $n = 16$), tertiary units in specialist hospitals ($n = 13$) and community children's nursing teams ($n = 10$). A further breakdown of the responses was attempted with regard to the patient population, but the results proved somewhat inconclusive as many units indicated that they fell into more than one of the categories listed in the questionnaire (see Appendix 18.1, q.1b).

A second question asked about the procedures and models used for planning discharge. It was apparent from the responses that many sites did not utilise any form of planning or model. While most indicated their awareness of the importance of a planned approach, the questionnaire stimulated many to question their practice on this aspect. This provided the researchers with justification for the study.

Main findings and discussion of results

The literature review will be linked to some of the data, illustrating key issues from the studies and reports in order to assess how the data compare with the literature. As a consequence of limited research on the topic of discharge planning, it has been necessary to take a more lateral and liberal perspective with the associated material. The results will concentrate on the substantive evidence extracted from the responses.

A historical reflection illustrated the context within which the literature evolved. Communication and teaching are explored as key elements in discharge planning. The psychological component is reviewed and linked to co-ordination and continuing care issues for children and their families. In conclusion, the authors reflect on the study and make recommendations for future work.

An examination of the data will illustrate the complexities of the planning process and factors that impinge upon family satisfaction. The discussion will be linked to the questionnaire with the responses used in order to illustrate common practice within the population used.

A number of responses can be compared with the recommendations outlined in the proposals made by the DoH (1989).

First, it was recommended that:

There is a definition of the responsibility of all those involved.

The questionnaire asked respondents to state who prepares children and families for discharge. A range of people are involved, including the named nurse, the doctor, the dietician, the pharmacist and the community outreach team, reflecting some of the DoH groups of health care professionals detailed in the 1989 report. However, a less comprehensive list was detailed in the sample, although the actual question may not have elicited the information needed for valid comparison. It is probable that others thought to have a stake in the discharge process did not appear relevant for respondents to detail. It is, however, important that key personnel are consulted to provide continuing care as a failure to do so could result in difficulties in practice. There were other personnel detailed in the sample responses, demonstrating the range of associated people who can be involved in the process.

The second element in the DoH (1989) paper states that:

There is a need for timely communication between the staff involved, which is clear in the arrangements for discharge. (DoH, 1989).

The survey detailed the time at which discharge planning was commenced and illustrates that this was, for the most part, very early in the admission process. In the group responding from the

DGHs, 75 per cent recorded this as being between zero and 12 hours. Approximately 50 per cent of those from tertiary units recorded 0–12 hours, the remaining responses not stipulating a time period. Those responding from community practice did not complete this section informatively.

The question to pose, however, is whether this continues for the duration of the admission or whether it is only refocused as the child's discharge draws near. Further investigation will elicit whether a systematic approach was used in practice.

The third and final recommendation from the DoH (1989) states that:

There should be allocation of responsibility for discharge planning to a named person who can ensure that all procedures have been completed before a patient is discharged.

The study illustrated that there was in most cases the probability of a named nurse or primary nurse being a key player in the process. Overall, the named or primary nurse was identified by 54 per cent of the DGH group, although the medical team was detailed in 36 per cent of responses. Similar evidence was demonstrated in the tertiary and community sample group, but this was less easy to quantify as a percentage.

Respondents were asked to outline the factors influencing the commencement of discharge planning, and some interesting data were revealed (Figure 18.1).

It is clear that the nature of the admission will influence the planning process, and evidence from the tertiary units illustrated a co-ordinated approach. Similarly, in some day units, planning is carefully linked to the pre-admission period, and all aspects of continuing care are considered in the process.

Respondents from the questionnaire detailed the ways in which information was presented to the family: 51 per cent presented verbal information, 46 per cent written information and 3 per cent other methods, including, for example, videos (Appendix 18.1, q. 8).

Respondents sent examples of their discharge information. These included hospital generated leaflets on, for example:

- post-operative care at home for a child with grommets
- the care of sutures
- the application of plaster of Paris
- care of the child with a temperature
- chest physiotherapy for the child with asthma.

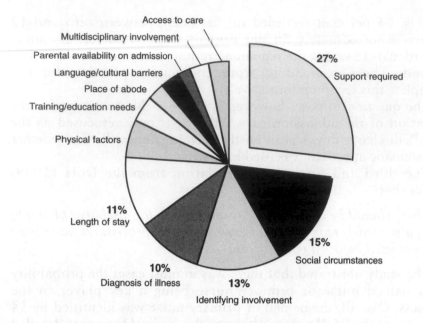

Figure 18.1   Factors influencing the
commencement of discharge planning

Some units utilised information sheets from journals, such as on diar-
rhoea and vomiting, on immunisation, specifically designed to copy
for families.

It is clear from the literature that communication is crucial for
families, but none of it will be effective if the written leaflets and
packages available are not used by those people in the best position
to give them out. Further work should be geared toward this element
to assess whether these items were used constructively – or not, as
Cox (1992) found in her study.

In the study undertaken, the personnel in the primary health care
team were identified. Respondents stated those likely to be contacted
with regard to discharge and the time frame for this to occur. Many
respondents identified a number of key people who would be
involved. The health visitor was named by 95 per cent, the GP by 90
per cent and the school nurse by 50 per cent; 40 per cent identified
others but did not specify who. This group of personnel needs to be
more clearly defined in future research (Appendix 18.1, q. 9 and 10).

Similarly, links with the children's community teams were detailed,
illustrating the establishment of a comprehensive link in 75 per cent
of respondents. It is, however, important to note that this may be

more to do with the sample used in the study and the fact that 47 per cent did not respond. The results may not thus be truly representative and should be viewed with caution.

A consideration of the needs of families from culturally diverse populations was included, but the responses returned did not provide significant information to analyse for this aspect. Many of those responding did not feel that this was a particular issue for them, which was interesting as the communities targeted certainly included many inner-city locations, which would include significant populations of these families. This is an important aspect to develop and crucial to ask families with regard to assessing individual need. It is, however, outside the scope of this initial study, although it will be more specifically developed in any further research.

As Thornes (1993) reports, the use of telephone, letter or personal communication to facilitate handover is essential. In some complex cases, a liaison discharge officer may be involved. However, evidence that parents experience difficulty in obtaining the equipment and supplies required for continuing care was not confirmed in the study, even though the issue was included. Thornes indicated that this was more likely to occur following discharge from tertiary centres (Thornes, 1993). An examination of the responses from tertiary centres included in the questionnaire indicates that planning meetings and the co-ordination of the discharge are likely to be part of the process for children with complex care needs. Indeed, one respondent identified that planning discussions were held for all children at a twice-weekly psychosocial meeting.

This study did not seek the views of the family, but it is imperative that parental concerns are identified and incorporated into the discharge planning to ensure that the child's home care is successful. These concerns may at times not be articulated or realised until the family are within their own environment providing care and have become aware of gaps in their knowledge (Hill, 1993). The opportunity for the child and family to reassess, with a children's community nurse, the child's care needs, alongside a recognition of any knowledge deficit, is an essential part of the discharge planning process. This is particularly important as the hospitalisation experience moves towards discharge home.

In the questionnaire, the authors asked respondents to identify the ways in which parents and families were involved in the discharge planning process (Appendix 18.1, q. 20). The evidence detailed indicated that discussions and meetings were utilised, along with verbal advice. Surveys and information sheets were detailed as a source, and indicators were given to support the involvement of parents and families in the whole process. It would be pertinent to establish from the parents' point of view whether this was indeed the case; anecdotal evidence suggests otherwise.

Within the triad of doctor, parent and child, the child is often afforded minimal status. He may be excluded, therefore, from receiving relevant information about his health care needs (Mayall, 1995). Just like parents, children are more compliant if they have a better understanding of their own health care needs and treatment patterns (Alderson, 1990). Sadly, old habits die hard, and the child's voice is often unheard or dismissed. This area, however, was not explored in the survey. Subsequent research on discharge planning must include the child's perspective.

At each point of the care cycle, discharge planning must be considered and re-affirmed. Families may need to develop an insight into the role of the primary health care team and whom to approach for advice, support, information or resources at any given point. It may be appropriate to assign a key person in order to limit families' confusion and anxiety (Thornes, 1993). This is especially important where care management is shared across a range of health care professionals. It was anticipated that models of good practice would emerge from the data collected from the questionnaire, but responses to this question were singularly absent or negative. Further research on this topic should consider this aspect.

Similarly, an evaluation and audit of the discharge planning process is important, and the quest for some supporting evidence was sadly lacking, although, as mentioned earlier, respondents did comment that it had raised their awareness of the relevance of this with regard to good practice.

Conclusions and recommendations for clinical practice

A number of issues have so far been identified and explored, illustrating the complexities of the discharge planning process. It is clear that ineffective communication and co-ordination lead to dissatisfaction. It is imperative to allocate responsibility for discharge planning to a named nurse. The named nurse must, by the very nature of the role, be cognisant of the multifaceted components of discharge planning. The principles detailed in Thornes' (1993) study identify the knowledge and skills essential for the implementation of the planning process. Furthermore, Siarkowski-Amer and Pidgeon (1991) suggest that documentation may be the weak link in the discharge planning process and state that efficiency in documentation may equate with a higher standard of care. Indeed, the data from the survey that is referred to in this chapter highlight the lack of use of a theory or model for discharge planning in those responding to the questionnaire, another area warranting more comprehensive evaluation.

It is evident from the literature that a discharge plan is the key element for facilitating effective and efficient transfer from secondary to primary care. The interface between all partners in the continuing care process needs to be clearly identified, the communication network being fitted together rather like a jigsaw (Figure 18.2). The child is the central core of the puzzle, and it is essential that full co-operation be facilitated between a number of other key players in the process, who, how and what being dictated by individual need and circumstance. What is very clear from the literature and from the information gathered in the study is that many of the gaps in service provision may be associated with the loss of an important piece of the picture. Furthermore, completion of the puzzle may at times be compromised by a lack of vision of the totality of the interfaces needed.

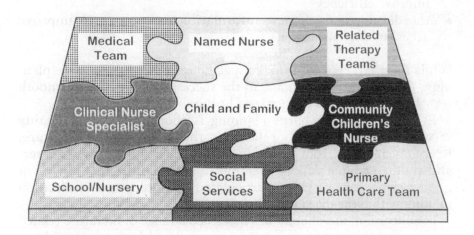

Figure 18.2   A co-ordinated approach to discharge planning

Clearly, the literature explored identifies the issues associated with planning continuing care for children and their families. Effective discharge planning is dependent upon an explicit consideration of all its complexities. The literature, however, also indicates that the process is in reality often fragmented, disjointed and poorly managed. Much of the material is outdated or not based on UK health care practice; this needs addressing.

In a recent publication, the then Secretary of State for Health of the UK (DoH, 1996b) identified four key principles on which to base health care practice across the political spectrum. These focused on the NHS being universal in its reach, of high quality, available on the basis of clinical need and responsive. While these principles belong to a previous government's White Paper, they undoubtedly remain relevant within the field of discharge planning. However, the new White Paper, *The New NHS: Modern, Dependable* (DoH, 1997), re-affirms the historical principles of the NHS.

The current UK government's vision for driving change within the NHS focuses on quality and efficiency. Key targets included in an evidence-based framework are:

- the promotion of clinical cost-effectiveness through clinical excellence
- the development of primary care groups to promote the delivery of services
- the devolution of responsibility to primary care groups in order to improve efficiency
- the development of new information technology to improve access to documentation.

While these targets do not make specific reference to discharge planning, they are clearly germane to the success of a timely and smooth transition at the interface between hospital and home.

Evidence-based discharge planning is about providing a quality service and is not simply related to the delivery of health care. Recommendations from the study include seeking the views of carers and children from a wider geographical area in order that models of good practice can be clearly articulated and utilised in all decision making within the discharge planning arena.

In conclusion, this chapter has described a range of literature related to examining the interface between hospital and home, and evidence from the exploratory study has been used to illustrate practice within a small geographical location in the South of England. The objectives of the study have been addressed through a number of areas. In particular, the research illustrates the critical nature of communication and information for families. It is clear that the ability to meet the holistic health care needs of the child is dependent upon collaboration and co-ordination between all parties. Recommendations for further enquiry have been made as the chapter has evolved. It is necessary to set this work within the wider context of international health care, comparing practice across continents in order to ensure that the best evidence is used to inform decision making for the sick child and his or her family.

Appendix 18.1

Discharge planning

Examining the interface between hospital and home

Please ✓ the relevant box below

1. Please identify the type of unit you are working on:

    (a)   District general hospital ☐   (b)   Medical   ☐

          Tertiary hospital   ☐   Surgical   ☐

          Community   ☐   Day care   ☐

          Other (please state)   ☐   Other (please state) ☐

2. Within your Unit, is there a formalised discharge planning procedure?

                              Yes ☐   No ☐

    Comments:

3. Identify the stage in the child's admission when discharge planning commences:

                      Within 0–12 hours from admission   ☐

                      Within 12–24 hours from admission   ☐

                      Within 24–48 hours from admission   ☐

                              Other (please state)   ☐

    Comments:

4. Outline the factors influencing the commencement of discharge planning:

5. Who instigates discharge planning?

    Primary nurse   ☐   Ward sister/Charge nurse   ☐

    Named nurse   ☐   Doctor: SHO/registrar/consultant ☐

                                    Other (please specify below)   ☐

6. Who co-ordinates the following elements?

    ● Transport   ● Dressings
    ● Pharmacological products   ● Equipment

7.   Who prepares the child and family for discharge? (Please list all personnel involved):

8.   In what ways is information presented to the family?

Verbal	☐
Written	☐
Other (please specify below)	☐

Comments:

(NOTE: We would welcome copies of discharge information used in your Unit)

9.   At what stage in the discharge planning process is the Primary Health Care Team (PHCT) informed of the child's discharge?

10.   Which personnel would be contacted?

Health visitor	☐	GP	☐
School nurse	☐	Other (please specify below)	☐

11.   Do you have links with a Children's Community Team (CCT)?

Yes ☐   No ☐

12.   At what stage are they informed of the child's discharge?

13.   For which group of children are discharge planning meetings held?

14.   Identify the personnel involved in the meetings:

15.   How is information disseminated to PHCT/CCT?

16. What discharge planning facilities exist for families from ethnic minority backgrounds?

Interpreters ☐   Advocates ☐

Written information ☐   Family health workers ☐

Videos ☐   Other (please state) ☐

Comments:

17. Can you outline the ways in which you would like to enhance your discharge process?

18. How is the discharge planning process evaluated/audited?

19. Does your discharge planning process use a specific theory/model?

Yes ☐   No ☐

Please outline:

20. Identify the ways in which parents/families are involved in the discharge planning process.

Thank you for your time in completing this questionnaire. A brief synopsis of our findings can be obtained if desired.

344 *Margaret Lane and Sarah Baker*

References

Alderson P. (1990) *Choosing for Children: Parents Consent to Surgery*, Oxford, Oxford University Press.

Arthur V. (1995) 'Written patient information: a review of the literature', *Journal of Advanced Nursing* 21: 1081–6.

Audit Commission (1993) *Children First: A Study of Hospital Services*, HMSO.

Botting B. (1995) *The Health of our Children*, OPCS.

Bradford R. and Singer J. (1991) 'Support and information for parents', *Paediatric Nursing* May: 18–20.

Coombes R. (1995) 'From parent to expert', *Child Health* 2(6): 237–40.

Cox B. (1992) 'Research into practice', *Paediatric Nursing* 4(10): 24–6.

Darbyshire P. (1994) *Living with a Sick Child in Hospital*, London, Chapman & Hall.

Department of Health (1976) *Fit for the Future*, Report of the Committee on Child Health Services (Court Report), London, HMSO.

Department of Health (1989) *Discharge of Patients from Hospital*. HC(89)5, London, DoH.

Department of Health (1991) *The Welfare of Children and Young People in Hospital*, London, HMSO.

Department of Health (1992) *The Patient's Charter*, London, HMSO.

Department of Health (1996a) *The Patient's Charter: Services for Children and Young People*, London, HMSO.

Department of Health (1996b) *Child Health in the Community*, NHS Executive, London, HMSO.

Department of Health (1997) *The New NHS: Modern, Dependable*, London, Stationery Office.

Ellerton M. and Merriam C. (1994) 'Preparing children and families psychologically for day surgery: an evaluation', *Journal of Advanced Nursing* 19(6): 1057–62.

Glasper E. and Straddling P. (1989) 'Preparing children for admission', *Paediatric Nursing* 1(5): 18–20.

Glazebrook C. and Sheard C. (1994) 'A prospective study of factors associated with delayed discharge in school-aged children undergoing ward based minor surgery', *International Journal of Nursing Studies* 31(6): 487–97.

Gray J. Muir (1997) *Evidence-based Healthcare. How To Make Policy and Management Decisions*, London, Churchill Livingstone.

Hayes V. E. and Knox J. E. (1984) 'The experience of stress in parents of children hospitalised with long-term disability', *Journal of Advanced Nursing* 9(2): 333–43.

Hill D. (1993) 'Coordinating a multidisciplinary discharge for the technology-dependent child based on parental needs', *Issues in Comprehensive Pediatric Nursing* 16: 229–37.

Jennings P. (1994) 'Learning through experience: an evaluation of "hospital at home"', *Journal of Advanced Nursing* 19: 905–11.

Jessner L., Blom X., Gaston E. and Waldfogel S. (1952) 'Emotional implications of tonsilectomy and adenoidectomy on children'. In Eissler R. S. (ed.)

Psycho-analytic Study of the Child, New York, International Universities Press.

Kanneh A. (1991) 'Communicating with care', *Paediatric Nursing* 3(3): 24–7.

Kelly M., Alexander C. and Morris N. (1991) 'Maternal satisfaction with primary care for children with selected chronic conditions', *Journal of Community Health* 16: 213–24.

Kelly P., Taylor C. and Tatman M. (1995) 'Hospital outreach or community nursing?', *Paediatric Home Care and Child Health* 2(4): 160–3.

Kongelbeck S. (1990) 'Discharge planning for the child with infantile spasms', *Journal of Neuroscience Nursing* 22(4): 238–44.

Leonard B., Brust J. and Nelson R. (1993) 'Parental distress: caring for medically fragile children at home', *Journal of Pediatric Nursing* 8(1): 22–30.

McClowry S. (1993) 'Pediatric nursing psycho-social care: a vision beyond hospitalisation', *Pediatric Nursing* 19(2): 146–8.

McGibbon G. (1997) 'How to avoid the pitfalls of questionnaire design', *Nursing Times* 93(19): 49–51.

Mayall B. (1995) 'The changing context of childhood: children's perspectives on health care resources including services'. In Botting B. (ed.) *The Health of our Children*, OPCS.

Ministry of Health (1959) *The Welfare of Children in Hospital*, Report of the Platt Committee, London, HMSO.

Morgan M., Calnan M. and Manning N. (1988) *Sociological Approaches to Health and Medicine*, London, Routledge.

Morse J. and Field P. (1996) *Nursing Research. The Application of Qualitative Approaches*, London, Chapman & Hall.

Polit D. and Hungler B. (1983) *Nursing Research Principles and Methods*, Philadelphia, J.B. Lippincott.

Siarkowski-Amer K. and Pidgeon V. (1991) 'Documentation of discharge teaching before and after use of a discharge teaching tool', *Journal of Pediatric Nursing* 6(5): 296–301.

Smith F. (1995) *Children's Nursing in Practice*, London, Blackwell.

Snowden A. and Kane D. (1995) 'Parental needs following the discharge of a hospitalised child', *Pediatric Nursing* 21(5): 425–8.

Stacey M. (1991) *The Sociology of Health and Healing*, London, Routledge.

Stationery Office (1996) *National Health Service: A Service with Ambition*.

Thornes R. (1993) *Bridging the Gaps,* London, Action for Sick Children.

Vernon D., Shulman J. and Foley J. (1966) 'Changes in children's behaviour after hospitalisation', *American Journal of Diseases in Childhood* 111: 581–93.

Visintainer M. and Wolfer J. (1975) 'Psychological preparation for surgical patients: the effect on children and parents stress responses and adjustments', *Pediatrics* 11(56): 187–202.

Waltz C., Strickland O. and Lenz E. (1991) *Measurement in Nursing Research*, Philadelphia, F.A. Davis.

While A. (1992) 'Consumer views of health care: a comparison of hospital and home care', *Child: Care, Health and Development* 18: 107–16.

Whyte D. A. (1994) *Family Nursing: The Case for Cystic Fibrosis*, Aldershot, Avebury.

19 *Intravenous antibiotics at home: a parents' perspective*

Claire Ruskin

Introduction

Family-centred care and parental participation in care are essential aspects of paediatric nursing and are crucial in the care of the child with a chronic illness. It is, therefore, logical that the insights and experiences of parents are used as a source of evidence for our practice.

This chapter focuses on the experience of parents of children with cystic fibrosis (CF) who administer intravenous (IV) antibiotics to their child at home. Information was obtained through informal interviews undertaken with a small group of parents. A literature review is followed by a presentation of findings, which are discussed in relation to current literature. Common themes emerged that related to the parents' initial experiences and their perceptions of normality and control and of the advantages offered by home-based IV therapy. The chapter uses these findings to raise awareness of the education and support required by parents who administer IV therapy to their children. Recommendations for practice based on the findings are described; these include parent-to-parent support and a need for 24-hour support for parents who engage in this scheme.

At the hospital used in this study, parents are offered the opportunity to administer IV antibiotics at home by the CF liaison nurses. The selection of parents for whom this may be appropriate is based on a careful assessment made by the multidisciplinary team. Parents are required to show an understanding of the procedure involved and be deemed competent to undertake this role in the home. The home environment itself must be conducive to carrying out the procedure, providing a clean and safe area for the preparation of the antibiotics. Parents are initially trained on the ward under supervision; then, when the parents feel confident, they can then carry out the procedure at home with support. The CF liaison nurse supervises the initial home administration, and further visits are made, allowing for continuous assessment and support. The frequency of visits is dependent upon individual requirements.

346

Experience as an undergraduate student had generated a special interest in the care of children with CF and led to an awareness that few studies existed that directly explored parental perceptions of caring for a chronically ill child. The aim of the study was thus to investigate the feelings and perceptions of parents in their experience of administering IV antibiotics to their child within their home environment.

Literature review

The majority of the literature available that relates to the home-based administration of IV antibiotics is concerned with the description of procedures and guidelines for care. There appears to be a paucity of research examining this aspect of care, a point also identified by Gill (1993), Coyne (1995) and Neill (1996). There is, however, a wealth of literature and policy documents that endorse home-based care. These illuminate the philosophy that underpins the home-based administration of IV antibiotics and the subsequent evolution of parental roles.

There has been a growing shift from the provision of hospital-based care towards the delivery of home-based care within paediatric nursing. Formal paediatric home care schemes are evolving and becoming more widely accepted. This movement has been influenced by the high cost of inpatient care, the development of new techniques that make sophisticated home care feasible, patient preference and a belief in the greater benefits of home nursing (Lessing and Tatman, 1991).

Based on their experience of working at the Regional Paediatric CF Unit in Leeds, McLaughlin and Hasse (1994) assert that home care is an essential component of quality care. Their belief is that a home service gives optimum treatment with minimum disruption to the family but must be accompanied by a strong home support system and comprehensive monitoring.

Kendrick (1993) endorses that home care is congruent with normal family life and focuses on the importance of teaching parents to assume new roles. Stephenson (1989) describes a scheme for teaching parents to undertake IV therapy for children with CF. The key components are set criteria that parents must meet prior to training.

Cluroe (1989) discusses the benefits of home care and in her article portrays the experience and feelings of a small number of parents. Dialogue from the parents is included in the text, thus giving a more descriptive insight into their experience of home care. The parents mentioned in Cluroe's paper appeared to find home care a positive experience and acknowledged the benefits for the child in terms of reduced admission to hospital.

Other studies have also indicated the benefits of home care (Donati *et al.*, 1987; Gilbert *et al.*, 1988; van Aalderen *et al.*, 1995). Advantages highlighted include a reduction in the number of hospital admission days, an increased independence from hospital and a decreased risk of cross-infection (van Aalderen *et al.*, 1995).

Whyte (1992) carried out a longitudinal ethnographic study over 5 years into the professional support of the family with CF cared for at home, the primary aim of the research being to gain a deeper understanding of the feelings, experiences and interactions of parents. Whyte describes the chronic burden of care that can precipitate family crises, interaction patterns and the coping responses of families. A study over such a timescale can uncover a great deal of information regarding the experience of parents, and such detail can give a more accurate account of problems that can occur and how families cope.

Nuttall and Nicholes (1992) conducted 32 semi-structured interviews (40 questions) with the purpose of describing the concerns of mothers and of adolescents with CF regarding hospital and home care. The authors found that, in terms of health care management at home (including intravenous therapy), a major concern expressed by 50 per cent of the mothers related to the time constraints in the morning of giving treatment prior to school. Fifty eight per cent of mothers also mentioned that the major burden for the child's care fell on them.

These latter studies highlight that there are disadvantages of home care that may often be overlooked or minimised.

Methodology

Design

The methodological perspective pertaining to this small study is qualitative in nature as the study seeks to investigate the experiences and perceptions of parents. On the topic of the use of qualitative research, Streubert and Carpenter (1995) assert that although qualitative research is a relatively newly accepted form of creating nursing knowledge, it is still essential that nurses continue to advance nursing knowledge. Qualitative studies can help professionals to become sensitised to the viewpoint of a family through an accurate and full description of their experiences (Deatrick *et al.*, 1993). The use of this method offers the possibility of permitting families to set and follow their own agenda in terms of which topics are explored rather than confining them to an agenda set by the preconceptions either of the researcher or based on existing literature.

Setting

The study was carried out in the field; interviews took place in the CF clinic at a local children's hospital. This provided what was for these parents a familiar and natural environment to discuss the care of their child.

Sample

Qualitative research typically focuses on relatively small samples selected purposefully; the aim is to illuminate the area of study, and there is greater concern for information richness than for representativeness (Morse, 1991). The sample was chosen from a target population of attendants of the CF clinic on a random day.

Eligibility criteria for selection were that the participants must have had at least one experience of administering IV antibiotics to their child. Saturation of the data was achieved with six participants, this being the point at which the researcher believes that he or she is not hearing anything new and any subsequent interviews will not reveal any new information (Morse, 1991).

Informed consent

At the start of the clinic, the CF liaison nurse issued parents with a letter from the researcher explaining the nature of the study. Any interested parents were subsequently introduced to the researcher, and a further explanation of the study was given, highlighting confidentiality and anonymity, before the parents agreed to talk about their experiences. Assurance was given that the parents could withdraw from the study at any time. In retrospect, a letter given in advance would have given parents more time to consider participation, and written consent would be obtained.

Subjects

Of the six subjects interviewed (one father and five mothers), all had a variety of experiences and had been giving IV antibiotics at home for varying lengths of time. The range of experience was from 4 weeks to 8 years, and the number of times that antibiotics had been administered varied accordingly.

Data collection and analysis

Tape-recorded semi-structured interviews were used as the method of data collection. The aim of the interview was to allow the parents to describe their own experiences in their own way at their own pace, thus resembling normal conversation. The benefits of such a technique have previously been noted (Mishler, 1991; Jerrett, 1994; Darbyshire, 1995; Callery and Luker, 1996).

Discourse analysis took place employing manifest analysis, whereby explicit words, terms and phrases were identified (Masterson, 1998). This was used in conjunction with a modification of Spiegelberg's 1975 Descriptive Phenomenology model, as cited in Streubert and Carpenter (1995). The three steps of the model – intuiting, analysing and describing – were followed. Content analysis occurred during the interview while listening to the descriptions and during the transcription phase. Once transcribed, the recorded tapes were then played back and compared with the script on disk to improve accuracy, thus allowing for analysis to take place throughout the study. The major stage of analysis occurred while re-reading the transcripts, highlighting common themes and experiences, identifying any significant statements and therefore grouping phenomena.

Findings

In order to provide an element for discussion, details of selected themes will be described. The following themes were selected on the basis that they would give an insight into the common experiences of parents: initial experiences, normality and control, and training and support. To appreciate the relevance of the study regarding current practice, the findings will be discussed in relation to existing research and literature.

Initial experiences

When asked about their initial experiences, parents described numerous feelings, the predominant one being that of nervousness. As one parent expressed it:

> I was worried, frightened actually, because you know I might make a mess... I thought I was never going to be able to do this but it were all right.

Another parent held a similar view of her first experiences:

> I mean it is all right just doing it in hospital while there is somebody there saying no don't do that; it was a bit nerve wracking at first but you, er, get used to it.

Parents are understandably worried about carrying out the procedure despite the training and assessment of their capabilities. Parents initially express doubt and lack faith in their abilities, as one mother stated:

> it is frightening because, all said and done, you are just a parent.

This indicates that parents do need support and encouragement in terms of their capacity to participate in their child's care. Not only are parents taking on an extended role, but they must also come to terms with the fact that they may, as a consequence of their actions, potentially harm their child. This additional concern was expressed by all but one of the parents.

Current literature supports the initial experiences expressed by parents in this small study. Stephenson (1989) describes a home care scheme and states that all parents find the first day nerve-wracking, quoting one parent's reaction: 'Can I really cope on my own?' Stephenson (1989) answers 'yes', although she does go on to say that even some experienced parents still find home therapy quite stressful. Despite this finding, such parents still find it preferable to hospital admission. Catchpole (1989), in describing a home care scheme, stated that families were capable of management at home and found that their confidence grew in time.

Carrying out clinical skills is obviously daunting at first for parents, but as the literature indicates, they quickly become familiar with the procedures. Donati *et al.* (1987) found that in their research, observed skill and confidence were demonstrated by most patients and families after 3–5 days of managing home treatment.

Normality and control

Despite such feelings of nervousness and concern, it is evident that, following their initial experiences, parents did become used to the procedure and accepted it in day-to-day functioning. Four parents described the procedure as being 'second nature' to them, the admirable point being that their confidence did eventually grow and they were able to develop their skills. After 8 years' experience, one mother stated:

> I mean as the years go on, I mean it's just second nature; I mean you just do it, don't you?

This is also indicated when parents talk of the locations in which they have administered IV medications: in a caravan and a car on a day trip, for example. Neither of these parents commented on being concerned or perturbed by the sight of shocked onlookers. All but one of the parents commented on the apparent ease of the procedure. Another theme common to all parents was the fact that the Port-a-cath (a permanent venous access device) had made the procedure simpler and had made life easier for the child. Cluroe (1989) also describes central lines as being advantageous for families.

The parents appeared to find the involvement in their child's care a positive experience, such active participation providing an element of control for the parents. One parent expressed it thus:

> It makes you feel like you are doing something positive as well,

another stating:

> I mean I'm quite independent and quite happy being in control of his life.

The theme that occurred most frequently for all parents was that of normality and the flexibility that it gives both parents and children. One of the parents stated the following advantages:

> your child stays within the normal routine, the sleep pattern is not so disturbed, the day to day routine stays the same, you know, at meal times, going to school...

Other benefits highlighted included the possibility for siblings and other family members to become involved, and for the child to become involved in his or her own care by helping. One parent pointed out that the latter would help the children to familiarise them-selves with the procedure, preparing them for future independence.

A sense of 'normality' is achieved through the ability to stay at home rather than spend lengthy periods in hospital and all the parents stated, at least twice in their conversations, that they all preferred home care to hospital care. Some disadvantages of hospital care that emerged included a disturbed routine and sleep, waiting around, the possibility of hospital-acquired infection, and the distance and time spent travelling to hospital, although one parent did point out that, on the contrary, her son actually enjoyed going to hospital.

Despite such disadvantages, one parent did note the advantage of nurses administering the antibiotics in hospital at antisocial times. One mother also noted that it can become tiring at home and commented on the fact that her day revolved around her child's 'injections'.

It is significant that parents find the experience positive and benefit personally from the home care scheme. Whyte (1992) found that parents perceived a successful accommodation into overall family life, this in turn giving them a positive self-image. Stephenson (1989) also states that when parents have a greater input into their child's treatment, it gives them a great deal of satisfaction. These reactions are more specific to the care of the chronically ill child at home and compare with those of the child in hospital for a short stay. As Neill (1996) states, although parents found involvement in care a very positive experience, the parents of short-stay children in a hospital setting often preferred professionals to carry out clinical care. Jerret (1994) asserts that active involvement and personal discovery are beneficial learned methods for parents to deal with their child's illness management. Therefore, it can be seen that participation at various levels of care can be beneficial for both child and parent.

As the present study indicated, the overall experience was positive in nature. Despite this, some parents did describe some disadvan-tages. Van Aalderen *et al.* (1995) have highlighted two disadvantages of home care: the therapeutic burden at home, and the fact that patients may not have the discipline to comply. Although the authors have identified areas of concern in the home care scheme, they still hold the overall conclusion that home care is beneficial. The basis for this conclusion derives from their personal experience of setting up a home care programme. Box (1993) found that school-age children preferred the social side of being in hospital and that home care can cause additional stress on the family. Other possible disadvantages have been highlighted by Youngblut *et al.* (1994), these being day-today problems of coping and the negative psychosocial impact on the family. There are obviously going to be disadvantages to such schemes, indicating the need for continuous assessment and support that will identify any such problems before they escalate.

Training and support

A major theme that emerged was that of parents appreciating the nursing staff's confidence in their ability to carry out the procedure at home. This aspect was identified by all but one parent. All parents appreciated the availability of 24-hour support on the phone to contact either the ward or the liaison nurse during working hours.

All but one parent indicated that the training received was in general sufficient. Three parents suggested the need for clearer language in the teaching process and argued that nursing and medical terminology should not be used. A suggestion made by two parents was the use of some sort of a 'test' that should be given on the ward, followed with a certificate. Four parents mentioned that a booklet or formal written information guide could be given and would prove useful, having it at home to refer to whenever they lacked confidence or forgot anything.

A suggestion made by two of the parents was that it would be useful to talk to other parents who had already commenced home care. They believed that it would provide them with support and increase their confidence by hearing that other parents were carrying out the procedure at home. As for advice to other parents who are offered the chance to administer IV antibiotics to their child at home, the overwhelming advice from the parents interviewed would be to recommend it.

There is a need to consider the training and support given to parents as both contribute to the parents' total experience. As the parents in this study have indicated, it is an essential requirement that ample support and training is made available.

A variety of training methods were identified from a review of the available literature. McLaughlin and Haase (1994) describe a home care scheme whose training programme includes an informal study evening covering the drugs used, the safe disposal of equipment, potential complications and side-effects, and methods of administration. A teaching folder is also provided. The next stage comprises practical teaching and then a home visit on the first day to supervise administration.

Cluroe (1989) identifies the need for a teaching programme undertaken by one nurse, and geared to individual needs. Kendrick (1993), in discussing a home care scheme, emphasises the use of a study night and the need for practical training and continued education. It is difficult to ascertain any optimum method of training, but it appears that a more structured programme with frequent updates is beneficial.

Whyte (1992) carried out a study of four families caring for a child with CF, the focus being on the nursing contribution to the support of the family. Using an ethnographic perspective, Whyte discovered that parents describe nursing support in various forms: providing information, explaining the meaning of investigations, answering questions, listening, providing a link between the clinic and the home and between the home and school, and providing help with child care.

Gow and Ridgway (1993) argue that illnesses such as CF can be successfully managed at home on the basis that sufficient support can be planned and provided. Donati *et al.* (1987) also found that home treatment works for parents if they have back-up and support readily available from nursing and medical staff. The literature has clearly indicated that home visits are a vital part of ongoing support.

It is essential that support and training be viewed as an ongoing process. Parents may not always be able to cope with administering the antibiotics at home; it is thus valuable for parents to recognise their limitations and that they can always rely on alternative or extra support and assistance without feeling that they have failed. As Kendrick (1993) points out, there should always be the option for flexibility between home and hospital treatment. It is essential that the concept of negotiation of care is adopted, as Coyne (1995) states that the parents, as primary carers, should not be neglected.

Conclusions and recommendations for practice

The conclusions reached from the research conducted confirm what existing literature has described regarding IV antibiotic home care for children with CF. The conclusions drawn from this particular study are outlined below:

1. Most parents in the study appeared to be nervous when first carrying out the procedure at home. In our role of supporting and educating, we, as nurses, should offer parents considerable support in their training and during their first experiences at home. Support should be an ongoing process, and education should be updated.

2. After some experience, most parents stated that the procedure became 'second nature'. This finding indicates that parents can eventually feel at ease and confident in their actions.

3. Parents liked the sense of being in control. As children's nurses, we should acknowledge this fact, and if parents are involved in the care of their child, we should support them and let them continue to do so as much as possible, respecting them in their actions (by negotiating levels of participation).

4. It is apparent that parents prefer to care for their child at home if they are given the opportunity to do so. As nurses, we should value parents' contribution to their child's health care and accept that they are capable of performing such clinical procedures as administering IV antibiotics.

5. 24-hour contact and home visits were of value to the parents and also boosted their confidence.

6. Although the parents did not complain about the method of training, they did offer some suggestions, namely;

   - the use of a booklet
   - that all instructions should be given in lay terms and avoid using 'nursing language'
   - a certificate at the end of training
   - being able to talk to other parents who had commenced the home care scheme.

7. The use of a Port-a-cath appeared to help in the home administration of IV antibiotics.

Further research

The results of this piece of research provide only a partial picture of the experiences of parents. A longitudinal study, ethnographic in nature, combining interviews with participant observation during the training process, and following parents through their 'career' in administering IV antibiotics may provide a more detailed picture. It would also be beneficial to: (a) compare parents' experiences of administering IV antibiotics in hospital and at home; (b) investigate the child's experience; and (c) gain an insight into the views of other family members. With regard to training and support, further research could investigate a cross-section of programmes across the country in order to review the variety of training methods and support available; optimal training and support could then be highlighted.

References

Box J. (1993) 'A family affair', *Nursing Times* 89(39): 36–7.

Callery P. and Luker K. (1996) 'The use of qualitative methods in the study of parents' experiences of care on a children's surgical ward', *Journal of Advanced Nursing* 23(2): 338–45.

Catchpole A. (1989) 'Cystic fibrosis: intravenous antibiotics at home', *Nursing Times* 85(12): 40–2.

Cluroe S. (1989) 'Parental involvement in intravenous therapy', *Nursing Times* 85(9): 42–3.

Coyne I. T. (1995) 'Parental participation in care: a critical review of the literature', *Journal of Advanced Nursing* 21(4): 716–22.

Darbyshire P. (1995) 'Family-centred care within contemporary British paediatric nursing', *British Journal of Nursing* 4(1): 31–3.

Deatrick J. A., Faux S. A. and Moore C. M. (1993) 'The contribution of qualitative research to the study of families' experiences with childhood illnesses'. In Feetham S. L., Meister S. B., Bell J. M. and Gilliss C. L. (eds) *The Nursing of Families: Theory, Research Education and Practice*, London, Sage.

Donati M. A., Guenette G. and Auerbach H. (1987) 'Prospective controlled study of home and hospital therapy of cystic fibrosis pulmonary disease', *Journal of Paediatrics* 111(1): 28–33.

Gilbert J., Robinson T. and Littlewood J. M. (1988) 'Home intravenous antibiotic treatment in cystic fibrosis', *Archives of Diseases in Childhood* 63: 512–17.

Gill S. (1993) 'Home administration of intravenous antibiotics to children with cystic fibrosis', *British Journal of Nursing* 15(2): 767–70.

Gow P. and Ridgway G. (1993) 'The development of a paediatric community service'. In Glasper E. A. and Tucker A. (eds) *Advances in Child Health Nursing*, Harrow, Scutari Press.

Jerrett M. D. (1994) 'Parent's experiences of coming to know the care of a chronically ill child', *Journal of Advanced Nursing* 19(6): 1050–6.

Kendrick R. (1993) 'Teaching children with cystic fibrosis and their families to give IV therapy', *Paediatric Nursing* 5(1): 22–4.

Lessing D. and Tatman M. A. (1991) 'Paediatric home care in the 1990s', *Archives of Diseases in Childhood* 66: 994–6.

McLaughlin S. and Haase L. (1994) 'Home is where the heart is', *CF News*. Winter: 8–9.

Masterson A. (1998) 'Discourse analysis: a tool for change in nursing policy, practice and research'. In Smith P. (ed.) *Nursing Research – Setting New Agendas*, Arnold.

Mishler G. E. (1991) *Research Interviewing – Context and Narrative*, London, Harvard University Press.

Morse J. M. (1991) 'Strategies of sampling'. In Morse J. M. (ed.) *Qualitative Nursing Research – A Contemporary Dialogue* (rev. edn), London, Sage.

Neill S. J. (1996) 'Parent participation, 2: Findings and their implications for practice', *British Journal of Nursing* 5(2): 110–17.

Nuttall P. and Nicholes P. (1992) 'Cystic fibrosis: adolescent and maternal concerns about hospital and home care', *Issues in Comprehensive Pediatric Nursing* 15: 199–213.

Stephenson K. (1989) 'Giving antibiotics at home', *Nursing Standard* 40(3): 24–5.

Streubert H. J. and Carpenter D. R. (1995) *Qualitative Research in Nursing – Advancing the Humanistic Imperative*, Philadelphia, J. B. Lippincott.

van Aalderen W. M. C., Mannes G. P. M., Bosma E. S., Roorda R. J. and Heymans H. S. A. (1995) 'Home care in cystic fibrosis patients', *European Respiratory Journal* 8(1): 172–5.

Whyte D. A. (1992) 'A family approach to the care of a child with cystic fibrosis', *Journal of Advanced Nursing* 17(3): 317–27.

Youngblut Y. M., Flatley-Brennan P. and Swegart H. (1994) 'Families with medically fragile children: an exploratory study', *Pediatric Nursing* 20(5): 463–8.

Further reading

Darbyshire P. (1994). *Living with a Sick Child in Hospital – the Experiences of Parents and Nurses*, London, Chapman & Hall.

Feetham S. L., Meister S. B., Bell J. M. and Gilliss C. L. (1993) *The Nursing of Families: Theory, Research, Education and Practice*, London, Sage.

Polit D. F. and Hungler B. P. (1993) *Essentials of Nursing Research – Methods, Appraisal, and Utilisation* (3rd edn), Philadelphia, J. B. Lippincott.

20 *There's a whole family hurting: the experience of living with a child with chronic pain*

Bernadette Carter

It's... a terrible, *terrible* thing to see a child in pain. (Mother, interview)

Introduction

Chronic pain, like acute pain, is in the individual child's head – that is to say, only he or she can experience that pain. This does not mean that the pain is not real: it is real to the child experiencing it even if it is difficult for those outside this individual experience to validate it. This study, undertaken with three children and their families, explores their experiences of living with chronic pain. It provides an insight into their perspective of the way in which pain impacts on their life. The stress experienced as a result of not being believed and of feeling different is explored. The effects of pain in terms of the feelings engendered and the restrictions imposed are considered and reflect that families are not passively giving in to the pain but are active in their attempts to deal with it. The difficulties experienced when interfacing with professionals are presented.

This study arose out of concerns for the impact that living with chronic pain has on children and their families. Chronic pain is a hidden issue and is often denied (Teasell, 1997). Personal discussion and experience suggested that many children experiencing chronic pain are poorly managed and their experiences little understood. This chapter focuses on the findings of the study and the implications for practice. Sections on the methodology of the study and the analysis of the data are presented only in outline. The narratives are compelling, and through these, the experiences of the children and their parents unfold. This story demands that professionals take notice of what is truly a family experience.

359

Literature review

Background issues

Chronic pain, like acute pain, is in the individual child's head – that is to say, only that child can experience his or her pain. This does not mean that the pain is not real; it is real to the child experiencing it even if it is difficult for those outside the child's individual experience to validate it (Carter, 1994, 1998). People with chronic pain are all too often seen as being 'at fault' in some way (DeGood and Kleinman, 1996). Emotional variables, including anxiety, depression and poor self-esteem, are all associated with chronic pain, and there is evidence that these all impact on patients' experiences (Elton, 1987; Robinson *et al.*, 1990). The relative paucity of literature focusing on children's experience of chronic pain means that, when appropriate, adult literature has been drawn on.

The factors involved are hierarchical and have interdependent relationships. Chronic pain in adults is often seen in terms of its financial consequences (Horn and Munafó, 1997). In children, the loss could be equated with lost schooling and a potential loss of future earnings. Broadly speaking, paediatric chronic pain literature focuses on a number of key areas:

- conditions in which there is an obvious pathology and where there is some expectation of pain, such as juvenile rheumatoid arthritis (JRA);
- conditions in which there is some difficulty identifying an obvious pathology, and when it can be identified, there is room for discrepancy between the child's report of pain and the medical diagnosis, such as migraine;
- the effect of familial pain on children's pain experiences.

Anthropological literature acknowledges the way in which the person who has pain interacts in-and-with his or her world (Good *et al.*, 1992; Bendelow and Williams, 1995). This literature informs our understanding of children's pain and demonstrates the increasing importance of understanding, preventing and effectively mediating children's chronic pain.

Defining chronic pain

There is no universal definition of chronic pain, although a number of different definitions or categories of chronic pain have been proposed (see, for example, McGrath *et al.*, 1990; Schechter *et al.*, 1993; Varni *et al.*, 1996). Chronic pain is always acknowledged as being complex, difficult to deal with, resistant to treatment and often associated with the notion of somatic fixation. Schulz and Masek (1996) highlight this complexity when they state:

> that the etiological processes that originally initiated the pain experience may not be the same as the processes that maintain pain over time. (p. 124)

This is an important difference to note, but, it is equally important to remember that the pain may feel the same (or worse) to the person experiencing it regardless of whether the processes are the same or not. Schulz and Masek (1996) further state:

> the multiple levels of chronic pain point to the scientific difficulty of dividing pain conditions into those that are caused by organic pathology and those that are considered to be caused by psychological factors. (pp. 124–5)

In the past, pain tended to be categorised as either organic (real) or non-organic (not real) pain. Both *feel* real and therefore *are* real, and it is often impossible for health care professionals to differentiate between pain with or without an organic cause.

Models of chronic pain

There are a number of different models of chronic pain that contribute to an understanding of the plasticity and individuality of the experience; two models will be briefly outlined. Covelman *et al.* (1990) present a model, derived from their work in a child guidance centre, that considers issues such as the child's vulnerability and identifies the interrelationship between factors that result in increased symptom expression and a dysfunctional adaptation to pain. This has merit but seems to focus on the fact that children do not cope well with pain and therefore adapt dysfunctionally. An element of blame perhaps comes through this model, although this is undoubtedly not the intention of the authors.

Brodwin and Kleinman (1987) present an anthropological (adult-orientated) perspective that is useful to consider in relation to children's chronic pain. It examines the social meanings of pain in relation to 'family, ethnic/cultural community, work site, and health care organisation' (p. 109). Brodwin and Kleinman (1987) propose that chronic pain has two anthropological forms: pain disease and pain illness. These represent two separate domains of knowledge about, and behavioural response to, pain. When these perspectives meet conflict may result.

Pain disease reflects the doctors' perspective on patients' suffering, is biomedically orientated and is concerned with identifying pathologies or symptom clusters. Pain illness, however, is culturally grounded and reflects the patients' account of their experience of chronic pain, such as changes to their lifestyle, as well as their emotional responses. These aspects guide patients in treatment decisions. Both the disease and illness domains offer different explanatory models for aetiology, onset of symptoms, pathophysiology, course of illness and treatment. The following list, adapted from Brodwin and Kleinman (1987), demonstrates how many factors affect the way in which pain is interpreted and communicated:

- Children's pain symptoms are experienced in the context of their social world
- The child's experience of pain depends on stressors in his or her socio-cultural environment
- Environment affects the personal meaning that children and their families attribute to pain
- Different professionals offer differing perspectives, which shape their interpretation of pain
- The meaning of pain and the emotional responses to it are highly idiosyncratic and not easily understood by people outside the experience. Children communicate their pain illness using shared *idioms of distress*, which allows their pain to be understood by others.

The interplay of these factors results in specific personal meanings within the child's 'life-world'. It is vital that health care professionals understand and incorporate these 'illness meanings' into their management strategies.

The meaning of pain and the child's attributes

The meaning of pain is a crucial factor to take into consideration, even though the focus has mostly been on the impact of acute pain on the family (Watt-Watson *et al.*, 1990; Mathews *et al.*, 1993). Beales *et al.* (1983) and Page (1991) have shown that children with JRA attribute different meanings to their pain depending on their age and that this affects intensity of pain experience and emotional response. Varni *et al.* (1996) found that higher perceived pain intensity was associated with higher depressive and anxiety symptoms, lower general self-esteem and more behavioural problems. The family and close friends provide a crucial context for chronic pain, and their responses affect its trajectory.

Children who experience chronic pain are sometimes described as being somehow less resilient than non-chronic pain children, an implication of this being that they are poor copers, are manipulative and use pain for secondary gain. They are often described as being ambitious over-achievers who are also vulnerable, anxious and more likely to become depressed than their non-chronic pain counterparts (Robinson *et al.*, 1990).

The methodological strength of some of the early studies has, however, been questioned, and more recent studies are beginning to question their claims. Koval and Pritchard's (1990) study on children with headaches showed that they demonstrated more psychosomatic problems and behavioural disturbances than controls, and their parents had a lower expectation of achievement. Robinson *et al.* (1990) showed that children with chronic pain are described by parents as being anxious or apprehensive, lacking in communication and not really having anyone in whom to confide. It is interesting to note many studies on childhood chronic pain draw data from the parents rather than from the children or young people involved.

Modelling and familial patterns

Familial patterns or modelling are cited by many writers (for example, Dura and Beck, 1988; Rickard, 1988; Mikail and von Bayer, 1990; Robinson *et al.*, 1990; Roy *et al.*, 1994; Segal-Andrews *et al.*, 1995, Kotchick *et al.*, 1996). Pain families are said to create pain children who present their idiom of distress in line with the familial model. The family acts as a source of advice, interpretation, negotiation and so on about treatment and the meaning of pain, pain behaviour becoming embedded in the family dynamics (Edwards *et al.*, 1985).

The children of chronic pain patients are more adversely affected than the children of healthy parents or parents with other chronic medical conditions (for example, diabetes) and often seen to be more somatically focused. Children often mirror their parents in relation to coping strategies, negative thinking and adherence (Gil *et al.*, 1991). The children of chronic pain patients are often more psychologically disturbed, have a greater level of external locus of control, and present more complaints and more episodes of seeking help. Roy *et al.* (1994), however, suggest caution should be adopted since:

> a priori that chronic pain in a parent is more harmful to the child than normal control groups and other medical conditions is premature... The notion that parents with chronic pain endangers the well-being of their children should be viewed with caution. (p. 25)

Triggers and journeys

Robinson *et al.* (1990) propose that certain triggers or life events can result in the generation of symptoms that emerge unconsciously. They describe a 'threshold surface' that has to be breached for symptoms, specific to the individual, to emerge, this being affected by psychosocial and treatment effects.

The notion of the stressful 'journey to diagnosis' is evident within the general child chronic illness literature (for example, Knafl *et al.*, 1995). There is often an increasing somatic fixation as the child and the family focus on trying to identify the cause of pain. As the family and the health care professionals 'dance' around the issue of 'what's wrong', conflict often arises, and the family can easily be seen to be over-anxious and the cause of the child's pain. Brodwin and Kleinman (1987) state:

> Thus, the trajectory of somatic amplification is frequently a transactional result of doctor–patient relationships. (p. 116)

Increasing conflict can contribute to increasing somatisation and can result in the child's pain being labelled 'psychosomatic' and thus not really deserving of medical attention. The final referral in the 'journey' is often to the child psychiatrist, which families may see as the medical (cure) system finally failing and giving up on them. Children and their families generally prefer to have a medical label than the associated stigma of a mental health label for the cause of the pain.

Approaches to care and management

Pharmacological approaches (Zeltzer and Zeltzer, 1989), as well as a range of non-pharmacological therapies, are employed in managing chronic pain (McGrath and Humphreys, 1989), and early rather than late intervention is likely to provide a better outcome

(Greipp, 1988). McGrath *et al.* (1990) propose a series of clinical guidelines for the effective management of children with chronic pain. While the pain itself must be respected and treated (often pharmacologically), this may not get to the heart of the problem, which has gone beyond the initial pathology.

Medical crisis counselling (MCC) and its role is discussed by Schulz and Masek (1996) as a means of legitimising the children's pain and pain illness and decreasing his or her suffering. They state that the focus is on the children moving from a state of 'passive disability to a state of empowered control over their lives' (p. 125). They suggest that this can be achieved through good communication, explanation and multidisciplinary working, which acknowledges the biopsychosocial aspects of chronic pain and could improve the trajectory of chronic pain. Eight core issues of MCC relate to fears of:

- becoming isolated
- being stigmatised
- becoming dependent
- being abandoned
- dying
- expressing one's anger
- changes in self-image
- losing control over life.

Conclusion

It can thus be seen from the reviewed literature that progress is being made in relation to understanding chronic pain and children. Models have been proposed that help to frame the way in which professionals approach and consider the management of the child with chronic pain. An exploration of the attributes of the child and the family have been explored, although further study is obviously needed to provide an explanation that will satisfy many of the families, of why their child is experiencing chronic pain. However, there is little literature that actively explores how the experience of chronic pain feels for the child and his or her family, and how this experience impacts on their lives.

Methodology

Statement of intent

The intention of this study was to explore the feelings, perceptions and experiences of families living with a child experiencing chronic pain.

Aims of the study

The aims of the study were to:

1.   explore how children feel about their pain
2.   develop a critical appreciation of how children's lives are affected by pain
3.   determine the impact that children's pain has on the daily lives of (close) family members
4.   explore how families cope with this impact
5.   consider the role of professionals in family support (including pain management).

Methodological approaches

A constructivist, collaborative, strongly qualitative approach under-pinned the research, the children and their families being seen as partners in the study rather than respondents (Schwandt, 1994; Nespor, 1998). The study was exploratory in nature and drew on the lived experiences of the children and their families. The term 'family' is taken to include anyone whom the child sees as being special to them; thus, aunts, uncles, neighbours, teachers and school friends could be included. Data were generated through interviews and jour-nals. A staged developmental approach was used (Table 20.1).

Sample

A purposive sample of three families was drawn from families nomi-nated and previously approached by the Pain Nurse Practitioner from the Starship Hospital. Asking the Pain Nurse Practitioner to identify and make initial contact with potential families minimised the possibility of families feeling pressured to take part in the study. The following inclusion criteria were identified:

●   The child should meet the criteria for the 'diagnosis' of chronic pain
●   The child should be aged between 7 and 13 years
●   The child should show cognitive achievements appropriate for his or her age
●   The family as a unit should be in agreement to take part in the study.

Chronic pain or chronic persistent pain is prolonged, persists past the normal time of healing and is generally agreed to last 3 months or longer (Schechter *et al.*, 1993). Implicit in this definition is that factors apart from nociception caused by injury are probably involved (Merskey and Bogduk, 1994). Within this study, a child who had experienced pain for 3 months or longer, from whatever cause, would be deemed to meet the first inclusion criterion.

Table 20.1   Overview of stages of the study

Stage 1

- Initial contact with families by researcher
- Informed consent gained
- Families received information sheets and journals
- Families made entries to journal for a 4-week period

Stage 2

- Informal interviews with families based on issues arising from journals

Stage 3

- Heuristic analysis of all data (journals and interview tapes)

Stage 4

- Write report and feed back to study centre
- Distribute report to families, study centre and Scholarship Committee
- Generate articles for publications and conferences

Ethical considerations

The child's rights were paramount throughout the study. While this study was not directly therapeutic for the children, the opportunity to discuss their pain was seen as being potentially beneficial. A commitment was made to withdraw from a family at any time should they so wish. Ethical clearance was sought and gained from the North Health Ethics Committee. All care was taken to protect those participating in the study.

Contacting the families and generating the data

The initial contact with the family was by letter and/or telephone, outlining the research study. Informed consent was gained after an appropriate dialogue with the family and the child, and was confirmed in writing. The family received a package containing information sheets and journals for them to complete. The journals were open, unstructured notebooks that allowed the family to make entries as they felt appropriate. The children received their own journal that they could complete to reflect their own individual experiences and feelings. There was no format imposed for the completion of the journal, although guidelines indicated issues that might be included and suggestions for when the families might make their entries. It was hoped that each journal would be a personalised reflection of their individual experiences. The journals were distributed to the families about 6 weeks prior to the interview stage.

During the interview stage, the researcher visited each family. The interviews were loosely structured and developed from the materials that the families included in their journals. They took place in a variety of settings that were seen by the families and researcher to be appropriate, including the family home, a hotel and the hospital. This aimed to minimise the disruption to family life. The families could elect to be interviewed separately or as a family unit.

Data analysis

All data were analysed using the heuristic method (basically, a discovery-orientated method of analysis). This involved each of the families being considered both as a separate unit and then as one of the units within the entire study (Table 20.2).

Transcripts of all the audiotaped interviews and journals were made. Detailed field notes of the non-taped conversations were taken, with the families' permission. Each line of transcript was assigned a code, these being used to help to structure and 'index' the material. A total of nine diaries and seven interviews were transcribed and analysed (Tables 20.3 and 20.4). To structure the findings and recommendations, themes were identified from the data. A model was then developed to provide structure and meaning to the analysis and has been used to present the findings.

Table 20.2   Overview of the children in the study

Family	Gender and age	Primary site of pain (no diagnosis of cause)
Family 1	Girl, aged 13 years	Knee pain
Family 2	Girl, aged 13 years	Abdominal pain
Family 3	Boy, aged 12 years	Back pain

Table 20.3   Overview of interviews

Interview	Audio-taped	People present	Duration (minutes)	Number of words
1	✓	Mother, father and child	60	5674
2	✓	Mother, father and child	60	9759
3	x	Mother and child	30	n/a
4	✓	Mother and child	60	6072
5	x	Mother, father and child	40	n/a
6	✓	Mother	60	10,953
7	✓	Child	45	5586

Table 20.4   Overview of diaries

Family diary	People who contributed	Number of words
1	Mother, father and child	3523
2	Mother, father, grandmother and child	2822
3	Mother and child	1355

Much of the data were generated by the children and their mothers, some fathers tending to take a background role even though their concern and support were evident.

Main findings

Five main themes, all inextricably interlinked, emerged from the data. The findings will be presented and discussed within each of these five areas (Figure 20.1). The quotations are taken either from the interview transcripts, from the journals, or from field notes.

Sub-themes also emerged in the analysis; these have been identified within the text but, because of a lack of space, have not been allocated separate subheadings.

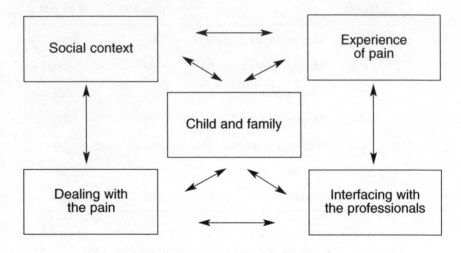

Figure 20.1   Model of chronic pain

The child and the family

The family emerged as the most important theme for all of the participants, although the greatest focus on the life of the family came from the parents. This theme received greater attention than the child's personal experience of pain. Two sub-themes were identified:

- the concerns and desires of the child and the family
- the feelings and tension or stress experienced by the family as a result of the child's pain.

It is important to note at this point that each family presented a unique portrait of their experiences and of their own family concerns, desires, feelings and stressors. Despite the uniqueness of each family, there were resonances between the different narratives. What was apparent from all the families was the balancing act they felt that they were performing with their lives and the stresses that this created for them. An example of this was the need to balance protecting their child with the need to push them to 'keep them going'. One mother stated:

> I'm trying hard to encourage him to keep going and I'm aware that he sees this as callousness on my part. I'd love to know where to draw the line on sympathy without being mean! (Mother, diary)

All of the children in the study were at a stage at which they had achieved some degree of control over their lives and desperately wanted more independence; they resisted over-protection and being treated as younger children. The alienation of the child within the family was presented as an issue by the families. The child's role and function within the family had been changed subtly or more dramatically by the experience of pain. For the family, the effects went beyond those affecting the child and their parents and included the child's siblings.

None of the children interviewed believed that their siblings really understood their pain. In some cases, siblings were seen to be an important, stabilising and secure influence, whereas one child felt that her siblings did not want to get involved. While many of these tensions are interesting to pursue, it should be remembered that the children experiencing the pain were going through adolescence. Their parents recognised this but felt that the changes were related to their child's pain.

The notion of the family being accused of, or being the source of, their child's pain was incredibly difficult for parents to deal with and an accusation they firmly rejected. The parents' usual roles were confused or challenged by the child's pain. They were confronted with issues and problems with which they felt ill equipped to deal. Their belief in themselves had been challenged, and they resented the way in which they were being scrutinised for ineffective parenting, discipline and so on. They resented being judged by experts who had no real understanding of how *their* family worked.

The child's pain had not only impacted on internal family functioning, but also on the way in which parents managed external links such as work. The randomness of the 'bad' days (when the child needed care at home) and the unpredictable course of the child's pain increased the difficulties for parents juggling the demands of employment and their responsibility for their child.

All parents wanted to be able to cope better or to change their way of coping. One mother expressed this when stating:

> I think, I'd just change our way of dealing with [the pain]… deal with him in a non-stressful way… or become more unstressed about the whole thing. (Mother, interview)

Immense stress was a central issue of the families' narratives. They remembered their 'pre-pain family' as one in which there were small everyday stresses but the current extreme tensions did not exist. Powerlessness and helplessness were evident in the parents' descriptions; they saw themselves as onlookers to their child's pain. Thus, parents reported the devastation that their child's pain had had on their lives. One mother stated:

> you're made to feel a bit of a freak and your child's a freak, and your family's a bit of a freak. And it's really not. (Mother, interview)

Despite these often unrecognised pressures, however, the families were 'determined to survive' regardless of how tough life became.

The experience of pain

This theme can be broadly divided into two sub-themes:

- the effects of pain
- the feelings engendered by the pain.

The individuality of each child's experience of pain was evidenced from their narratives. The physical experience was related to the type of pain. One child described his pain as being 'deep inside' him and:

> when I get stabbing pain I can, can sort of be paralysed for a couple of seconds… sort of not be able to move… maybe not because I can't but because I don't want to because it makes it worse. (Child, interview)

Despite obvious differences in the type of pain the feelings engendered by it had much in common. The children and the families all had degrees of concern that the pain might go on forever. One child stated that she felt 'trapped', 'fearful' and 'scared', and said that she used to worry about dying from the pain.

The children and their parents knew what exacerbated the pain. Examples of this were eating, getting edgy, getting overtired and moving too much. The children found that pain made them feel profoundly tired. One child reported 'only *just* making it [through the day]'. Tiredness meant that the children found it harder to deal with their pain, and this contributed to their mood change. Parents also experienced devastating tiredness.

None of the children or families dwelt on the pain itself, and they all had a fairly pragmatic approach to it. One of the children said that it was pointless describing it because people either 'didn't really believe you or if they did they couldn't help much, so why bother?'

Dealing with pain

This theme can broadly be divided into two reasonably distinct sub-themes:

- strategies for coping with pain (including medication)
- the restrictions that the pain created.

These sub-themes have been drawn together as they provide examples of when families were using good coping skills – which meant that the pain did not really restrict their lives – and when coping was very problematic – which resulted in the pain restricting their lives. In presenting the findings in this manner, there is no wish to imply that restrictions reflected the families' inability to cope. The families faced real difficulties everyday and, by their *own* estimation, generally coped well. They were strong, loving families facing a seemingly awful situation with courage. It is important to note that the children and families spent more time considering the strategies they used to manage the pain rather than the restrictions that it imposed.

All of the children had been prescribed analgesics, which they found did little to shift their background pain. The analgesics were generally simple, readily available, over-the-counter remedies that were not the answer to the families' prayers. The children did their best to focus on things apart from their pain. Each did this in his or her own way through activities that were important to them, such as being with their friends, singing or using the computer, as well as sport in a more limited way. Other distractions, such as creative visualisation, self-hypnosis and positive thinking, were less valued by the children: one girl said that she had little time for 'any of that hippy stuff'. Other strategies used tended to be passive and involved 'time out' activities such as relaxing and trying to sleep. Strategies that had been 'given' to the children by the hospital were sometimes a source of contention. Relaxation exercises were used occasionally by the children, although all reported they had difficulty in relaxing, especially when they were stressed or in pain. Physiotherapy was not viewed positively, one girl saying that physiotherapists were:

> just sick in the mind... and they stand there with a smile on the face while they're doing it... they'll have a *big* grin and they say 'I know this hurts' but they don't really... you feel like they're just saying it. (Child, interview)

The child did not see the outcome of greater mobility as being worth the pain that had to be borne to achieve it.

Transcutaneous electrical nerve stimulation was used by one child, but only to help him to get through crises of pain at school; he rarely used it at home. Another child had been prescribed analgesic patches, which helped but also made her feel ill – 'like totally dazed out' – when she first started using them. Despite the use of painkillers, the children were somewhat suspicious of them. One girl said:

> We're learning about drug abuse at school and I've discovered painkillers can kill my liver. So much for helping me!!!! (Child, interview)

The children, however, were generally sanguine about taking them even if they felt that they were not strong enough when the pain was really bad.

Each family had considered options outside mainstream practice. One mother reported one visit when she was 'desperate to try anything': she had been urged to take her son to see a Chinese herbalist, and she described it as a 'huge mistake' as:

> He [her son] was really angry. He didn't want to go and I *made* him. And I really regret making him go because he didn't like the guy... And didn't trust him. And told me that he felt unsafe. And as soon as he said that I felt *really* bad. (Mother, interview)

The urge to turn to someone outside both the family and the existing services offered by conventional approaches was strong. All the parents voiced the need for more help, some definitive answers and an end to the pain.

Despite the impact of pain, the families did *not* really describe their lives as being restricted. The children keenly felt their loss of independence, which made them different from their peers. All the parents expressed some level of fear for the future and were worried that life would always have these restrictions. Overall, the parents and children were remarkably optimistic and positive despite the real difficulties imposed by a child experiencing chronic pain.

Social context

Within this theme two sub-themes were apparent:

- the school and friends
- other people.

'Other people' included colleagues of the parents, employers and friends. The school was inextricably bound up with the children's social life, their role in their community, and their network of friends.

School was a focus of the children's lives; they were bright, motivated and generally successful at school. All were concerned about the amount of time they had been forced to miss. This meant that they were missing both school work *and* the social aspects, such as school trips and after-school activities. Missed school meant that they had to catch up on the work, and this 'puts a strain on you'. All of the schools had been supportive, flexible and accommodating. Individual teachers were seen to be 'good', while some teachers were criticised for thinking that they 'know best even when they don't!' Friends were really important and 'the best bit of school'. All the children stated that they would never bring the subject of their pain up with their friends as they wanted to fit in and not bore them. One child stated, 'I normally prefer them to think that I don't have pain'.

Other people provided a source of worry as well as support. Parents had to battle with the ongoing questions of what was wrong with their child, what the treatment was, whether the child was better and so on. Parents found themselves sick of repeating the same things, especially when they felt that they had no answers and neither did anyone else. One mother, for example, stressed the difficulties:

The relatives especially, expected you to justify what the medical experts were telling you and at times the doctors themselves didn't know what was going on! (Mother, diary)

Interfacing with professionals

Within this theme, two sub-themes are described:

- encounters with the professionals
- the quest for a diagnosis and/or cause of the child's pain.

While the parents acknowledged the difficulties of finding a diagnosis and the efforts made, they did feel that 'things' had 'gone on and on'. They had real difficulties coming to terms with the fact that the doctors were unable to answer the question 'why?'. None of the parents or children knew why their child had this pain. One father described the feeling that his daughter's pain had gone on for so long that 'she was being put in the too hard basket' and her mother felt that they were being 'written off'. The lack of a diagnosis was a major concern. The children also felt that there was sometimes nothing positive to 'hang on to'. Indeed, one child was told that her pain would not disable her, despite her being on two crutches at the time. The whole lack of a diagnosis meant that management seemed uncertain and directionless. This coloured much of their dealing with professionals.

Prior to being referred to the pain experts, all of the families had experienced problems dealing with a variety of other doctors. Doctors were the focus of these traumatic experiences as these were the people the families expected would sort things out. Nurses gained very little attention in relation to this: they were generally seen to be supportive, kind but rather peripheral. All of the parents felt that they and their child had been disbelieved and judged by the professionals. Some parents told particularly difficult stories about bad experiences in this respect. One child wrote in her diary that:

> a couple of the doctors treated me like I was faking. I was 11 and knew that I was being accused of lying. This made me really angry, because it didn't help the pain (it actually got worse) and it really hurt me to be called a liar when the pain was very real. (Child, diary)

The children and their families had seen many different specialists and felt that communication between them was generally poor: each new contact felt like starting all over again. Referral fatigue was obvious. One mother explained how it made her feel:

> That's why I really felt like thumping people. I got so angry... I'd say.. 'Haven't you read his notes? ...'No, I haven't got to them yet, I'll get to them later'... I'm sure there's a reason and in some respects they want to

create their own impressions first but they've got to realise asking the same questions a million times is so unsettling for the child, *really* frustrating for the parent. (Mother, interview)

Another aspect of communication was mentioned by one child who felt that the doctors ought to 'talk to me more not just my mum'. The listening aspect of communication was seen to be as important as information giving. One child said:

Listen!!!!! ...*Listen* to what the people [with chronic pain] have to say *and take notice* of it. Treat them as people no matter how young they are... [The doctors] get really patronising... I just get *really* fed up with it. (Child, interview)

Some parents had experienced clashes with health professionals that had been extremely emotionally draining. This seemed to occur when parents who were very stressed were patronised by doctors and told not to worry as 'not much was wrong'. On other occasions, parents felt accused of being the (dysfunctional) cause of the child's problems, which was why medicine could not help.

The psychological issues, impacted on many interactions with medical staff, were seen to be something that had to be borne. The children's notes bore the sticker of the Child and Family Unit, which, they felt, implied to some doctors that the pain problem was entirely psychological and not something needing physical support. This led to a number of misunderstandings.

Considering the faith that the families placed in the pain team, they were still reluctant to disclose any stresses. They felt that any family troubles were private and not something they would necessarily discuss. In addition, parents had learnt to be cautious about disclosing things as they could easily be misinterpreted, adding to the supposed evidence of a dysfunctional family. Overall, the pain team were seen to be busy 'saviours': parents were eternally grateful for the support, belief and help that they gained from them. They were seen to be 'different' from the sort of the professionals with whom they normally came into contact. They 'worked as a team' and had the families' interests at heart.

Conclusions

The overwhelming conclusion from this small study is the huge toll that living with a child experiencing chronic pain has on the family.

The challenges are both emotional and pragmatic, and appear to go largely unrecognised by the professionals to whom the families turn for help. By the time the families reach expert and appropriate help, they appear to be disillusioned, physically drained and emotionally exhausted. The referral fatigue experienced on their journey through the experts does not reflect well on the health professionals they have encountered en route. Even when in the haven of being cared for by people whom they acknowledge as believing them and offering support, they still feel isolated, anxious and occasionally abandoned. To say that families cope in spite of, rather than because of, professional intervention is, perhaps, to put the case too strongly. However, it appears to be the families' determination that helps them to survive so that they can continue to ask questions, challenge decisions and demand to be heard.

The child's pain has repercussions far beyond the child, affecting every aspect of family life. Health care professionals tend to underestimate the stress and tension engendered by the awfulness of caring for a child whose pain is apparently undiagnosed. Families need to be understood on their own rather than on professional terms. They need to be believed rather than disregarded, accepted rather than judged. They need their concerns and anxieties accepted and not dismissed as demented, hysterical outbursts.

The words of a researcher can tell only a partial story. The words of a child sum up much of what living with chronic pan is about: 'not just my burden... it's my brother's and family's as well'. Surely it is our responsibility as professionals to help to share that burden by acknowledging its existence and providing solutions to relieve it.

Recommendations for professionals caring for children with chronic pain

These are necessarily general recommendations made in the light of the small sample of this study:

1. Families with a child experiencing chronic pain are in crisis. Indeed, the most appropriate description would perhaps be a 'chronic crisis', although this does create a linguistic paradox. Appropriate, individually tailored support needs to be offered and established to meet the unique needs of each family.
2. Referral of the child to expert pain care as early as possible in the child's pain 'career' is crucial.

3. Communication between professionals must be improved, and the child's notes should be seen as a valuable resource.
4. The family must be listened to and believed; they are the experts on their child's pain.
5. Children need to be offered an appropriate level of explanation and information that is directed specifically at them.
6. Families need to have a plan for the future to help them to deal with any new pain crises that arise.

Acknowledgements

This study was made possible through the Nestlé Charitable Scholarship awarded through the Florence Nightingale Foundation. My thanks are extended to the families who took part in the study and to the professionals working at Starship Children's Health, Auckland, New Zealand.

References

Beales J. G., Keen K. J. and Holt P. J. L. (1983) 'The child's perception of the disease and the experience of pain in juvenile chronic arthritis', *Journal of Rheumatology* 10(1):61–5.

Bendelow G. and Williams S. (1995) 'Transcending the dualisms: towards a sociology of pain', *Sociology of Health and Illness* 17: 139–65.

Brodwin P. E. and Kleinman A. (1987) 'The social meanings of chronic pain'. In Burrows G., Elton D. and Stanley G. V. (eds) *Handbook of Chronic Pain Management*, BV, Elsevier Science.

Carter B. (1994) *Child and Infant Pain: Principles of Nursing Care and Management*, London, Chapman & Hall.

Carter B. (1998) *Perspectives on Pain: Mapping the Territory*, London, Arnold.

Covelman K., Scott S., Buchanan B. and Rosman B. (1990) 'Pediatric pain control: a family systems model'. In Tyler D. C. and Krane E. J. (eds) *Advances in Pain Research Therapy*, vol. 15, New York, Raven Press.

DeGood D. E. and Kleinman B. (1996) 'Perception of fault in patients with chronic pain', *Pain* 64: 153–9.

Dura J. and Beck S. A. (1988) 'A comparison of family function when mothers have chronic pain', *Pain* 35: 79–89.

Edwards P. W., Zeichner A., Kuczmeirczyk A. R. and Boczkowski J. (1985) 'Familial pain models: the relationship between family history of pain and current pain experience', *Pain* 21: 379–84.

Elton D. (1987) 'Emotional variables and chronic pain'. In Burrows G., Elton D. and Stanley G. V. (eds) *Handbook of Chronic Pain Management*, BV, Elsevier Science.

Gil K. M., Williams D. A., Thompson R. J. and Kinney T. R. (1991) 'Sickle cell disease in children and adolescents: the relation of child and parent pain coping strategies to adjustment', *Journal of Pediatric Psychology* **16**(5): 643–63.

Good M. J. D., Brodwin P. E., Good B. J. and Kleinman A. (1992) *Pain as Human Experience. An Anthropological Perspective*, California, University of California Press.

Greipp M. E. (1988) 'Reflex sympathetic dystrophy syndrome in children', *Pediatric Nursing* **14**(5): 369–72.

Horn S. and Munafó M. (1997) *Pain. Theory, Research and Intervention*, Buckingham, Open University Press.

Knafl K. A., Ayres L., Gallo A. M., Zoeller L. H. and Breitmayer B. J. (1995) 'Learning from stories: parents' accounts of the pathway to diagnosis', *Pediatric Nursing* **21**(5): 411–15.

Kotchick B. A., Forehand R., Armistead L., Klein K. and Wierson M. (1996) 'Coping with illness: interrelationships across family members and predictors of psychological adjustment', *Journal of Family Psychology* **10**(3): 358–70.

Koval A. and Pritchard D. (1990) 'Psychological characteristics of children who suffer from headache: a research note', *Journal of Child Psychology and Psychiatry* **31**(4): 637–49.

McGrath P. J. and Humphreys P. (1989) 'Recurrent headaches in children and adolescents: diagnosis and treatment', *Pediatrician* **16**: 71–7.

McGrath P. J., Unruh A. M. and Branson S. M. (1990) 'Chronic nonmalignant pain with disability'. In Tyler D. C. and Krane E. J. (eds) *Advances in Pain Research Therapy*, vol. 15, New York, Raven Press.

Mathews J. R., McGrath P. J. and Pigeon H. (1993) 'Assessment and measurement of pain in children'. In Schechter N. L., Berde C. B. and Yaster M. (eds) *Pain in Infants, Children and Adolescents*, Baltimore, Williams & Wilkins.

Merskey H. and Bogduk N. (1994) *Classification of Chronic Pain*, 2nd edn, Seattle, IASP Task Force on Taxonomy, IASP Press.

Mikail S. and von Bayer C. (1990) 'Pain, somatic focus and emotional adjustment in children of chronic headache sufferers and controls', *Social Science Medicine* **31**: 51–9.

Nespor J. (1998) 'The meanings of research: kids as subjects and kids as inquirers', *Qualitative Inquiry* **4**(4): 369–88.

Page G. G. (1991) 'Chronic pain and the child with juvenile rheumatoid arthritis', *Journal of Pediatric Health Care* **5**: 18–23.

Rickard K. (1988) 'The occurrence of maladaptive health-related behaviors and teacher-rated conduct problems in children of chronic low back pain patients', *Journal of Behavioral Medicine* **11**: 107–16.

Robinson J. O., Alverez J. H. and Dodge J. A. (1990) 'Life events and family history in children with recurrent abdominal pain', *Journal of Psychosomatic Research* **34**(2): 171–80.

Roy R., Thomas M., Mogilevsky I. and Cook A. (1994) 'Influence of parental chronic pain on children: preliminary observations', *Headache Quarterly, Current Treatment and Research* **5**(1): 20–6.

Schechter N. L., Berde C. B. and Yaster M. (eds) (1993) *Pain in Infants, Children and Adolescents*, Baltimore, Williams & Wilkins.

Schulz M. S. and Masek B. J. (1996) 'Medical crisis intervention with children and adolescents with chronic pain', *Professional Psychology: Research and Practice* 27(2): 121–9.

Schwandt T. A. (1994) 'Constructivist, interpretivist approaches to human inquiry'. In Denzin N. K. and Lincoln Y. S. (eds) *Handbook of Qualitative Research*, Thousand Oaks, CA, Sage.

Segal-Andrews A. M., Alschuler S. M. and Harkness S. E. (1995) 'Chronic abdominal pain: treating the meaning of pain', *Family Systems Medicine* 13: 233–43.

Teasell R. W. (1997) 'The denial of chronic pain', *Pain Research and Management* 2(2). Located via Internet search at http://www.pulsus.com/pain/02_02/teas_ed.htm

Varni J. W., Rapoff M. A., Waldron S. A., Gragg R. A., Bernstein B. H. and Lindsley C. B. (1996) 'Chronic pain and emotional distress in children and adolescents', *Developmental and Behavioral Pediatrics* 17(3): 154–61.

Watt-Watson J. H., Evernden C. and Lawson C. (1990) 'Parents' perceptions of their child's acute pain experience', *Journal of Pediatric Nursing* 5(5): 344–9.

Zeltzer L. K. and Zeltzer P. M. (1989) 'Clinical assessment and pharmacologic treatment of pain in children: cancer as a model for the management of chronic or persistent pain', *Pediatrician* 16: 64–70.

21 *A collaborative approach to evidence-based child health nursing practice*

Sue Nagy

Introduction

Evidence from Australia, the UK and the USA suggests that while research output has increased, clinical nurses make limited use of the findings to improve patient care (Funk *et al.*, 1991; Stetler and DiMaggio, 1991; Capra *et al.*, 1992; Nagy *et al.*, 1992; Webb and Mackenzie, 1993; Pearcey, 1995).

Indeed, Baessler *et al.* (1994) found that research reported in professional journals was the *least common* method by which nurses obtained practice knowledge, patient information, personal experience, nursing school information and 'what has worked for years' being the *most common* methods.

The results of studies aimed at identifying factors that inhibit the development of evidence-based practice have suggested that the main problems seem to be that:

- clinical nurses have neither the time to locate research reports nor the skills to evaluate them
- they tend to regard many research reports as having limited relevance for clinical practice
- many nurses do not believe that they have the autonomy to incorporate research-based evidence into their patient care.

These problems may be overcome if all levels of child health nurse (clinicians, researchers, educators and managers) collaborate to advance evidence-based practice.

Nursing is, therefore, still a long way from the achievement of evidence-based practice. However, a failure to apply research findings to practice is not a problem confined to nursing. Concerns about research utilisation plague most of the practice professions, for example medicine (Haines and Jones, 1994), psychology (Simionato, 1991) and occupational therapy (Ottenbacher *et al.*, 1986).

The problems that practice professions encounter in accessing and using research literature centre around busy clinicians' lack of time to develop and maintain critiquing skills and to keep up with the sheer volume of research reports that are published each year. In nursing, additional problems include a limited amount of clinically relevant research and a failure of health care organisations to commit resources for the establishment of evidence-based nursing practice.

This chapter will outline an initiative designed to overcome the problems of implementing evidence-based practice in child health nursing. Based on a collaboration between nurses, this initiative aims to advance evidence-based nursing practice in Australian child health centres.

The aims of the chapter are:

- to examine the conditions that must exist for nurses to be able to apply research findings to their practice, and to evaluate the extent to which obstacles prevent these conditions being met
- to propose a model that will overcome such obstacles so that evidence-based clinical guidelines can be developed and implemented.

A number of studies in Australia (Wright *et al.*, 1996; Nagy *et al.*, 1997), the UK (Webb and Mackenzie, 1993; Pearcey, 1995) and North America (Funk *et al.*, 1991; Pettengill *et al.*, 1994) have surveyed nurses on the reasons why they do not apply the results of research to their practice. These studies have in general used large samples, and most have good response rates (Table 21.1). Furthermore, there has been remarkable consistency in the findings.

Table 21.1 Nurses' views of evidence-based practice in three countries

Investigators	Country	Sample child health nurses	Response rate %
Nagy *et al.* (1997)	Australia	267	65
Wright *et al.* (1996)	Australia	350	82
Hicks (1996)	UK	230	46
Pearcey (1995)	UK	398	67
Webb and Mackenzie (1993)	UK	94	not stated
Funk *et al.* (1991)	USA	1989	40
Pettengill *et al.* (1994)	USA	404	74

In the next section of this chapter, the findings of these studies are examined in order to evaluate the extent to which the conditions necessary for evidence-based practice are currently met within nursing, and to identify the factors that prevent these conditions being met.

Conditions necessary for nurses to be able to apply the findings of research to their practice

For evidence-based practice to be established, several conditions are necessary. First, a body of clinically relevant and rigorously conducted research must be available on which practice decisions can be based. Second, nurses must be aware of the potential for scientific evidence to contribute to patient care. Third, nurses must have the skills to locate and evaluate clinical research reports. Fourth, they must have time away from the patient's bedside to obtain, read and evaluate research reports. Finally, employing organisations must be prepared to commit the resources necessary for the implementation of evidence-based practice.

A body of clinically relevant research evidence

The body of nursing research has increased considerably in recent times. For example, in 1952, when the first edition of *Nursing Research* went to press in the USA, it was the only journal devoted to publishing research papers, and in that year only 14 studies were published. The 1985 edition of *Nursing Research* published 95 studies, and by this time there were also four other journals specialising in the publication of nursing research (Brown *et al.*, 1984). Since 1985, there has been an even greater proliferation of nursing research journals all over the world, several of which are now devoted specifically to child health nursing research. Especially encouraging is the publication of *Evidence-based Nursing*, a new journal that publishes abstracts and critiques of rigorously conducted and clinically relevant nursing research.

Child health nursing research is also increasing. In Australia, for example, the number of research papers presented to recent paediatric nursing conferences reflects a steady growth. At the conference convened by the Australian Council of Paediatric Nurses in 1990, for example, eight research papers were presented, which represented 22 per cent of the total number of papers. By 1994, the number had climbed to 24 research papers, representing 41 per cent of the total. This figure was maintained at the conference held in 1996, where 29 research reports were presented, representing 40 per cent of all papers.

For evidence-based practice to become widespread, nurses must have access to research that meets their clinical needs. While we can be encouraged by the growth of child health research, there also remain many areas of nursing practice for which there is no supporting evidence (MacGuire, 1990; Brown, 1995; Mulhall, 1995). We can not therefore, afford to become complacent about the kind of child health research that is currently being conducted.

A lack of clinical relevance of the existing research has been shown to be a problem for evidence-based child health nursing (Funk *et al.*, 1991; Hicks, 1996). In an Australian study conducted by the University of Western Sydney (Nagy *et al.*, 1997), as many as 80 per cent of Australian child health nurses have been found to believe that existing research has limited usefulness for clinical nursing decisions. These findings reflect the current situation in Australia, where research has tended to focus more on the development of nursing as an academic discipline than on solutions to problems faced by clinical nurses (Pearson *et al.*, 1997). It is now imperative that nursing turn its research efforts to the investigation of clinical problems in order to improve the delivery of nursing care. Such investigations are no less than can be expected of professional and accountable child health nurses.

To achieve these goals, mechanisms need to be set in place so that questions of clinical importance are identified and made readily available to researchers. These mechanisms require greater collaboration between clinical nurses and academic nurses than has been the case in the past.

Nurses' recognition of the potential for scientific evidence to contribute to patient care

The Australian studies and one British study (Pearcey, 1995) have reported that at least 80 per cent of nurses believed research to be a potentially important way of improving the quality of nursing care. An earlier study in the USA (Funk *et al.*, 1991) reported a figure of 65 per cent. These results demonstrate that, despite their misgivings about the clinical usefulness of much research, nurses are aware of the value of scientific research for patient care. We can no longer attribute the lack of evidence-based practice to clinical nurses' failure to value research. Instead, we have to look elsewhere for an explanation.

Nurses' skills in locating and evaluating clinical research reports

Clinical practice cannot be based on rigorously obtained evidence unless nurses have the skills and experience to conduct computerised searches, to locate the research reports in the library and to discriminate between good- and poor-quality research. Nurses must be aware of the need for further research when there are insufficient, inconclusive or conflicting results.

While nurses appear to be satisfied with their ability to locate research reports, data from the USA (Funk *et al.*, 1991) and Australia (Nagy *et al.*, 1997) show that most nurses (59 per cent in the USA and 64 per cent in Australia) are not confident about their ability to evaluate research reports. This work revealed that nurses were even less confident about their ability to interpret statistical results. The evaluation of research is an advanced skill that may begin in the classroom, but to be fully developed, additional assistance, such as continuing education, the accumulation of experience and the support of skilled mentors, is necessary.

Time available to obtain, read and evaluate research reports

Having the time to read and evaluate research reports and implement changes to practice is a continuing problem in nursing in both Australia and North America. A recent North American study (Pettengill *et al.*, 1994) found that lack of time was the strongest form of discouragement in the implementation of evidence-based practice. In addition, Nagy *et al.* (1997) found that 75 per cent of child health nurses regarded the volume of research reports as being too large to be able to maintain currency. Evidence-based practice can be advanced if nurses have some time free of patient care responsibilities to be able to read the literature. While this may be difficult to achieve in times of increasing health care costs, it is absolutely essential to the implementation of nursing care of the highest quality.

As most clinical nurses are required to spend 100 per cent of their working time with their patients, one solution is to use their off-duty time. Only 15 per cent of child health nurses surveyed in Nagy *et al.*'s (1997) study indicated that they were prepared to read and evaluate research reports in their off-duty hours. However, when they were asked about their willingness to do so if they were also able to use *on-duty* time, the percentage who were willing to contribute changed to 45 per cent.

These results suggest that many nurses are willing to put in personal time and effort to do the work necessary to support evidence-based practice. However, they also want the employing organisations to recognise that the delivery of professional nursing care (as with medical and allied health care) requires more than just attendance at the patient's bedside.

Organisational support to implement evidence-based practice

The support of organisational management is also necessary to foster a climate in which innovation is encouraged and nurses feel that they have the autonomy to make evidence-based changes (Lynn, 1990). Nagy *et al.* (1997) asked child health nurses in a specialist paediatric hospital to indicate who they thought would be supportive in upper and middle management. Nurse unit managers were seen as the most supportive group (endorsed by 54 per cent of respondents), followed by nursing administrators (44 per cent) and finally hospital senior management (18 per cent). These results are interesting considering that senior management at the same hospital had already committed a large amount of funds and resources for the advancement of evidence-based nursing practice. Perhaps these results are more of a reflection of the respondents' lack of personal knowledge of senior hospital managers than of any genuine lack of support. A similar situation has been noted by Funk *et al.* (1995), who found that clinical nurses did not view administrators as willing to support evidence-based practice. The administrators, however, saw themselves as being highly encouraging and supportive.

Pettengill *et al.* (1994) found that while having insufficient time was the greatest barrier, a lack of support from nursing administration was regarded as the next most discouraging factor in the application of research to practice. It is, therefore, important that senior managers not only commit resources to evidence-based practice, but must also be perceived by nurses to value innovative behaviour and unequivocally to recognise the autonomy of clinical nurses to incorporate the results of high-quality research into their practice.

Even when presented with research findings that have been clearly recommended, nurses have been reluctant to apply findings (Funk *et al.*, 1991; Capra *et al.*, 1992; McCurren, 1995). This reluctance often occurs because nurses do not believe that they have the power to make changes without approval from power holders within the organisation.

Summary

In summary, the evidence is that most nurses recognise the value of research for patient care but lack the resources necessary to implement evidence-based practice. In order to advance evidence-based practice, it is necessary:

• to identify areas in which evidence is non-existent, inconclusive or of little value
• to encourage and facilitate research in these areas
• to provide instruction and mentorship to enable nurses to develop fully their research evaluation skills
• to provide time away from the patients' bedside for nurses to locate and review research literature
• for management to both support, and be seen to support, evidence-based practice in their organisation.

An organisationally driven model for evidence-based nursing practice

There have been many models, strategies and plans designed to promote the use of research in nursing practice. Models include the Research Utilization Program (Funk *et al.*, 1989) and the Iowa Model of Research in Practice (Titler *et al.*, 1994) and strategies for the establishment of adjunct and joint appointments between universities and clinical institutions, as well as the improved education of nurses in the importance and use of research (see also Janken *et al.*, 1988; Umlauf and Gray, 1991; Grinspun *et al.*, 1993; Barnsteiner *et al.*, 1995; Dufault, 1995). Despite these initiatives, we still can not claim that our practice is based on empirical research.

Many previous models have focused primarily on the individual nurse rather than co-ordinating efforts throughout the organisation (for example, Hunt, 1987; Brown, 1995). These attempts tend to have a 'hit-and-miss' quality that depends on individuals having the skills and time to access and evaluate reports, and on the extent of their confidence in their own decisions. The research reviewed in this chapter suggests that formal mechanisms co-ordinated at organisational level and including continuing education are those most likely to be successful. Kitson (1996: p. 432) accurately identified a major problem when she argued that:

> Action emerging from informal attempts to change practice may be unsystematic, poorly thought through and neither contribute to a deeper understanding of the intervention being investigated nor the process of introducing that change.

The Royal Alexandra Hospital for Children model for evidence-based practice

The Royal Alexandra Hospital for Children in Sydney, Australia, is currently establishing organisationally co-ordinated centres for evidence-based paediatric practice in nursing and medicine. Similar centres are planned for allied health and management.

The Centre for Evidence-based Paediatric Practice-Nursing (CEPP-N) is based on a model that has the capacity to involve the collaboration of *all* nursing staff within the organisation. The aim of the CEPP-N is to co-ordinate the combined efforts of the hospital nursing staff in achieving evidence-based practice. The CEPP-N works closely with two hospital committees: the Clinical Practice Committee, which oversees all nursing clinical issues, and the Policy and Procedure Committee, which is responsible for writing clinical policies and guidelines.

The model consists of two parallel processes: (a) the writing of systematic reviews with recommendations for the development of evidence-based clinical guidelines, and (b) the continuing education of all nurses in the organisation in the evaluation of research reports and in the implementation of new evidence-based clinical guidelines (Figure 21.1). In the next section, details of the way in which the model operates are described.

The parallel processes of evaluation and education

Clinical topics are selected on which systematic reviews and evidence-based guidelines are to be written (Figure 21.1). These topics are selected jointly by the hospital's Clinical Practice Committee and the staff of the CEPP-N. All the nursing staff are encouraged to express their views to members of these committees regarding priorities for topics to be investigated. Topics may focus on nursing procedures (for example, the delivery of oxygen therapy), the

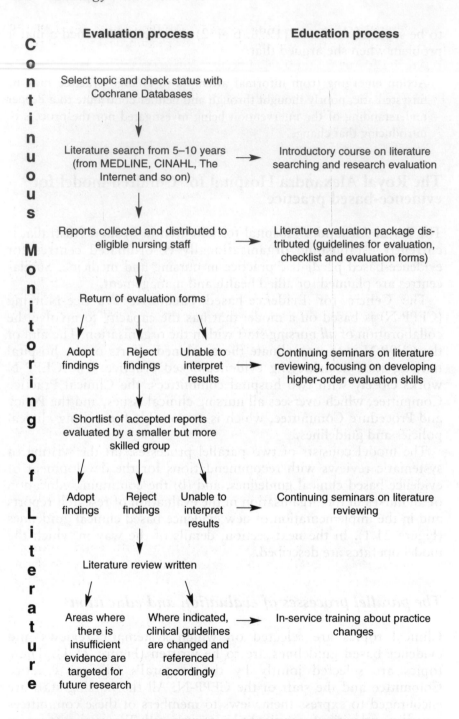

Figure 21.1   Royal Alexandra Hospital for Children model
for the adoption of evidence-based practice

management of clinical problems (for example, nappy rash) or the care of children with a specific disorder (for example, cystic fibrosis) or group of disorders (for example, neoplastic disease).

Once a topic has been selected, checks are then made with databases such as the Cochrane Collaboration and the York Centre for Reviews and Dissemination to locate any similar or related reviews. In cases where such reviews exist, the results are incorporated into the recommended guidelines. However, while the Cochrane Collaboration reviews only randomised controlled trials, the CEPP-N reviews all research designs.

The review process commences with a thorough search for published and unpublished research literature. The collected research reports are distributed to all staff who have been through an accreditation process. Accreditation as a 'novice evaluator' requires the completion of an introductory course on research evaluation. It is intended that all registered nurses employed in the hospital will ultimately complete the introductory course. In this way, the burden of literature evaluation will be spread among all the nurses. As staff become more skilled, they may complete advanced courses and become accredited at higher levels.

Novice evaluators provide the first line of evaluation. They read reports and make recommendations about the usefulness of the findings based on the presence or absence of major design flaws. Reports that survive this evaluation round are referred to 'advanced evaluators' for a second round.

A literature evaluation package is also distributed to each evaluator. This package consists of a set of guidelines for evaluation, an evaluation checklist and forms on which evaluators can write their evaluations. Completed evaluation forms are returned to the CEPP-N. The evaluation forms ask reviewers to select from three possible review outcomes:

1. That the research was conducted in a sufficiently rigorous manner for the findings to be recommended for adoption. Evaluators are required to describe the strengths of the research methods that lead to their recommendation.

2. That the research contained sufficient flaws for doubt to be thrown on the usefulness of the findings. Evaluators are required to describe the nature of these flaws. Such articles are not subjected to further consideration but are documented in the completed literature review.

3. That the reviewer did not have the skills necessary for this particular report. In this case, evaluators are required to indicate

the areas of the report where they encountered a problem. Ways of handling such problems are then addressed in future evaluation seminars and thereby become part of the continuing education process.

The resulting shortlist of reports is further reviewed by evaluators who have been accredited at a higher level. The outcomes of this round of evaluations are the same as those used for the previous round of reviews.

When all the reports have been evaluated, the CEPP-N staff write a literature review that includes recommendations for changes to clinical guidelines, references to support these changes and, where there is insufficient evidence to guide practice, suggestions for topics for future research. The identification of such topics should help researchers to focus on questions that are both clinically relevant and of a high priority.

The CEPP-N staff provide in-service sessions to inform nursing staff of the changes to clinical guidelines and the associated systematic literature review. As each literature review is completed, the CEPP-N continues to monitor that literature and to update reviews and associated guidelines as new evidence becomes available.

Conclusion

The central position in this chapter is that, irrespective of the discipline, evidence-based practice cannot become a reality if the responsibility for it remains only at the level of the individual practitioner. Evidence-based practice can best be promoted when it is undertaken as a co-ordinated effort at the organisational level. As the CEPP-N becomes fully established, links will be made with other national and international child health centres in order to instigate collaboration in order to reduce duplication of effort in producing evidence-based clinical guidelines. While the CEPP-N focuses on the organisation, it is not limited to it.

The model described in this paper addresses most of the barriers to evidence-based practice that have been identified in the literature. It provides for all nurses in an organisation to be involved in the reviewing of literature, thereby reducing the workload on individual nurses. This model also gives considerable emphasis to the development of educational processes and to the identification of priorities for child health nursing research.

The CEPP-N is part of a larger plan in the Royal Alexandra Hospital for Children for centres of evidence-based practice in nursing, medicine, allied health and management. The centres for nursing and medicine are currently being established; those for allied health and management are planned. It is expected that such a network will ensure that practice at the Royal Alexandra Hospital will be based on multidisciplinary co-operation and empirical evidence.

References

Baessler C .A., Blumberg M., Cunningham J. S. *et al.* (1994) 'Medical-surgical nurses' utilization of research methods and products', *MEDSURG Nursing* 3: 113–14.

Barnsteiner J., Ford N. and Howe C. (1995) 'Research utilization in a metropolitan children's hospital', *Nursing Clinics of North America* 30: 447–55.

Brown G. (1995) 'Understanding the barriers to basing nursing practice upon research: a communication model approach', *Journal of Advanced Nursing* 21: 154–7.

Brown J. S., Tanner C. A. and Padrick K. P. (1984) 'Nursing's search for scientific knowledge', *Nursing Research* 33: 26–32.

Capra M., Houghton S. and Hattie J. (1992) 'RNs' utilisation of research findings', *Australian Journal of Advanced Nursing* 16: 21–5.

Dufault M. (1995) 'A collaborative model for research development and utilization', *Journal of Nursing Staff Development* 11: 139–44.

Funk S. G., Tornquist E. M. and Champagne M. T. (1989) 'A model for improving the dissemination of nursing research', *Western Journal of Nursing Research* 11: 361–7.

Funk S. G., Champagne M. T., Wiese R. A. and Tornquist E. M. (1991) 'Barriers to using research findings in practice: the clinician's perspective', *Applied Nursing Research* 4: 90–5.

Funk S. G., Champagne M. T., Tornquist E. M. and Wiese R. (1995) 'Administrators' views on barriers to research utilization', *Applied Nursing Research* 8: 44–9.

Grinspun D., Macmillan K., Nichol H. and Shields-Poe D. (1993) 'Using research findings in the hospital', *Canadian Nurse* Jan.: 46–8.

Haines A. and Jones R. (1994) 'Implementing findings of research', *British Medical Journal* 308: 1488–92.

Hicks C. (1996) 'A study of nurses' attitudes towards research: a factor analytic approach', *Journal of Advanced Nursing* 23: 373–9.

Hunt M. (1987) 'The process of translating research findings into nursing practice', *Journal of Advanced Nursing* 6: 189–94.

Janken J. K., Dufault M. A. and Yeaw E. M. S. (1988) 'Research round tables: increasing student/staff awareness of the relevancy of research to practice', *Journal of Professional Nursing* 4: 186–91.

Kitson A. (1996) 'From research to practice: one organizational model for promoting research-based practice', *Journal of Advanced Nursing* 23: 430–40.

Lynn M. R. (1990) 'Research commitment starts at the top', *Journal of Pediatric Nursing* 5: 136–7.

McCurren C. D. (1995) 'Research utilization: meeting the challenge', *Geriatric Nursing* 16: 132–5.

MacGuire J. (1990) 'Putting research findings into practice: research utilization as an aspect of the management of change', *Journal of Advanced Nursing* 15: 614–20.

Mulhall A. (1995) 'Nursing research: what difference does it make?', *Journal of Advanced Nursing* 21: 576–83.

Nagy S., Crisp J. and Brodie L. (1992) 'Journal reading practices of RNs in NSW Public Hospitals', *Australian Journal of Advanced Nursing* 9: 29–33.

Nagy S., Lumby S., McKinley S. and Macfarlane C. (1997) 'Paediatric nurses' use of research findings'. Unpublished report, Sydney, University of Western Sydney, Nepean.

Ottenbacher K. J., Barris R. and Van Deusen J. (1986) 'Some issue related to research utilisation in occupational therapy', *American Journal of Occupational Therapy* 40: 111–16.

Pearcey P. A. (1995) 'Achieving research-based nursing practice', *Journal of Advanced Nursing* 22: 33–9.

Pearson A., Borbasi S., Fitzgerald M., Kowanko I. and Walsh K. (1997) 'Evidence based nursing: an examination of the role of nursing within the international evidence based health care practice movement'. Discussion paper No. 1, ACT, Canberra, Royal College of Nursing.

Pettengill M. M., Gillies D. A. and Clark C. C. (1994) 'Factors encouraging and discouraging the use of nursing research findings', *Image: Journal of Nursing Scholarship* 26: 143–7.

Simionato R. (1991) 'The link between empirical research, epistemic values, and psychological practice', *Australian Psychologist* 26: 123–7.

Stetler C. B. and DiMaggio G. (1991) 'Research utilization among clinical nurse specialists', *Clinical Nurse Specialist* 5: 151–5.

Titler M. G., Kleiber C., Steelman V. *et al.* (1994) 'Infusing research into practice to promote quality care', *Nursing Research* 43: 307–13.

Umlauf M. G. and Gray A. (1991) 'Building a model for utilizing nursing research in the clinical setting', *Gerontology and Geriatrics Education* 12: 93–103.

Webb C. and Mackenzie, J. (1993) 'Where are we now? Research mindedness in the 1990s', *Journal of Clinical Nursing* 2: 129–33.

Wright A., Brown P. and Sloman R. (1996) 'Nurses' perceptions of the value of nursing research for practice', *Australian Journal of Advanced Nursing* 13: 15–18.

Index

A

A&E departments
  accident prevention role 144–5
  children attending 128
  nurses in 144
  nurses' qualifications 143
ability, to use evidence 49–50
academic aspirations 8–9
access to evidence 48–9, 50–1
  see also journals
accidents
  accident prevention strategies
    128–9, 140–2
  definition 131–2
  factors influencing 129–30
  gender and social class 129–30
  Injury Minimisation Programme
    141
  statistics 129–30
accident surveillance study 128–47
  accident statistics 129–30
  age groups of participants 135
  aim of study 128
  background literature 129–32
  bias prevention 139–40
  conclusion 145–6
  consent to research 134
  data collection 130–1
    procedure 133–4
    structured interviews 139,
      142
    structured questionnaire 133
  discussion 138–45
    accident prevention
      strategies 140–2
    implications for nursing
      practice 142–5
    limitations of study 138–40
    methodological issues
      138–40

  ethical considerations 134
  ethnic origin of participants 136
  future developments 146
  methodology 133–4
  objectives of study 132
  post-accident support visits 143
  research question 132
  results 135–8
    accident details 136–8
    analysis 135
    demographic and social
      information 135–6
  sampling 133–4
acetaminophen, *see* paracetamol
acetanilid 266
Achieving Effective Practice (NHS
  directive) 1
acquired immune deficiency
  syndrome, *see* HIV/AIDS
Action for Sick Children 166
Added Power and Understanding in
  Sex Education, *see* A PAUSE
adolescent patients
  popularity/unpopularity of
    249–50, 255
  standards for 250
adolescent sexual activity 205–6
adolescent sexual health 185–202
  literature review 187–8
    acquiring sexual health
      knowledge and skills 187
    professionals' role in
      education 188
    rational decision making *v.*
      self-efficacy 187–8
  need for promotion of 186
  research study 188–99
    aims of study 188–9
    bias 190
    'bracketing' 189
    conclusion 198–9

contraception 193, 208
data analysis 191
discussion 195–8
findings 191–4
GPs and family planning
    clinic consultations 192
implications for practice
    195–8
methodology 190–1
nurses' role 190–1, 193–4,
    197–8
pilot study 190
relationship skills 192–3
sample 189
sexual knowledge learning
    process 191–2, 195–6
sexual self-efficacy 192–3,
    196–7, 209
adult intensive care units (AICUs)
    225
    paediatric training 235
adult patients, popularity of 244
advocacy 5, 9, 10, 29, 160
    school nurses 122
AIDS, *see* HIV/AIDS
anatomy, children's knowledge of,
    research study 148–62, 168
    background 148
    conclusions 160
    consent to research 153
    data analysis 156–7
    discussion 157–9
    ethical considerations 153
    limitations of study 159–60
    literature review 148–52
    methodology 152–6
        grid scoring system 155–6
        projective drawing method
            153, 154, 159
        prompted technique 153,
            154–5
        unprompted technique 153,
            154
    recommendations 160
    results 156–7
    sampling 152

antibiotics, *see* intravenous
    antibiotic administration
antipyretics 262–3, 264, 265, 269,
    281
    administration to comply with
        parents' wishes 270
    nurse education in use of 282
    in prevention of febrile
        convulsions 270–2
    see also paracetamol
A PAUSE (Added Power and
    Understanding in Sex
    Education) 195, 203–23
    adult/peer-led partnerships
        219–20
    background 204–10
    future developments 218–20
    future funding 219
    recommendations 218–20
    research project 210–12
        results 210–12
    service provision 212–18
        extension of service 212
        facilitators 213–15
        funding 212
        gender balance 216
        peer-led sessions 216–18
        programme content 212–13
        role of school nurse 213,
            214–15, 218, 220
    see also sex education
arachidonic acid 263
aspirin 266, 268
assessment
    clinical/academic staff roles
        15–18
    Research Assessment Exercise
        43
    of theory, grid of marking
        criteria 19
    see also clinical assessment
Australian Council of Paediatric
    Nurses, conference 384
autonomy, in use of evidence 50

B

BA (Hons) in Paediatric Nursing,
  see nursing graduates
bathing, tepid/warm 271, 282
Bayer (pharmaceutical company) 9
body temperature
  bathing and sponging to reduce
    271, 282
  circadian rhythms 266, 278
  in febrile convulsions 270–2
  in fever 265–6
  thermoregulation 263–4
bradykinin 268
A Bridge to the Future 224, 232
Bristol Children's Hospital 4
British Journal of Nursing 43
British Medical Journal 112
British Paediatric Association (BPA)
    112
  dependency level definitions 241
  survey and report on intensive
    care 224, 227
Brook Advisory Service 215

C

care
  client-centred 26, 30–2, 33,
    37–8
  documentation of 21–2
'care by nursing' (CBN) units 69
'care by parent' (CBP) units 69, 70
Care of Critically Ill Children (BPA
    report) 227
caring, *v.* research 3
Center for Disease Control, USA 10
Centre for Evidence-based
  Paediatric Practice Nursing
  (CEPP-N) 389–93
*Child: Care Growth and
  Development* 47
Child Health in the Community
  (DoH report) 164, 325

children
  competent decision-makers on
    own health 124
  passive subjects or social actors?
    110–13
  see also views of children on
    local health services
Children Act 1989 112, 149
Children's Charter *(Patient's
  Charter: Services for Children
  and Young People)* 112, 149,
  163, 164, 322, 325
chronic pain, research study
  359–81
  aims of study 366
  background 359
  conclusions 377–9
  coping strategies 373–4
  data analysis 368–70
  data collection 368
  definition 360–1
  ethical considerations 367
  findings 370–7
    child's and family's concerns
      370–2
    conclusion 365
    dealing with pain 373–5
    experience of pain 372–3
    interfacing with
      professionals 376–7
    social context 375
    stress 371, 372
  literature review 360–5
    approaches to care and
      management 364–5
    background issues 360
    defining chronic pain 360–1
    key areas 360
    meaning of pain and child's
      attributes 362–3
    modelling and familial
      patterns 363–4
    models of chronic pain
      361–2
    triggers and journeys 364

methodology 365–8
  methodological approaches
    366
  stages of study 367
models of chronic pain 361–2,
  370
pain process, initiation *v.*
  maintenance 361
recommendations for
  professionals 378–9
restrictions created by 373–5
sample 366–7
statement of intent 365
CINAHL 61
circadian rhythms 266, 277–8
client-centred care 26, 30–2, 33,
  37–8
clinical assessment 16
  collecting evidence 19–24
  commentary in practice 20–1
  conclusion 54–5
  critical incident analysis 20
  data sources 19
  discussion of practice in general
    22–3
  documentation of care 21–2
  incessant? 22
  'inform-change-monitor' 18
  means of 18–19
  observation of nurse in practice
    22
  outcomes 23–4
  reflective diary extracts 21
  tripartite relationship 13, 15–18
  written evidence 23
clinical governance 1, 4, 39
clinical nurse teachers 15
clinics, for teenagers 125
Cochrane Centre database 22, 48,
  61, 391
cognition, hypothetico-deductive
  model 309
commentary in practice 20–1
communication
  in discharge planning 326–7
  in local health services,
    children's views on 115–17

see also information *entries*
community care, decision making
  in transfer from hospital to
  home care, *see* decision analysis
community practice teachers 15–16
conferences
  Australian Council of Paediatric
    Nurses 384
  International Evidence-based
    Child Health Nursing
    Conference 2
consent, to research 7, 10, 134,
  153
  proxy consent 7, 10–11
continuous negative extra thoracic
  pressure (CNEP) ventilators 10
contraception 193, 208
coping strategies
  in chronic pain 373–4
  mothers of children in intensive
    care units 92
counselling
  medical crisis counselling
    (MCC) 365
  for parents and nurses of
    children in intensive care
    units 104–5
Court Report 324
critical incident analysis 20
critically ill children
  transport of 228
  see also intensive care; intensive
    care units
cryogens 263, 264
cystic fibrosis, *see* intravenous
  antibiotic administration

D

Database of Abstracts of Reviews
  of Effectiveness (DARE) 61
data collection
  for clinical assessment 19–24
  see also under individual studies
decision analysis
  applications 310

assumptions 316–18
cognitive process continuum
    308
concept map 309
decision flow diagram 311
limitations 316–18
model and process 310–12
sensitivity analysis 317
in transfer from hospital to
    home care 306–21
    aim of decision analysis 312
    background 306–7
    case example 312–16
    clinical judgements 308–9
    iatrogenic morbidity 313–14
    implications for practice
        318–19
    maximum expected utility
        (MEU) 315–16
    objectives of decision
        analysis 312
    stages in decision analysis
        312–16
    variables affecting decision-
        making process 308–10
decision making, on basis of
    evidence 49–50
Declaration of Helsinki 7
dependency level definitions 241
depression, in mothers of children
    in intensive care units 99–100,
    105
Descriptive Phenomenology model
    350
diabetes, PDSN role evaluation
    285–305
    age-banded education sessions
        300–1
        discussion 300–1
        evaluation approach 300
        evaluation results 300–1
    aim of hospital service 285
    background 285–7
    clinic attendance 297–300
        clinic reminder cards 298,
            299

discussion 299–300
evaluation approach 298
evaluation results 298–9
non-attendance (DNA) rate
    298, 299–300
teenagers' questionnaire on
    service 300
conclusion 301–2
home management for newly
    diagnosed children 287–94
    advantages 287–8, 293
    availability of community
        services 287
    background 287–8
    clinical condition at
        presentation 293–4
    cost effectiveness 287, 292–3
    dietary education 289
    discussion 292–4
    emergency on-call service
        289
    evaluation approach 290
    evaluation results 290–1
    family education 288–9, 296
    information booklets 289
    practical skills for families
        288, 289
readmission of children with
    established diabetes 294–7
    discussion 296–7
    evaluation approach 294
    evaluation results 294–6
    psychological support 297
    psychosocial issues 296–7
recommendations for practice
    302
role justification objectives 286
diazepam 272
*Discharge of Patients from
    Hospital* (DoH report) 324,
    334–5
discharge planning, research study
    322–45
    aims of study 323, 331
    conclusions 338–41
    cultural aspects 337

data analysis 333
documentation in discharge
    planning process 338–9
DoH recommendations for
    discharge procedure 324,
    334–5
ethical considerations 333
findings and discussion 333–8
    factors influencing discharge
        planning 335, 336
    information leaflets 335–6
literature review 323–31
    communication 326–7
    co-ordinating discharge and
        continuing care 330–1
    early discharge and hospital
        costs 325
    historical overview 323–5
    psychological issues 328–9
    teaching 327–8
methodology 331–3
objectives of study 332
questionnaire 332, 342–4
recommendations for clinical
    practice 338–41
responsibility for 334, 335, 338
sample 332–3
success criteria 330–1
see also under decision analysis
discourse analysis 350
discussion, of practice in general
    22–3
distress, idioms of 362
doctors *v.* nurses, children's views
    122–3, 124
documentation of care 21–2
drop-in clinics 125
Dunblane massacre 10

E

Economic and Social Research
    Council 111

education
    curriculum development model
        51–4
    in making judgements/decisions
        49–50
    mandatory research modules 6
    post-registration 6
    pre-registration programme
        aims 39
    promoting evidence-based care
        through 51–4
    see also higher education
Education Act 1993, sex education
    191
empowerment 164
ENB Open Learning Pack 197
enjoyment of nurses in caring, *see*
    popularity of child patients
environment, influencing nurses'
    approaches to care 29
ethics
    ethical dimensions of research
        9–10
    unethical HIV drug trials 10
    see also consent; *and under*
        individual studies
evidence-based medicine, definition
    2
Evidence-based Nursing 44, 384
evidence-based nursing practice
    clinical assessment, *see* clinical
        assessment
    collaborative approach 382,
        389, 392, 393
    conclusion 392–3
    conditions for applications of
        research findings to practice
        384–8
        clinically relevant research
            evidence 384–5
        decision to use evidence
            48–50
        locating and evaluating
            research reports, skills
            for 386

organisational support 387–8
recognition of potential of
    evidence 385
summary 388
time availability 386–7
implementation 55, 382–94
nurses' views 383
organisationally driven model
    388–9
reasons for non-development of
    382
research problems 59–60
research questions 59
Royal Alexandra Hospital
    model 389–93
    evaluation and education
        processes 389–92
sources of practice knowledge
    382

F

families
    family needs v. research 9
    nurses' partnerships with
        254–5, 257–8
    unpopular parents 257, 258
    see also parents
family planning clinics 125
febrile convulsions
    antipyretics in prevention of
        270–2
    body temperature in 270–2
    management strategies 262
    paracetamol administration to
        prevent 280
    see also fever *entries*
fever
    body temperature in 265–6
    definitions 263, 276–8
        inconsistencies in 266,
            276–8
    endotoxin-induced 266–7
    interpretation of 265–6, 281–2
    nature of 263–5

positive immunological role
    262, 264, 265, 281
signs and symptoms 277
see also febrile convulsions
fever, nurses' management of,
    research study 262–84
conclusion 281–2
findings 276–80
    administration of
        paracetamol to prevent
        febrile seizures 280
    fever definitions 276–8
    reasons for administration of
        paracetamol 273, 274,
        279–80
    understanding of
        paracetamol action 278
implications for clinical practice
    280–1
literature review 263–72
    antipyretics in prevention of
        febrile convulsions 270–2
    interpretation of fever
        265–6, 280–1
    nature of fever 263–5
    paracetamol action 266–8
    paracetamol because of
        parents' wishes 270
    paracetamol to provide
        comfort 268–9
methodology 272–6
    triangulation 274
purpose of study 262
questionnaire 273, 274

G

Getting Evidence into Practice
    (NHS bulletin) 11
Gillick competence 7, 10
Gillick judgement 148
Graduate Diploma in Child Health
    Nursing 14
graduate level practice 13
    level 3 practice 19

nature of 19
need for nursing as graduate
    activity 14–15
tripartite relationship 13, 15–18
see also nursing graduates
Grantham and Kesteven General
    Hospital 3

H

Health of the Nation
    accidents as target area 128,
        129, 130
    sexual health strategy 206
health services
    clinics for teenagers 125
    views of children, *see* views of
        children on local health
        services
Health Visitors' Association 112
higher education
    academic aspirations 8–9
    legacy of graduate training 26,
        27
    move into 1, 3, 5
    nursing integrated into 9
    programmes of study 13–14
    shift from teaching into research
        5
    see also education; nursing
        graduates
Higher Education Quality Council
    19
HIV, unethical drug trials 10
HIV/AIDS 204
Home Accidents Surveillance
    System 130–1
home care 309–10
    family concerns 348
    v. hospital care, cost-
        effectiveness 325
    transfer from hospital, *see*
        decision analysis

home care schemes
    advantages and disadvantages
        347–8
    evolution of 347
homosexuality 218
hospitals
    'care by nursing' (CBN) units
        69
    'care by parent' (CBP) units 69,
        70
    changing nature of admissions
        325
    children's concepts of 167–9
    discharge, *see* discharge
        planning
    home care *v.* hospital care, cost-
        effectiveness 325
    preparation for, *see* information
        leaflets *entries*
    see also parental participation in
        care of hospitalised children
human immunodeficiency virus, *see*
    HIV/AIDS
hyperalgesia 268
hypothetico-deductive model of
    cognition 309

I

iatrogenic morbidity 313–14
ibuprofen 262, 266, 278–9, 282
    v. paracetamol 267–8
idioms of distress 362
illness, children's
    conceptions/misconceptions of
        167–9
implementation, of evidence-based
    practice 55, 382–94
inclination, to use evidence 48
information accessibility in local
    health services 121–2
    need for 124–5
    see also communication; *and*
        information leaflets *entries*

information leaflets/booklets 50
  burns and scalds 326–7
  for diabetes management 289
  on discharge from hospital
      335–6
  intravenous antibiotic
      administration 354
information leaflets, in preparing
  children for hospital admission,
  research study 163–84
  aim of study 169
  average reading age 176
  background 163–4
  conclusion 182
  discussion 180
  implications for clinical practice
      181–2
  leaflets
      design and content 169–71,
          172–5, 177, 178–9
      evaluation 172
      parent views 176–80
      piloting 172
      readability 171–2
      SMOG testing 175
      specifically for children? 181
  limitations of study 180–1
  literature review 164–9
      children's concepts of
          hospital and illness 167–9
      information giving 164–5
      information leaflets/booklets
          166, 167, 169
      parental dissatisfaction with
          information provision
          165–6
      preparing children 166–7
      who prepares children? 169
  methodology 169
  needs assessment 171, 175
  pilot study 176
  recommendations for clinical
      practice 181–2
  results 177–80
      age group suitability 179–80
      leaflet content 178–9

  leaflet design 177
  parents' preparation
      methods 179
  sample characteristics 177
'inform-change-monitor' 18
informed consent, *see* consent
Injury Minimisation Programme 141
intensive care, provision and
  outcome, research study 224–43
  aims of study 231
  background 224–5
  conclusion 240
  design of study 238–9
  literature review 225–7
  methodology 228–31
  mortality risk 227, 233–5
  objectives 232
  outcome evaluation 228–31
  outcome measures 231
  pilot study 233–5
  questions to be considered 232
  research questions 231
  sample 235–7
      inclusion criteria 236–7,
          237, 241
  tertiary care units 224, 226,
      227, 228
  time schedule 239
intensive care units, mothers of
  children in, research study
  90–109
  aim of study 92–3
  'burnt-out' nurses 103, 105
  care and treatment information
      96
  concern for the child 96–7
      altered body image 97
      environment 97
      fear of death or permanent
          brain damage 96–7
  conclusion 107
  coping, *see* support and coping
      below
  counselling for parents and
      nurses 104–5
  critical illness 91

discussion of fears with nurses
    97
findings
    discussion of 93–104
    summary of 103–4
impact on mothers 95
implications for nursing practice
    104–5
implications for nursing
    research 105–6
initial experience 94
initial shock and crisis 94
initial stabilisation 95
    availability of nurse for
        parents 104, 105
literature review 91–2
methodology 93
parent as carer 96–7, 100
perception of doctors 103
perception of nursing 100–3
    befriending 102
    competent care 101–2
    humour 102–3
    individualised nursing care
        101
    mothers' perceptions of
        nurses 102
    parental education 102
research questions 90, 92–3
stress and stressors 92, 95
support and coping 98–100
    coping strategies 92
    depression 99–100, 105
    impact on the family 98–9
    siblings 98
waiting and reflecting 94–5
International Evidence-based Child
    Health Nursing Conference 2
*International Journal of Nursing
    Studies* 43
intravenous antibiotic
    administration at home in cystic
    fibrosis, research study 346–58
    aim of study 347
    background 346–7
    conclusions 355–6

findings 350–5
    advantages/
        disadvantages for
        families 352–4
    flexibility between home and
        hospital treatment 355
    initial experiences 351
    normality and control 352–4
    parental concerns 351, 355
    Port-a-cath 352, 356
    training and support for
        parents 354–5, 355, 356
    further research 356–7
    literature review 347–8
    methodology 348–50
        data collection and analysis
            350
        design 348–9
        informed consent 349
        sample 349
        setting 349
        subjects 350
    recommendations for practice
        355–6
Iowa Model of Research in Practice
    388

J

Joseph Rowntree Foundation 111
Journal of Advanced Nursing 43,
    44, 47
*Journal of Child and Family
    Nursing* 44
Journal of Child Health Care 47
Journal of Clinical Nursing 43
*Journal of Pediatric Oncology
    Nursing* 43
journals
    academic 43, 44
    clinical 43
    evidence available in 46–8
    evidence-based 43–4
    nursing journals 43–51
    on-line access 49

role in promoting evidence-
    based care 42–56
weekly magazines 43
see also individual journal titles
juvenile rheumatoid arthritis (JRA)
    362–3

L

language, overcomplicated
    terminology 116–17
leaflets, *see* information leaflets
lecturer practitioners 1, 5, 15
Local Government Act 1988 218
Local Voices 112

M

manifest analysis 350
Marc goes to Hospital (film) 166
mastery experience model 196
medical crisis counselling (MCC)
    365
medication
    form of 116
    UKCC standards for
        administration of 278
medicine/nursing overlap 45
MEDLINE 61
menarche, age of 204–5
Mengele, Dr Josef 9
Mental Health Practice 43
mothers, *see* intensive care units,
    mothers of children in

N

named nurse 253
National Institute for Clinical
    Excellence 4
NHS, key targets 340

NHS Centre for Reviews and
    Dissemination 11, 61, 145, 203,
    391
Nightingale, Florence 2–3
Nuremberg trials 7, 10
nurses
    v. doctors, children's views
        122–3, 124
    named nurse 253
    see also school nurses
nursing graduates, research study
    26–41
    ability to challenge *status quo*
        34, 35–6, 38, 39
    acquisition of practical skills 33,
        35, 36
    assimilation and shaping of
        beliefs and values 30–3
    background 27–8
    conclusion 38–9
    data analysis 29–30
    discussion 38–9
    impressions of being graduates
        34–6
    influence of preparation for
        practice 30–3
    literature review 28–9
    main themes 30–8
    methodology 29–30
    practice styles 37–8
    usefulness of theoretical basis of
        course 32–3
    see also graduate level practice;
        higher education
nursing/medicine overlap 45
nursing profession, academic
    aspirations 8–9
nursing research, paucity of 2
Nursing Research 384
nursing roles, expanded 2–3
nursing/social work overlap 45
Nursing Standard 43
Nursing Times 43, 44

O

observation, as data collection
    technique 22
outcomes, in clinical assessment
    23–4
outreach clinics 125

P

paediatric diabetes specialist nurse
    (PDSN) role, *see* diabetes,
    PDSN role evaluation
*Paediatric Intensive Care: A
    Framework for the Future* 224,
    224–5, 232
paediatric intensive care units
    (PICUs) 224, 227
    definition 225
    see also intensive care; intensive
        care units
paediatric nursing
    applicability of other disciplines'
        research to 48
    definition 45
    focus of 46
    overlap with other disciplines
        45
Paediatric Nursing 43, 47
paediatric nursing research
    access to evidence 48–9, 50–1
    decision to use evidence 48–50
    defining the evidence base 45–6
    see also journals
pain
    organic/non-organic 361
    see also chronic pain
pain disease 362
pain families 363–4
pain illness 362
painkillers 374
pain management 45–6, 373–4
    pharmacological/non-
        pharmacological 364–5

RCN guidelines for pain
    recognition and assessment
    50
paracetamol 262–3
    administration of
        to comply with parents'
            wishes 270
        by nurses, questionnaire
            274, 275, 279–80
        to prevent febrile seizures
            280
        to provide comfort 268–9
        reasons for 273, 274,
            279–80
        routes of administration 267
    v. ibuprofen 267–8
    physiological action 266–8
    in reducing temperature 281–2
    understanding of
        pharmacodynamic action
        274–5, 278
    see also antipyretics
parental participation in care of
    hospitalised children, research
    review 57–89
    advantages/disadvantages 58,
        67, 70
    conclusions 73
    data extraction 63
    discharge decisions 307,
        309–10, 315, 318
    discussion 70–3
    effect on children 69–70, 71–2,
        84–6
        emotional and physical
            wellbeing 70, 84–6
    effect on parents 58–9, 65–9,
        70–1, 74–83
        control and decision making
            67, 74–83
        emotional status 68–9,
            74–83
        knowledge and competence
            67–8, 74–83
        roles and relationships 66–7,
            74–83

ethnic minorities 72, 73
literature review 58–61
  exclusion criteria 63
  inclusion criteria 62–3
  journals searched 62
  methods 61–3
overview of studies 74–86
  effects on children 84–6
  effects on parents 74–83
parents' role, nurses' *v.* parents'
  expectations of 66
participants' characteristics
  64–5
participation defined 57
promotion of 58–9
research question 60–1
research studies 57–89
results 64–70
study characteristics 64
Parental Stressor Scale 92
parents
  'care by parent' (CBP) units 69,
    70
  parental dissatisfaction with
    information provision 165–6
  unpopular 257, 258
  see also families; intensive care
    units; and parental
    participation *entries*
*Patient Partnership: Building a
Collaborative Strategy* 112
Patient's Charter 112
on patient information 172
*Patient's Charter: Services for
Children and Young People*
(Children's Charter) 112, 149,
163, 164, 322, 325
Pediatric Cerebral Performance
Category (PCPC) 231, 236
Pediatric Index of Mortality (PIM)
227, 230, 236
Pediatric Overall Performance
Category (POPC) 231, 236
Pediatric Risk of Mortality
(PRISM) 227, 229, 231, 236
phenacetin 266, 268

phenomenology 246–7
Descriptive Phenomenology
  model 350
Physiological Stability Index 229
physiology, children's knowledge of
  168
physiotherapy, in chronic pain 374
Piaget, Jean 149
Platt Report 257, 323
popularity of child patients 244–61
  literature review 245–6
    patient and situational
      factors 245
    physical attraction 245–6
    temperament theory 246
  research study
    age groups 249–50
    analysis framework 247
    conclusion 259
    conditions (illnesses) 251–2
    data analysis 248–58
    discussion 259
    effect of separation on
      children 249
    families 254–5, 257–8
    family conformance to ward
      routine 257, 259
    method 248
    negative feelings 256–7
    nurse–family partnership
      254–5, 257–8
    nurses' experiences 255–6
    nurses' expertise 253–5
    participants 248
    purpose and focus of study
      246–7
    relationships 252–3
    support for nurses 250
    unpopular parents 257, 258
popularity/unpopularity 246
  of adolescent patients 249–50,
    255
  of adult patients 244
  of child patients, *see* popularity
    of child patients
  of parents 257, 258

Port-a-cath venous access device
    352, 356
pregnancy terminations 205
professional bodies, role of 10–11
Project 2000 5
    pre-Project 2000 trained nurses
        6, 8
prostaglandins 263, 265, 266–7,
    268
proxy consent 7, 10–11
psychological trauma, children
    admitted to hospital 166–7
PSYCLIT 61
Public Health Research and
    Resource Centre 112–13
'publish or perish' 5, 8
pyrogens 263

R

randomised controlled trials 3–4,
    59, 60
readability formulae 171–2
    SMOG 175
referral fatigue 376, 378
reflection 26–7, 28, 32, 35
reflective diaries 21
relaxation, in chronic pain 374
research
    v. caring 3
    on *v.* with children 7
    conducting 6–7
    'data first/patient second'? 5
    ethical dimensions 9–10
    nurses' perspective of 4
    paucity of nursing research 2
    utilisation problems 382–3
Research Assessment Exercise 43
Research Utilization Program 388
rights of children in research 7,
    9–11
Royal Alexandra Hospital, Sydney,
    model for evidence-based
    nursing practice 389–93

evaluation and education
    processes 389–92
Royal College of Nursing 10
Royal College of Paediatrics and
    Child Health 10

S

school nurses
    as advisors and advocates 122
    role in A PAUSE (Added Power
        and Understanding in Sex
        Education) programme 213,
        214–15, 218, 220
School Nursing Service 196
schools, sex education in 187, 191,
    195, 206–7
    see also A PAUSE
self-efficacy 187–8, 208–9
    sexual 192–3, 196–7, 209
sex education 191–2
    future developments 218–20
    and gender 207, 216
    'Heineken principle' 208
    parents and 191–2, 195–6
    recommendations 218–20
    in schools 187, 191, 195, 206–7
    theoretical perspective 208–10
    see also A PAUSE
sexual health
    strategies 206–7
    see also adolescent sexual health
SMOG testing of literature 175
socialisation 27
social work/nursing overlap 45
societal changes 204–5
socio-economic inequalities
    affecting accidents 130
sponging, tepid 271
stress
    in chronic pain 371, 372
    mothers of children in intensive
        care units 92, 95
    Parental Stressor Scale 92

T

teenage sexual activity, *see*
    adolescent sexual activity;
    adolescent sexual health
temperament theory 246
temperature, *see* body temperature
terminology, overcomplicated
    116–17
tertiary care centres 226, 227, 228
    definition 224
theatre in education (TIE) 219
theory–practice gap 1, 4–6, 15
    investigation and report 5
Therapeutic Intervention Score
    System (TISS) 230, 231
'think-aloud' 20–1
tiredness, pain and 373
treatment procedures, children's
    views on 115–17
treatment settings, children's views
    on 115–17
triangulation 274

U

United Nations Convention 7
universities, research-led
    philosophy 5
    'publish or perish' 5, 8
University of York, *see* NHS Centre
    for Reviews and Dissemination
unpopularity of patients and
    others, *see*
    popularity/unpopularity

V

views of children on local health
    services, research study 110–27
    background 110–12
    conclusion 125
    discussion 123–5
    ethical considerations 113–14

findings 114–23
    access to information and
        advice 121–2
    communication issues
        115–17
    cure *v.* care 123
    doctors *v.* nurses 122–3, 124
    ignoring children and young
        people 115–16
    need for recognition of fears
        118–19
    overcomplicated terminology
        116–17
    role of health care
        professionals 122–3
    treatment procedures
        117–19
    treatment settings 119–21
    implications for practice 123–5
    literature review 111–12
    methodology 113–14
Vygotsky, L.S. 149–50, 159

W

*Welfare of Children and Young
    People in Hospital* (DoH report)
    112, 164, 324
World Wide Web 50